feb 2020

Neurological Emergencies

Alejandro A. Rabinstein
Editor

Neurological Emergencies

A Practical Approach

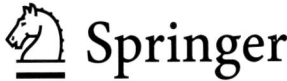 Springer

Editor
Alejandro A. Rabinstein
Mayo Clinic
Neuroscience ICU
Rochester, MN
USA

ISBN 978-3-030-28071-0   ISBN 978-3-030-28072-7 (eBook)
https://doi.org/10.1007/978-3-030-28072-7

© Springer Nature Switzerland AG 2020
This work is subject to copyright. All rights are reserved by the Publisher, whether the whole or part of the material is concerned, specifically the rights of translation, reprinting, reuse of illustrations, recitation, broadcasting, reproduction on microfilms or in any other physical way, and transmission or information storage and retrieval, electronic adaptation, computer software, or by similar or dissimilar methodology now known or hereafter developed.
The use of general descriptive names, registered names, trademarks, service marks, etc. in this publication does not imply, even in the absence of a specific statement, that such names are exempt from the relevant protective laws and regulations and therefore free for general use.
The publisher, the authors, and the editors are safe to assume that the advice and information in this book are believed to be true and accurate at the date of publication. Neither the publisher nor the authors or the editors give a warranty, expressed or implied, with respect to the material contained herein or for any errors or omissions that may have been made. The publisher remains neutral with regard to jurisdictional claims in published maps and institutional affiliations.

This Springer imprint is published by the registered company Springer Nature Switzerland AG
The registered company address is: Gewerbestrasse 11, 6330 Cham, Switzerland

*To Carlota, Hannah, and Joshua.
My reason for everything.*

Preface

I have dedicated my professional life to the care of patients with neurological emergencies, the research of ways to improve the diagnosis and management of these patients, and the training of residents and fellows of various medical disciplines on the recognition and treatment of acute and severe neurological problems. This book is a reflection of all those years of experience distilled in a practical format.

The book includes chapters on most of the acute neurological diagnoses encountered in the emergency department. Some may be found in the hospital, most commonly in the intensive care units. The list of topics covered cannot be complete, but it is quite comprehensive. It includes acute coma, dangerous causes of headache, seizures and status epilepticus, various acute cerebrovascular disorders, trauma to the brain and the spinal cord, tumors, severe central nervous system infections, and intoxications from prescription and recreational drugs. Neuro-ophthalmological and neuro-otological emergencies, always very challenging for nonspecialists, are specifically covered. The book also includes discussions on less common conditions, such as fulminant presentations of demyelinating diseases and severe presentations of movement disorders. Lastly, it incorporates chapters dedicated to neurological emergencies in specific populations, such as pregnant women and transplant patients.

Each chapter provides an updated overview of the topic while maintaining an eminently practical approach. A common pattern runs through the chapters by starting with short lists of diagnostic keys, treatment priorities, and crucial prognostic facts and concluding with cardinal messages to reinforce the most important concepts. Tables, figures, and algorithms are liberally used for illustration. By design, references are not overly abundant; only key articles are cited with a predilection for the most recent published information. My hope is that this book will serve its readers by increasing their understanding of the art and the science of caring for patients with acute neurological disease, not by explicating everything there is to know about each diagnosis, but actually by simplifying the approach to each condition.

It is a great pleasure for me that many of the authors of this book are some of my favorite former trainees. They have gone on to develop splendid academic careers and to become experts on their respective fields. I consider it a distinct privilege to have had them participate in this project. Their achievements make me truly proud for whatever degree of learning they may have acquired from me at some point in their training. Other authors are esteemed colleagues and established scholars without whose help this book would have never come to fruition. I thank every single one of the contributing authors for their diligence and generosity.

I also want to acknowledge and thank Barbara Lopez-Lucio for her invaluable editorial support throughout this process. Working with her made everything much easier.

Lastly, thanking the patients for allowing us to learn from them has become a bit trite. Yet, my gratitude to patients is genuine. Without practicing and teaching Medicine, my life would be much less fulfilling. And Medicine for me is about patients. Without them, it would be an abstraction.

Rochester, MN, USA   Alejandro A. Rabinstein

Contents

1. **Acute Coma** 1
   Alejandro A. Rabinstein

2. **Status Epilepticus** 15
   Michael D. Morris, Kent A. Owusu, and Carolina B. Maciel

3. **Headache Emergencies** 49
   Deena M. Nasr and Sherri A. Braksick

4. **Neuro-otologic Emergencies: A Practical Approach** 67
   Kiersten L. Gurley and Jonathan A. Edlow

5. **Neuro-ophthalmologic Urgencies and Emergencies** 85
   Devon A. Cohen and John J. Chen

6. **Neuro-Oncologic Emergencies** 107
   Michael W. Ruff and Alyx B. Porter

7. **Severe Infections of the Central Nervous System** 121
   Micah D. Yost and Michel Toledano

8. **Acute Neuromuscular Respiratory Failure** 151
   Katherine Schwartz and Christopher L. Kramer

9. **Acute Ischemic Stroke** 171
   Maximiliano A. Hawkes and Alejandro A. Rabinstein

10. **Acute Cerebral Venous Stroke** 189
    Catherine Arnold Fiebelkorn and Sherri A. Braksick

11. **Intraparenchymal Hemorrhage (Cerebral and Cerebellar)** 209
    David P. Lerner, Anil Ramineni, and Joseph D. Burns

12. **Aneurysmal Subarachnoid Hemorrhage** 231
    Sudhir Datar

13 **Management of Severe Traumatic Brain Injury: A Practical Approach** 245
  Daniel Agustin Godoy, Ahsan Ali Khan, and Andres M. Rubiano

14 **Traumatic Spinal Cord Injury** 271
  Alejandro A. Rabinstein

15 **Neurologic Emergencies from Recreational Substances** 281
  Kaitlyn Barkley and Christopher P. Robinson

16 **Neurological Emergencies from Prescription Drugs** 301
  Sherri A. Braksick and Deena M. Nasr

17 **Emergencies of Demyelinating Diseases** 319
  Shyamal C. Bir, Eduardo Gonzalez-Toledo, and Alireza Minagar

18 **Emergencies in Movement Disorders** 335
  Julieta E. Arena

19 **Neurologic Emergencies in Transplant Patients** 345
  Jeffrey Brent Peel and Lauren K. Ng

20 **Neurological Emergencies in Pregnant Patients** 357
  Jason Siegel

Index 377

Contributors

Editor

Alejandro A. Rabinstein, MD Department of Neurology, Mayo Clinic, Neuroscience ICU, Rochester, MN, USA

Authors

Julieta E. Arena, MD Movement Disorders Section, Neurology Department, Fleni, Buenos Aires, Argentina

Kaitlyn Barkley, MD Department of Neurosurgery, University of Florida, Gainesville, FL, USA

Shyamal C. Bir, MD, PhD Department of Neurology, LSU Health Sciences Center, Shreveport, LA, USA

Sherri A. Braksick, MD Department of Neurology, Mayo Clinic, Rochester, MN, USA

Joseph D. Burns, MD Department of Neurology, Lahey Hospital and Medical Center, Burlington, MA, USA

Department of Neurology, Tufts University School of Medicine, Boston, MA, USA

Department of Neurosurgery, Tufts University School of Medicine, Boston, MA, USA

John J. Chen, MD, PhD Department of Neurology, Mayo Clinic, Rochester, MN, USA

Department of Ophthalmology, Mayo Clinic, Rochester, MN, USA

Devon A. Cohen, MD Department of Neurology, Mayo Clinic, Rochester, MN, USA

Sudhir Datar, MD Department of Neurology, Wake Forest University Baptist Medical Center, Winston-Salem, NC, USA

Jonathan A. Edlow, MD Department of Emergency Medicine, Beth Israel Deaconess Medical Center and Harvard Medical School, Boston, MA, USA

Catherine Arnold Fiebelkorn, MD Department of Neurology, Mayo Clinic, Rochester, MN, USA

Daniel Agustin Godoy, MD Department of Critical Care, Hospital San Juan Bautista, Sanatorio Pasteur, Catamarca, Catamarca, Argentina

Neurointensive Care Unit, Sanatorio Pasteur, Catamarca, Catamarca, Argentina

Intensive Care Unit, Hospital San Juan Bautista, Catamarca, Catamarca, Argentina

Eduardo Gonzalez-Toledo, MD, PhD Departments of Radiology, Neurology, and Anesthesiology, Louisiana State University Health Sciences Center, Shreveport, LA, USA

Kiersten L. Gurley, MD Department of Emergency Medicine, Beth Israel Deaconess Medical Center/Harvard University School of Medicine, Boston, MA, USA

Maximiliano A. Hawkes, MD, FESO Departments of Neurology and Internal Medicine, FLENI, Buenos Aires, Argentina

Ahsan Ali Khan, MD Departments of Clinical Research and Neurotrauma, Meditech Foundation/Barrow Neurological Institute at PCH/University of Cambridge, Cali, Valle del Cauca, Colombia

Cristopher L. Kramer, MD Department of Neurology, University of Chicago, Chicago, IL, USA

David P. Lerner, MD Department of Neurology, Lahey Hospital and Medical Center, Burlington, MA, USA

Department of Neurology, Tufts University School of Medicine, Boston, MA, USA

Caroina B. Maciel, MD, MSCR Division of Neurocritical Care, Department of Neurology, University of Florida, McKnight Brain Institute, Gainesville, FL, USA

Alireza Minagar, MD, MBA Department of Neurology, Louisiana State University Health Sciences Center, Shreveport, LA, USA

Michael D. Morris, MD Department of Neurology, University of Florida, Gainesville, FL, USA

Deena M. Nasr, DO Department of Neurology, Mayo Clinic, Rochester, MN, USA

Lauren K. Ng, MD, MPH Department of Critical Care Medicine, Neurology, and Neurosurgery, Mayo Clinic, Jacksonville, FL, USA

Kent A. Owusu, PharmD Neurocritical Care, Department of Pharmacy, Yale New Haven Hospital, New Haven, CT, USA

Jeffrey Brent Peel, MD Department of Neurology, Mayo Clinic, Jacksonville, FL, USA

Alyx B. Porter, MD Department of Neurology, Mayo Clinic Arizona, Phoenix, AZ, USA

Anil Ramineni, MD Department of Neurology, Lahey Hospital and Medical Center, Burlington, MA, USA

Department of Neurology, Tufts University School of Medicine, Boston, MA, USA

Christopher P. Robinson, DO, MS Department of Neurology, University of Florida, Gainesville, FL, USA

Andres M. Rubiano, MD, PhD (c) Department of Clinical Research/Neurosciences Institute, El Bosque University/Meditech Foundation, Bogotá, Cundinamarca, Colombia

Michael W. Ruff, MD Department of Neurology, Mayo Clinic, Rochester, MN, USA

Katherine Schwartz, DO Department of Neurology, University of Chicago, Chicago, IL, USA

Jason Siegel, MD Departments of Neurology, Neurosurgery, and Critical Care Medicine, Mayo Clinic Florida, Jacksonville, FL, USA

Michel Toledano, MD Department of Neurology, Mayo Clinic, Rochester, MN, USA

Micah D. Yost, DO Department of Neurology, Mayo Clinic, Rochester, MN, USA

Chapter 1
Acute Coma

Alejandro A. Rabinstein

> **Diagnostic Keys**
> - When evaluating a patient with acute coma, exclude treatable causes first (such as basilar artery occlusion, deep cerebral venous thrombosis, infectious meningitis or encephalitis, autoimmune encephalitis, and nonconvulsive status epilepticus).
> - That said, the most common causes of coma in practice are toxic-metabolic (drugs, sepsis, renal and hepatic failure) and anoxic-ischemic.
> - Keeping a simple checklist can be extremely helpful to avoid missing important diagnoses.

> **Treatment Priorities**
> - Some causes of acute coma are eminently treatable as long as treatment is initiated without delay (e.g., basilar artery recanalization, antiepileptics for status epilepticus, antibacterials for fulminant meningitis, or acyclovir for herpes encephalitis).
> - Discontinuation of potentially culprit medications should always be attempted.
> - In many cases of coma from toxic-metabolic causes, the right management consists of waiting for the patient to recover spontaneously while avoiding secondary brain insults.

A. A. Rabinstein (✉)
Department of Neurology, Mayo Clinic, Neuroscience ICU, Rochester, MN, USA
e-mail: Rabinstein.alejandro@mayo.edu

> **Prognosis at a Glance**
> - The prognosis of acute coma is primarily dependent on the primary cause and whether there has been superimposed anoxic-ischemic brain injury.
> - Delayed recovery from coma is relatively common in daily practice.
> - Never rush to estimate the outcome of comatose patients, especially when no major structural brain injury is seen on imaging.

Introduction

Evaluating a comatose patient is always a challenge. The extent of the differential diagnoses and the gravity of missing a treatable disease can become overwhelming. However, relying on simple principles can greatly facilitate the task and prevent common mistakes. This chapter summarizes the primordial information that is necessary to know when evaluating coma and also provides advice from years of experience at the bedside. It is not meant as an exhaustive review of coma, but rather as a basic guide mixing basic concepts with practical recommendations.

Basic Pathophysiology

Coma is typically considered a result from bilateral cortical dysfunction or disorders affecting the ascending reticular activating pathways through the brainstem and diencephalon (i.e., thalamic and hypothalamic areas) [1]. It is common and pragmatically justified to discriminate causes of coma into structural and non-structural or diffuse. However, this definition cannot be strict. For instance, patients who become comatose from generalized seizures can subsequently developed permanent structural cortical injury if the seizures are not aborted in a timely manner. Similarly, patients with structural brain disease can also have superimposed metabolic or toxic causes to explain their coma [2]. Furthermore, while focal or lateralizing signs are characteristically observed in patients with structural brain damage, similar findings can occasionally be noted in patients with non-structural and fully reversible causes for the unresponsiveness, such as post-ictal deficits. In fact, heavy sedation and major metabolic abnormalities can even produce alterations of brainstem reflexes that would typically suggest either brain herniation or direct brainstem damage [1].

Diagnosis

The broad differential diagnosis of acute coma can be effectively trimmed by interpreting the information gained from a focused history and examination. Testing should be guided by this information. Table 1.1 shows a checklist that can be very useful to maximize the efficiency of the emergency evaluation of a comatose patient.

Table 1.1 Proposed checklist to streamline the evaluation of the acutely comatose patient

History
Acuteness of the unresponsiveness
Report of focal deficits or possible seizures
Previous recent symptoms
Comorbid conditions
Toxic exposures (recreational drugs, prescription medications, environmental)
Examination
General survey
Level of responsiveness (FOUR score)
Brainstem reflexes
Motor responses to pain (central and appendicular)
Meningeal signs
Muscle tone and clonus
Adventitious movements
Testing
Basic chemistry, including glucose
Toxicological screen, including alcohol[a]
Known prescription drugs[a]
Serum ammonia[a]
Arterial blood gases[a]
Brain imaging[a]
Non-contrast CT scan is sufficient for hemorrhage, extensive infarctions, and large masses
MRI is necessary for most other causes
Cerebrovascular imaging[b]
Noninvasive angiogram for basilar artery or intracranial carotid artery occlusion
Noninvasive venogram for cerebral venous thrombosis
Electroencephalogram to exclude non-convulsive status epilepticus
Spot EEG is sufficient in most cases when showing no epileptiform changes[a]
Continuous EEG is indicated when high suspicion for seizures or spot EEG with epileptiform changes[b]
Lumbar puncture to exclude meningitis/encephalitis
Testing for infection[a]
Autoimmune panel[b]

[a]When pertinent depending on history, initial examination, and clinical setting (i.e., emergency department vs ICU)
[b]More infrequently necessary

History

Although history is not always available in the Emergency Department, important information that one must try to elicit includes previous diseases, drug exposures, recent symptoms, characteristics of presentation if witnessed, and medications administered by paramedics in the field and en route. When evaluating comatose patients in the ICU, one should carefully review the course of the hospitalization, blood work results, and recent medications because this information very often provides valuable clues to identify the cause/s of the coma and factors that may be prolonging or deepening the unresponsiveness.

Physical Examination

The importance of an attentive, even if abbreviated, general survey should not be underestimated. This may uncover subtle signs of trauma (such as retroauricular ecchymosis), systemic signs of infectious or non-infectious vasculitis, stigmata of cirrhosis, needle marks suggestive of intravenous drug use, or clues to an underlying source of sepsis. Vital signs deserve special attention; they are not diagnostic per se except for severe hypothermia, but they can signal to possible causes (fever in cases of sepsis, serotonin syndrome, or neuroleptic malignant syndrome; hypotension in cases of sepsis, intoxication with tricyclic antidepressants or cyanide; hypertension in posterior reversible encephalopathy syndrome [PRES]; or various intoxications with recreational drugs such as methamphetamines, cocaine, or ecstasy).

A focused neurological examination should include an overall assessment of degree of responsiveness, brainstem reflexes, motor responses to pain, and breathing pattern. These features are included in the FOUR score (Fig. 1.1), which has been shown in various studies to be equal or superior to the Glasgow coma score in predicting the prognosis of neurocritical patients in the Emergency Department or the ICU [3–5].

Degree of Responsiveness

The degree of responsiveness should be described based on specific responses, rather than solely characterized by terms that may be misinterpreted, such as drowsiness or stupor. A patient who is truly comatose can have reflexive responses to external stimulation but without showing any sign of awareness.

Brainstem Reflexes

Evaluation of brainstem reflexes should include pupillary responses to a bright light, presence of blinking to corneal stimulation, eye movements to head turning (oculocephalic reflexes; they are preserved in a comatose patient when the eyes deviate in a conjugate fashion away from the direction of passive head rotation) or stimulation of the external auditory canal with cold water (oculocaloric reflexes; preserved in a comatose patient when the eyes respond with tonic deviation towards the irrigated ear), gag to pharyngeal stimulation, and cough to deep bronchial stimulation with a suction catheter. Presence and, when pertinent, asymmetry or responses should be noted. Unilateral non-reactive anisocoria should be considered a sign of brain tissue shift and uncal herniation with compression of the midbrain until proven otherwise by brain imaging. These "blown" pupils frequently acquire a slightly oval

1 Acute Coma

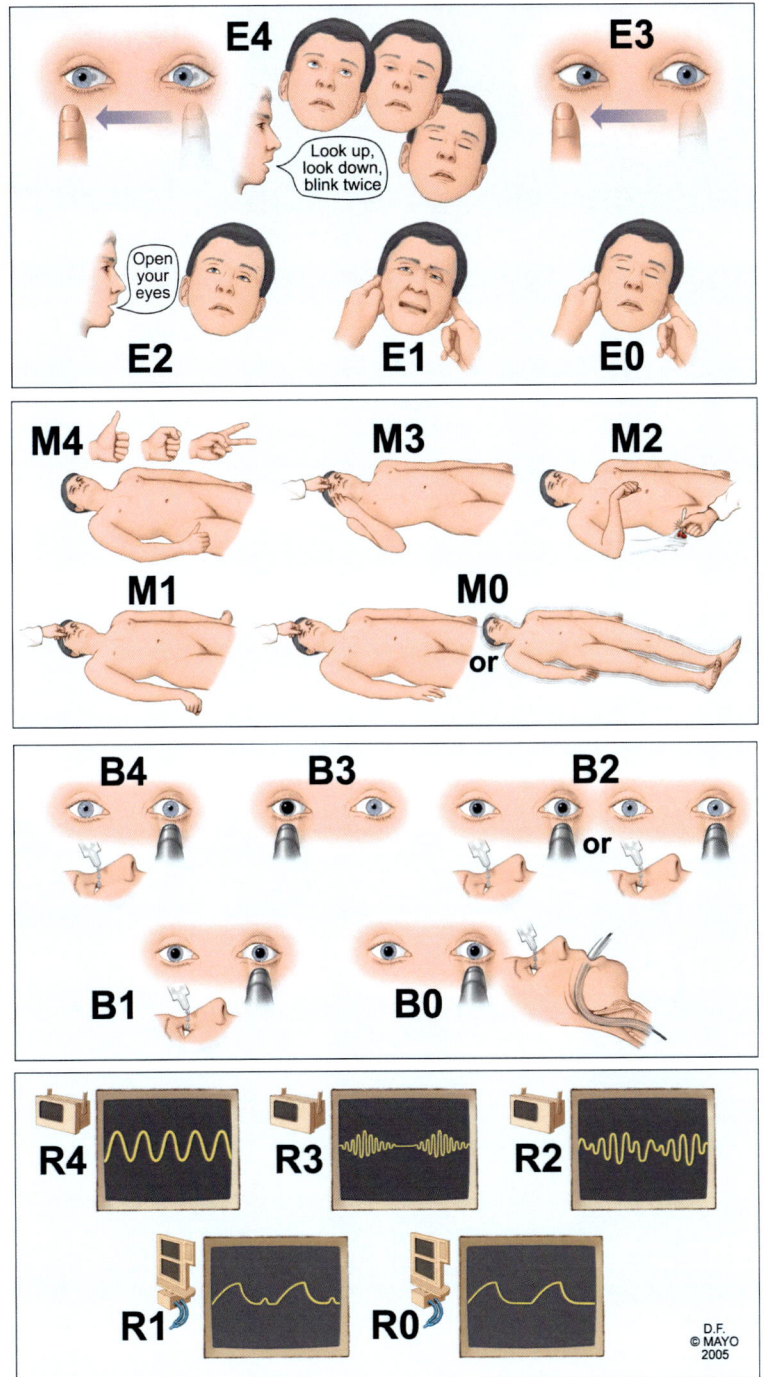

Fig. 1.1 The FOUR score. (Used with permission of Mayo Foundation for Medical Education and Research; all rights reserved)

shape but have smooth margins. Irregular margins are typically the result of previous surgery. Anisocoria with preserved reactivity may be entirely benign.

Motor Responses to Pain

Vigorous stimulation should be applied to determine the best motor response. Central stimulation (to temporomandibular joints, supraorbital notches, trapezii muscles, or sternum) serves to determine if localizing responses are present. Pressure on the nailbeds of fingers are useful to elicit withdrawal and to further assess for abnormal motor responses, either flexion or extensor (formerly known as decorticate or decerebrate). Pressure on the toes should also be applied to test for withdrawal responses of the legs and they should be differentiated from the triple flexion response, which represents a spinal reflex and denotes lack of higher-level inhibition. Abnormal flexion and extension responses as well as triple flexion responses are characterized by their consistent stereotypy (i.e., the response is always the same no matter how many times it is elicited). Asymmetry in motor responses should be carefully noted as it is the most common clue to the underlying presence of a unilateral brain lesion.

Additional Aspects of Neurological Examination

Presence of meningeal signs, muscle tone, and any adventitious movements (of the eyes, arms, or legs) should be noted. Difficulty flexing the neck is common in elderly patients and may simply be a consequence of degenerative changes of the cervical spine. However, flexion of the knees upon attempted flexion of the neck is a useful discriminating sign. Increased muscle tone is commonly seen with toxic encephalopathies; yet, when it preferentially affects the legs, one should suspect serotonin syndrome—particularly if associated with bilateral ankle clonus. Extreme whole body rigidity can be seen in neuroleptic malignant syndrome and certain forms of autoimmune encephalitis. Myoclonus and asterixis are frequently manifested in patients with various toxic and metabolic encephalopathies, and they carry limited prognostic significance in these cases. However, multi-segmental myoclonus can also be a sign of severe anoxic-ischemic brain injury after cardiorespiratory arrest [6].

Diagnostic Tests

Basic blood chemistry should be obtained in all cases. Searching for drug intoxication should always be considered, but the extent of the toxicological workup (recreational drugs, prescription medications, cyanide, etc.) should be guided by the history and examination [2]. Arterial blood gases, serum ammonia, and calculation of osmolar gap are also pertinent in many cases.

All other tests should be considered optional and adapted to the individual situation. Excluding treatable causes should be the guiding principle. An experienced clinician will have a mental checklist to determine if the following testing is necessary on each case (Table 1.1).

Brain Imaging

Although a non-contrast brain CT scan is often obtained in the Emergency Department or the ICU even prior to the neurological consultation, the yield of this investigation in comatose patients is relatively low except when acute basilar occlusion, subarachnoid hemorrhage, hydrocephalus, or mass lesions are strongly suspected. It is most useful for the detection of intracranial hemorrhage (subdural, subarachnoid, or intracerebral), large ischemic infarctions, and brain tumors. It may also show global brain edema in severe cases of anoxic-ischemic brain injury and in patients with severe hyperammonemia. However, it is insufficient to rule out structural brain damage. In many circumstances, a brain MRI is much more informative. Examples include herpes encephalitis, brainstem ischemia, PRES, extreme hypoglycemia, and fat embolism syndrome (Fig. 1.2). It is important to remember that even repeatedly negative MRIs do not exclude irreversible brain disease severe enough to keep the patient comatose, as it happens in some cases after cardiac arrest and in some cases of autoimmune encephalitis; in such cases the only telltale sign may be the progressive brain atrophy noticed on serial imaging. In some instances, it is necessary to obtain a noninvasive angiogram (suspected basilar artery occlusion) or venogram (cerebral venous thrombosis) of the intracranial circulation.

Electroencephalography

Patients who remain comatose after having clinical seizures should have an EEG to exclude non-convulsive status epilepticus as the cause of the persistent unresponsiveness [7]. While that indication is clear, there is debate in the literature regarding the indication of electroencephalography (EEG) in comatose patients without high suspicion of seizures. It is true that epileptiform abnormalities and even electrographic seizures are not infrequent among comatose patients without history of any clinical seizures [8, 9], but it is also true that it is unproven if treatment with antiseizure medications can improve the outcomes of these patients. I believe that clinical judgment should guide the decision whether to assess brain electrical activity in comatose patients without previous seizures. In these cases, nonspecific background abnormalities (slow wakes with low amplitude, sometimes with interspersed triphasic waves) are the most common finding—and this finding is inconsequential. If EEG is pursued, there is no question that continuous monitoring provides a higher diagnostic yield as compared with a 30-minute EEG [8]. Yet, the initial tracing has strong predictive value in regard to what more extensive monitoring will show [10].

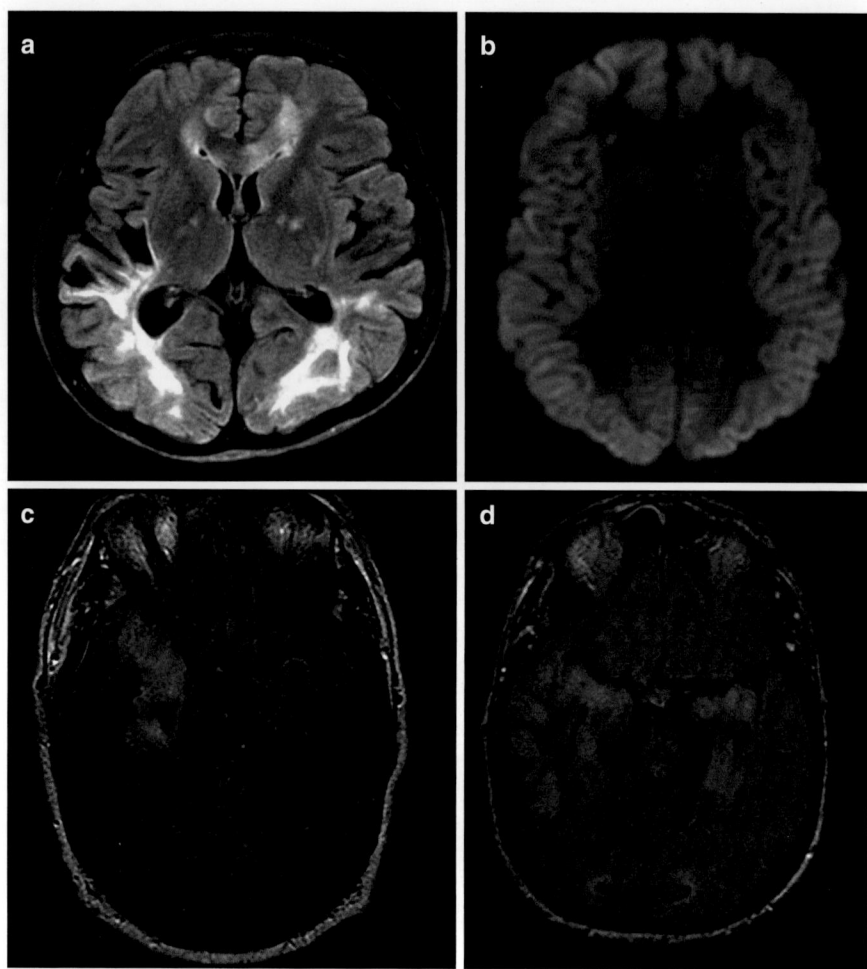

Fig. 1.2 Illustrative examples of various causes of coma documented by MRI. (**a**) Bilateral vasogenic edema predominantly affecting the occipital lobes in a patient with PRES (FLAIR sequence). (**b**) Severe anoxic cortical injury after cardiac arrest (DWI sequence). (**c**) Inflammatory changes affecting the right temporal lobe in a patient with HSV-1 encephalitis (FLAIR sequence). (**d**) Bilateral inflammatory changes predominantly affecting the limbic regions in a patient with paraneoplastic autoimmune encephalitis (FLAIR sequence)

Lumbar Puncture

Certainly not every comatose patient needs a lumbar puncture. On the other hand, when lumbar puncture is deemed indicated, it should be generally performed without delay. This statement is particularly true for suspected infectious etiologies of coma. Lumbar puncture should be considered indispensable in immunosuppressed patients with coma of unknown etiology. While cerebrospinal fluid analysis can provide supporting information for the diagnosis of non-infectious causes of coma, these other diagnoses can most often be made through noninvasive testing. Examples include acute subarachnoid hemorrhage (which causes xanthochromia, but is never a cause of coma with negative CT scan) [11], cerebral venous thrombosis (typically associated with increased opening pressure and some protein elevation), and PRES (protein elevation without increase in nucleated cells) [12]. A possible exception is intracranial hypotension, a disorder that produces some characteristic changes on gadolinium MRI (brain sagging, pachymeningeal enhancement), but must be confirmed by measurement of a low opening pressure upon lumbar puncture. It remains pertinent to remember that brain imaging (CT or MRI) is generally indicated before proceeding with lumbar puncture in comatose patients.

Treatment

The treatment of comatose patients is mainly determined by the underlying cause of the coma. Yet, some general concepts apply to most, if not all patients [13].

General Therapeutic Principles

Prompt stabilization of the airway and ensuring delivery of adequate oxygenation and blood perfusion remain cornerstones of the hyperacute treatment of any comatose patient. Administering intravenous thiamine before giving glucose remains best practice [2]. When trauma is known or deemed possible, the spine should be immobilized prior to transportation. If opiate or benzodiazepine intoxication is suspected, administration of naloxone and flumazenil may be attempted [2]. In patients with signs of acute brain herniation (e.g., anisocoric, mydriatic, non-reactive pupil), immediate hyperventilation and administration of an osmotic agent (hypertonic saline or mannitol) is indicated [14]. Beyond the hyperacute phase, the emphasis should shift towards avoiding secondary brain insults (including ongoing intracranial hypertension, nonconvulsive seizures, fever, hypoxia, dysglycemia, among others) and systemic complications (infections, venous thromboembolism, paroxysmal sympathetic hyperactivity, gastroduodenal ulcers, pressure sores, malnutrition, etc.)

Specific Treatments Based on Etiology

Table 1.2 lists causes of coma for which an effective treatment is available [1, 2, 14]. Notice that, in most cases, this treatment must be started emergently in order to be truly effective. Thus, therapeutic effectiveness greatly depends on timely recognition of the underlying etiology and implementation of the specific treatment without delay.

Table 1.2 Treatable causes of coma

Cause	Treatment	Emergency	Effectiveness
Cardiac arrest	Targeted temperature management (33° or 36 °C)	++	+
Basilar artery occlusion	Intravenous alteplase, mechanical thrombectomy	+++	++
Massive hemispheric infarction	Decompressive craniectomy	++	++
Status epilepticus	Anti-seizure medications	+++	+++
Intraparenchymal mass lesions	Surgery, osmotherapy, corticosteroids (if vasogenic edema)	++	++
Subdural or epidural hematoma	Surgery	+++	+++
Acute hydrocephalus	Ventricular drainage	+++	+++
Bacterial meningitis	Antibiotics and dexamethasone	+++	+++
Herpes simplex virus encephalitis	Acyclovir	+++	+++
Autoimmune encephalitis	Methylprednisolone, plasma exchange or intravenous immunoglobulin, rituximab	++	+++
Venous sinus thrombosis	Anticoagulation, consider local infusion of thrombolytic agent	+++	+++
Posterior reversible encephalopathy	Blood pressure control, discontinuation of possible culprit drugs, anti-seizure medications (if seizures)	+++	+++
Air embolism	Consider hyperbaric oxygen	+++	Possible
Drug intoxications	Antidotes when available	+++	Variable
Hypercapnia	Mechanical ventilation	+++	+++
Carbon monoxide poisoning	Normobaric or hyperbaric oxygen	+++	+++
Hypoglycemia	Dextrose	+++	+++
Diabetic coma	Insulin, fluids	+++	+++
Uremia	Dialysis	++	+++
Hyperammonemia	Lactulose, rifaximin	+++	+++
Pituitary apoplexy	Corticosteroids, +/−surgery	+++	+++
Myxedema	Thyroid hormone	++	+++
Wernicke's encephalopathy	Thiamine	+++	++
Extreme hypothermia	Slow rewarming	++	+++

The specific management of patients with acute intoxications from recreational substances or prescription drugs is discussed in detail in other chapters of this book.

Prognosis

The outcome of acute coma is dependent on the underlying cause of the unresponsiveness. Anoxic-ischemic brain injury has a worse prognosis, regardless of whether this injury was the original cause of the coma or occurred as a subsequent complication. It is difficult to make any generic statements about coma prognosis, but it is essential to keep in mind that many comatose patients experience delayed recovery, and therefore exercising caution is imperative when estimating prognosis in comatose patients, unless massive structural brain damage is documented.

Prognosis of coma has been most extensively studied in survivors of cardiac arrest. In such cases, multiple prognostic parameters have been validated, including the characteristics of the arrest (shockable vs non-shockable rhythm, quality of resuscitation), patient's comorbidities, physical findings (brainstem reflexes, myoclonus, motor responses to pain) on serial examinations without confounders, EEG (continuous vs discontinuous background, reactivity to external stimulation, presence of epileptiform discharges or seizures), somatosensory-evoked potentials (bilateral absence of cortical N20 responses on well-conducted testing remains the strongest indicator of poor prognosis), serum neuronal-specific enolase (released to the circulation after neuronal injury, but not as specific as the name suggests; it can also be released from erythrocytes after hemolysis), and brain imaging (global edema on CT scan, cortical and basal ganglia injury on MRI). All available parameters must be interpreted in combination before estimating a prognosis, and when there is inconsistency across the parameters (i.e., some indicating unfavorable prognosis but not others), one must acknowledge uncertainty and continue supporting the patient until the prognosis becomes clearer [15].

Coma after head trauma has a comparatively better prognosis, but neurological recovery may only become evident many days, weeks, or even months after the injury. Age is a major determinant of prognosis in patients with post-traumatic coma. Prognostic scores developed from data of large trials (CRASH, IMPACT) need to be interpreted with caution when applied to individual cases [16, 17]. When caring for young comatose patients after severe traumatic brain injury, it is highly advisable to continue long-term supportive care unless there is unquestionable evidence of devastating brainstem injury on physical examination and brain MRI.

Cardinal Messages
- Acute coma should be considered a treatable condition until treatable causes are adequately excluded.
- Keeping a mental or an actual checklist of the main diagnostic considerations is a practical way to ensure an efficient emergency evaluation of coma.
- Physical examination should focus on assessment of brainstem reflexes, motor responses to pain, muscle tone, meningeal signs, and adventitious movements.
- Testing should be rational and focused. While excluding treatable causes is an emergency, a shotgun approach to testing is inefficient and results may be potentially misguiding.
- When evaluating a comatose patient in the ICU, always review the ongoing and recent medication lists because drugs are often responsible for the state of unresponsiveness or major contributors to it.
- When available, specific treatments must be delivered without delay.

- Even when specific treatments are not available, optimal critical care may increase the chances of recovery.
- Prognosis should always be approached with caution and should never be delivered in a rush except when there is a need to discuss an emergency intervention.
- Prognosis after cardiac resuscitation should rely on multiple parameters and a poor prognosis should be communicated only when all parameters consistently portend an unfavorable outcome.
- In young patients with severe traumatic brain injury, even very prolonged coma may be compatible with meaningful neurological recovery.

References

1. Rabinstein AA. Coma and brain death. Continuum (Minneap Minn). 2018;24(6):1708–31.
2. Edlow JA, Rabinstein A, Traub SJ, Wijdicks EF. Diagnosis of reversible causes of coma. Lancet. 2014;384(9959):2064–76.
3. Wijdicks EF, Bamlet WR, Maramattom BV, Manno EM, McClelland RL. Validation of a new coma scale: the FOUR score. Ann Neurol. 2005;58(4):585–93.
4. Kevric J, Jelinek GA, Knott J, Weiland TJ. Validation of the Full Outline of Unresponsiveness (FOUR) Scale for conscious state in the emergency department: comparison against the Glasgow Coma Scale. Emerg Med J. 2011;28(6):486–90.
5. Wijdicks EF, Kramer AA, Rohs T Jr, et al. Comparison of the Full Outline of UnResponsiveness score and the Glasgow Coma Scale in predicting mortality in critically ill patients∗. Crit Care Med. 2015;43(2):439–44.
6. Wijdicks EF, Rabinstein AA. Myoclonus status and prognostication of postresuscitation coma: the bigger picture. Ann Neurol. 2016;80(2):173–4.
7. DeLorenzo RJ, Waterhouse EJ, Towne AR, et al. Persistent nonconvulsive status epilepticus after the control of convulsive status epilepticus. Epilepsia. 1998;39(8):833–40.
8. Pandian JD, Cascino GD, So EL, Manno E, Fulgham JR. Digital video-electroencephalographic monitoring in the neurological-neurosurgical intensive care unit: clinical features and outcome. Arch Neurol. 2004;61(7):1090–4.
9. Sutter R, Fuhr P, Grize L, Marsch S, Ruegg S. Continuous video-EEG monitoring increases detection rate of nonconvulsive status epilepticus in the ICU. Epilepsia. 2011;52(3):453–7.
10. Shafi MM, Westover MB, Cole AJ, Kilbride RD, Hoch DB, Cash SS. Absence of early epileptiform abnormalities predicts lack of seizures on continuous EEG. Neurology. 2012;79(17):1796–801.
11. Dupont SA, Wijdicks EF, Manno EM, Rabinstein AA. Thunderclap headache and normal computed tomographic results: value of cerebrospinal fluid analysis. Mayo Clin Proc. 2008;83(12):1326–31.
12. Datar S, Singh TD, Fugate JE, Mandrekar J, Rabinstein AA, Hocker S. Albuminocytologic dissociation in posterior reversible encephalopathy syndrome. Mayo Clin Proc. 2015;90(10):1366–71.
13. Hocker S, Rabinstein AA. Management of the patient with diminished responsiveness. Neurol Clin. 2012;30(1):1–9, vii.
14. Wijdicks EF. Management of the comatose patient. Handb Clin Neurol. 2017;140:117–29.
15. Rossetti AO, Rabinstein AA, Oddo M. Neurological prognostication of outcome in patients in coma after cardiac arrest. Lancet Neurol. 2016;15(6):597–609.

16. Charry JD, Tejada JH, Pinzon MA, et al. Predicted unfavorable neurologic outcome is overestimated by the Marshall Computed Tomography Score, Corticosteroid Randomization After Significant Head Injury (CRASH), and International Mission for Prognosis and Analysis of Clinical Trials in Traumatic Brain Injury (IMPACT) models in patients with severe traumatic brain injury managed with early decompressive craniectomy. World Neurosurg. 2017;101:554–8.
17. Maas AI, Lingsma HF, Roozenbeek B. Predicting outcome after traumatic brain injury. Handb Clin Neurol. 2015;128:455–74.

Chapter 2
Status Epilepticus

Michael D. Morris, Kent A. Owusu, and Carolina B. Maciel

Diagnostic Keys
- Maintain a high index of suspicion in at risk patient populations (history of epilepsy, structural brain abnormalities, meningoencephalitis, and intoxications) even in the absence of convulsive symptoms.
- Timely use of electroencephalography.
- Comprehensive history and physical examination targeting the identification of risk factors, triggers, toxic and infectious exposures, and comorbidities.
- Workup of etiology should be tailored to history and may include comprehensive metabolic panel and complete blood count, toxicologic screen, antiseizure drug levels, autoimmune and paraneoplastic panels, cerebrospinal fluid profile, and neuroimaging.

M. D. Morris
Department of Neurology, University of Florida, Gainesville, FL, USA

K. A. Owusu
Neurocritical Care, Department of Pharmacy, Yale New Haven Hospital, New Haven, CT, USA

C. B. Maciel (✉)
Division of Neurocritical Care, Department of Neurology, University of Florida, McKnight Brain Institute, Gainesville, FL, USA
e-mail: carolina.maciel@yale.edu; carolina.maciel@neurology.ufl.edu

Treatment Priorities
- ABCs: continuous assessment of airway patency, adequate ventilation, and stability of hemodynamic parameters prior to and during implementation of targeted therapy.
- Triaging to appropriate level of care.
- Prompt initiation of first-line treatment (benzodiazepines) followed by a stepwise approach to escalation of therapy.
- Monitoring drug response, drug-drug interactions, and systemic toxicity.
- Titration of subsequent individualized therapy based on EEG findings, comorbidities and most likely etiology.

Prognosis at a Glance
- Mortality rates vary widely and are intimately related to etiology, response to therapy, and age.
- Patients with post-anoxic SE have highest mortality (60–100%), followed by those with cerebrovascular disease-associated SE (20–60%) and those with metabolic disturbances (10–35%).
- Patients over the age of 50 years are also at increased risk for poor outcomes.
- Mortality rates are as high as 23–57% in refractory and super-refractory cases.
- Systemic complications are common, and include cardiac arrest, arrhythmias, hemodynamic collapse, hypoxemia, acid/base disturbances, and rhabdomyolysis.
- Multiple assessment tools are available and may be useful in gauging prognosis based on patient-specific factors.

Introduction

Status epilepticus (SE) affects 10–40 persons per 100,000 population every year in the United States, and results when the body fails to effectively employ seizure termination mechanisms or when ongoing processes lead to prolongation of seizures [1]. The rapid diagnosis and management of SE is of critical importance as seizure cessation is directly related to early initiation of seizure termination therapies. Further, SE is associated with prolonged hospital and intensive care lengths of stay and has annual direct inpatient costs estimated in $4 billion solely in the United States [1]. Prolonged SE can lead to permanent neurologic injury and is associated with a high morbidity and mortality. Despite its ominous consequences, patients are commonly undertreated on initial presentation [2, 3]. As such, this chapter is aimed at providing keys to the timely diagnosis and appropriate treatment of SE.

Definitions and Classifications

Status epilepticus is typically referred to using an operational definition describing greater than 5 minutes of continuous seizure activity or greater than two episodes without return to baseline; however, more descriptive definitions have been put forth in recent years to standardize the terminology used and facilitate the recognition of syndromes with distinct prognostic and therapeutic implications [4].

2015 International League Against Epilepsy

The 2015 International League Against Epilepsy (ILAE) [4] uses a conceptual definition utilizing operational time-based (T1 and T2 time points) classifications according to seizure type and likelihood of long-term consequences based on preclinical studies with animal models of epilepsy and clinical research.

- T1—abnormally prolonged seizures reflecting high likelihood of continuous seizure activity due to a) failure of physiologic mechanisms of seizure termination and/or b) overwhelming seizure initiation mechanisms.
  - Generalized convulsive SE: 5 minutes
  - Focal SE with impaired awareness: 10 minutes
  - Absence SE: 10–15 minutes
- T2—continuous seizure activity reflecting high likelihood of long-term consequences, such as neuronal irreversible injury (and death), modifications of neural networks, and potential neurologic deficits.
  - Generalized SE: 30 minutes
  - Focal SE with impaired consciousness: >60 minutes
  - Absence SE: Unknown

The 2015 ILAE taskforce also updated historical subclassifications of SE according to four subcategories (or axes) allowing for a framework to be used in the clinical diagnosis, individualized workup, and therapies.

- Axis I: Semiology of clinical presentation based on the presence or absence of prominent motor symptoms and extent of consciousness impairment
  - With prominent motor symptoms
    - Convulsive SE (commonly referred to tonic-clonic SE): marked abnormal muscle contractions, often bilateral, sustained or waxing and waning
      - Generalized convulsive
      - Focal onset with evolution to bilateral convulsive SE
      - Unknown

- Myoclonic SE (prominent cortical myoclonic jerks)
  - With coma
  - Without coma
- Focal motor
  - Repeated focal motor (Jacksonian)
  - Epilepsia partialis continua
  - Adversive status
  - Oculoclonic status
  - Ictal paresis (focal loss of function or inhibitory SE)
- Tonic status (prolonged tonic contractions of axial and/or appendicular musculature)
- Hyperkinetic SE

- Without prominent motor symptoms, i.e., nonconvulsive status epilepticus (NCSE)
  - NCSE with coma
  - NCSE without coma
    - Generalized
      - Typical absence status
      - Atypical absence status
      - Myoclonic absence status
    - Focal
      - Without impairment of consciousness (or aura continua, with any sensory symptoms including autonomic, visual, gustatory, emotional/psychic/experiential, tactile or auditory)
      - Aphasic status
      - With impaired consciousness
    - Unknown focal vs generalized
      - Autonomic SE
- Axis II: Etiology
  - Known or symptomatic (often a structural, metabolic, inflammatory, infectious, or genetic disorder)
    - Acute—acute insult to the brain
    - Remote—prior static structural abnormality regardless of cause
    - Progressive—progressive structural abnormalities
    - SE in defined electroclinical syndromes
  - Unknown or cryptogenic

Table 2.1 summarizes the many commonly encountered etiologies for SE. Among patients with new-onset status epilepticus (i.e., without previous history of epilepsy), the most common etiologies are cerebrovascular disease and tumors [5].

- Axis III: Electroencephalographic correlate (utilizing the American Clinical Neurophysiology Society terminology for critical care EEG) [6]
  - Location (main term 1: generalized, lateralized, bilateral independent, multifocal)
  - Pattern (main term 2: periodic discharges, rhythmic delta activity, spike-and-wave/sharp-and-wave)

Table 2.1 Etiologies of status epilepticus [4]

Hypoxic-ischemic brain injury Cardiac arrest	**Dementias** Alzheimer's disease Corticobasal degeneration Frontotemporal dementia Vascular dementia	**Trauma (acute or remote)** Closed head injury Epidural hematoma Open head injury Subarachnoid hemorrhage Subdural hematoma
Autoimmune ADEM Anti-GAD Anti-NMDA receptor encephalitis Anti-V-G K+ channel receptor encephalitis Cerebral lupus CREST Goodpasture syndrome Multiple sclerosis Paraneoplastic encephalitis Rasmussen encephalitis TTP	**Cerebrovascular disease** Aneurysmal subarachnoid hemorrhage Cavernous and arteriovenous malformations Cerebral venous thrombosis Intracerebral hemorrhage Ischemic stroke Posterior reversible leukoencephalopathy	**CNS anomalies** Dentate dysplasia Focal cortical dysplasia Lissencephaly Polymicrogyria Hydrocephalus
Central nervous system infections Bacterial meningoencephalitis Fungal infection Neurocysticercosis Prion disease Progressive multifocal leukoencephalopathy Protozoal infection Toxoplasmosis Viral encephalitis	**Metabolic derangement** Acidosis ↑ blood urea nitrogen Hepatic encephalopathy Hyperammonemia Hyperglycemia Hypernatremia Hypocalcemia Hypoglycemia Hypomagnesemia Hyponatremia Wernicke encephalopathy	**Genetic** Adrenoleukodystrophy Alexander disease Carnitine palmitoyltransferase deficiency Lafora disease Maple syrup urine disease Menkes disease Metachromatic leukodystrophy Porphyria Tuberous sclerosis complex Unverricht-Lundborg disease Wilson disease

(continued)

Table 2.1 (continued)

Mitochondrial disease	Intracranial tumor	Medications and toxins
Alpers disease	Dysembryoplastic neuroepithelial tumor	Alcohol intoxication and withdrawal
Leigh syndrome	Gangliogliomas	Alkylating agents
Mitochondrial encephalopathy, lactic acidosis, and stroke-like episodes	Gliomas	Baclofen intoxication and withdrawal
Myoclonic encephalopathy with ragged red fibers	Lymphoma	Benzodiazepine withdrawal
Neuropathy, ataxia, and retinitis pigmentosa	Meningioma	Beta-interferons
	Metastases	CAR-T
	Primitive neuroectodermal tumor	Carbapenems (imipenem in particular)
		Cephalosporin (cefepime in particular)
		Cyclosporine
		Digoxin
		Fentanyl
		Heavy metals
		Lidocaine
		Metronidazole
		Mexiletine
		Theophylline
		Tramadol
		Tacrolimus
		Subtherapeutic ASD levels

Although this list includes many of the recognized etiologies for SE, many less common etiologies may be excluded from this table

ADEM acute disseminated encephalomyelitis, *Anti-GAD* glutamic acid decarboxylase antibody, *NMDA* N-methyl-D-aspartate, *Anti-(V-G) K+ channel* voltage-gated potassium channel antibody, *CREST* calcinosis, Raynaud phenomenon, esophageal dysmotility, sclerodactyly, telangectasia syndrome, *TTP* thrombotic thrombocytopenic purpura, *CAR-T* chimeric antigen receptor T cell therapy, *ASD* antiseizure drug

- Morphology (sharpness, number of phases, absolute and relative amplitude, polarity)
- Time-related features (prevalence, frequency, duration, onset, dynamics, daily pattern duration and index)
- Modulation (stimulus-induced vs spontaneous)
- Effect of intervention on EEG

- Axis IV: Age
  - Neonatal (0 to 30 days)
  - Infancy (1 month to 2 years)
  - Childhood (>2 to 12 years)
  - Adolescence and adulthood (>12 to 59 years)
  - Elderly (60 years or older)

Other important definitions have been set forth to facilitate the recognition of important clinical syndromes and collaborations between centers for clinical research.

Nonconvulsive Status Epilepticus (NCSE)

NCSE is defined as prolonged or repetitive electrographic seizures without prominent motor manifestations. Clinical correlates may vary widely and are often subtle but have to last at least 10 minutes [4, 7]. Note that approximately 50% of patients with convulsive SE will go on to have nonconvulsive seizures.

The modified Salzburg Consensus Criteria is suggested to guide the diagnosis for all patients with disturbance of consciousness and suspicion of NCSE. It utilizes a combination of clinical and EEG data and has been demonstrated to have excellent inter-rater agreement [8].

- Clinical requirements.
  - Change from premorbid baseline state occurring within a relative short interval (minutes to hours).
  - Fluctuation of clinical course without rapid improvement (which would be more suggestive of post-ictal state).
  - Absent structural damage on neuroimaging accounting for depressed mental status and EEG pattern and clinical syndrome out of proportion to toxic/metabolic derangement.
- EEG requirements depend on the presence or absence of known epileptic encephalopathy, and electrographic findings must be present for at least 10 seconds (to meet the duration requirement of nonconvulsive seizures).
  - If no known epileptic encephalopathy, at least one of the following EEG criteria must be fulfilled:
    - Epileptiform discharges reaching frequencies >2.5 Hz.
    - Clear evolution of rhythmic (>0.5 Hz) or periodic patterns in frequency and space (spreading).
    - Any clinical correlate (even if subtle) associated with rhythmic (>0.5 Hz) or periodic patterns.
    - Clear electroclinical response within 10 minutes to intravenous antiseizure drug (ASD) therapy in patients with epileptiform discharges ≤2.5 Hz with fluctuation or rhythmic activity (>0.5 Hz) with or without fluctuation.
      - Clinical response is considered when patients improve in at least one of the following:
        - "Say your surname"
        - "Repeat 1, 2, 3"
        - "Raise your arms" (or to mimic if unable to follow commands)
        - Eye opening with stimulation from first three commands
        - Tracking examiner in response to first three commands.
      - If only EEG improvement is seen after intravenous ASD trial, the patient is considered to have "possible NCSE."

In patients with impaired consciousness in the setting of acute brain injuries, craniotomy, sepsis, renal or liver failure, or post convulsive seizure, there should be a high threshold of suspicion for NCSE. Clinical features that should raise concern include abnormal eye movements and facial myoclonus.

Refractory Status Epilepticus (RSE)

Ongoing SE requiring escalation of therapy beyond first-line (benzodiazepine) and another appropriately selected and dosed parenteral ASD (e.g., valproic acid, phenytoin, levetiracetam, lacosamide), regardless of the specific seizure duration. Refractory SE is not uncommon [9]. It can be seen in half of patients with new-onset SE [5].

Super Refractory Status Epilepticus (SRSE)

Ongoing SE lasting over 24 hours from initiation of therapeutic coma with anesthetic treatment. This includes cases where seizures persist through escalating doses of anesthetics and those that initially responded to treatment but recurred during or after weaning of anesthetic agents leading to their reintroduction [9].

Prolonged Refractory Status Epilepticus (PRSE)

RSE lasting over 7 days in spite of adequate escalating therapy with the exception of therapeutic coma with anesthetic agents [9].

Prolonged Super Refractory Status Epilepticus (PSRSE)

SRSE lasting over 7 days in spite of adequate escalating therapy including therapeutic coma with anesthetic agents [9].

New-Onset Refractory Status Epilepticus (NORSE)

A patient without known epilepsy or other neurologic process presenting with de novo refractory status epilepticus (RSE), in whom a clear culprit is not readily identified (no acute toxic exposure or structural brain abnormality or ongoing provoking metabolic derangement) [9]. This denomination does not indicate a specific diagnosis, but it is useful to facilitate the recognition of a syndrome and allow for multicenter research collaborations.

Febrile Infection-Related Epilepsy Syndrome (FIRES)

Considered a subcategory of NORSE, to further specify the subset of patients that presented with a prodrome of a febrile illness in the preceding RSE onset by a variable period of 2 weeks to 24 hours [9]. The onset of RSE may or may not be accompanied by a fever. In the past, this syndrome was commonly used in pediatric setting, but it is now applicable for all ages.

Pathophysiology

Seizure occurs in the setting of increased glutamatergic activity within the brain. Additionally, there is a decrease in the normal inhibitory signaling by gamma-aminobutyric acid A ($GABA_A$) receptors resulting in an overall excitatory state [10].

Progression to SE occurs initially with a cascade of changes within the brain. There are alterations in ion channel and neurotransmitter activity as well as changes in patterns of protein phosphorylation. A decrease in $GABA_A$ $\beta2/\beta3$ and $\gamma2$ receptor subunits (internalization of $GABA_A$ receptors) and an increase in excitatory N-methyl-D-aspartic acid (NMDA) receptors promote benzodiazepine resistance [10].

Epidemiology

Incidence of SE has been estimated between 10 and 41 per 100,000 persons annually in the United States [1]. Data from Centers for Disease Control and Nationwide Inpatient Sample suggest that SE was the underlying cause of death in approximately 2 per 100,000 persons. Recent trends suggest that population-standardized hospitalizations for status epilepticus have increased over 50% from 1999 to 2010, while age-standardized mortality remained relatively stable in this period. This relative disconnect between rising incidence with stable mortality suggest improvement in the detection (likely due to increased recognition of this condition and increased use of EEG monitoring) and accurate documentation as a coding diagnosis of SE [1, 11].

- Age stratification of incidence exhibits a U-shaped curve with higher incidences in the <10 years and >50 years age groups. The mean age of onset was 39.5 +/− 28.9 years.

- Mortality rates are lowest in the <10 year and highest in the ≥80 year age groups.
- Males have a higher incidence, earlier age of onset, and a higher mortality rate compared to females.
- Those of African descent have the highest incidence rates of SE, but lower mortality rates, when compared to other races.

Generalized convulsive SE is the most common type reaching 45–74% of all cases being admitted to the hospital [1]. However, the distribution of incidence according to the type of SE varies widely in the literature according to the type of study (retrospective or prospective, single center or multicenter, year of publication, level of care setting); thus, ascertaining true proportions of convulsive and nonconvulsive SE is difficult. Further, a significant proportion of patients with generalized convulsive SE will go on to have NCSE.

A 9-year prospective cohort registry reported that 1/3 of SE episodes were refractory (RSE), and <5% met criteria for super-refractory (SRSE). The overall mortality in this cohort was 15.5% but reached 24.5% in RSE and 37.9% in SRSE, while non-refractory cases were as low as 9.8% [12]. In another retrospective Finnish registry (excluding post-anoxic cases), lower hospital mortalities were seen in RSE at 7.4%; however, one-year mortality reached 25% and was associated with super-refractoriness of SE, dependence in others for activities of daily living, severity of organ dysfunction at admission, and older age [13].

- Factors independently associated with RSE were severe consciousness impairment, older age, and lack of known remote etiology for SE.
- Younger age and severe impairment of consciousness correlated with SRSE, but most cases were not predicted by these variables.

In a multicenter RSE registry including 44 participating countries, the majority of cases occurred in patients with a cryptogenic etiology and without a prior history of epilepsy. Mortalities reached 25% despite seizure control being achieved in 74% of cases. Favorable course was associated with younger age, prior history of epilepsy, and low number of anesthetic agents used [14].

Up to 58% of patients with SE have no history of epilepsy [11]. Autoimmune and infectious causes are relatively uncommon (<10% each), but are often refractory to initial treatment and are more frequently seen in younger patients [15].

A precise ascertainment of comorbid conditions is limited by potential underreporting in documentation and coding. Commonly reported conditions include seizures, stroke, congenital disease, and metabolic complications to be among the most common comorbid conditions; anoxia, central nervous system infection, and neoplasm convey the highest mortality rates [11].

Evaluation and Diagnosis

Status epilepticus is a medical emergency, and the approach to these patients start with a comprehensive but focused assessment with the following priorities:

- Stabilization of airway, breathing, and circulation (ABCs) and establishment of intravenous access for treatment, while prioritizing patient safety with aspiration precautions and safety bed padding in place. Prompt implementation of pulse oximetry, blood pressure, and cardiac monitoring are advised.
- Rapid exclusion of hypoglycemia with glucose fingerstick measurement.
- Basic laboratory workup: complete blood count and basic metabolic panel with magnesium and phosphorous, lactic acid, creatine phosphokinase, ammonia, liver function profile, blood and urine drug screen including alcohol, amphetamines, and cocaine.
  - Seizures and SE commonly lead to leukocytosis, which may be pronounced and not necessarily point towards infectious etiology of seizures.
  - Metabolic derangements may lower seizure threshold including hypo-/hypernatremia, hypomagnesemia, elevated blood urea nitrogen, hyperammonemia, hypo-/hyperglycemia, and hypo-/hypercalcemia.
  - Prolonged convulsions may lead to rhabdomyolysis and lactic acidosis. Rhabdomyolysis in turn can produce acute kidney injury from tubular damage.
- Expanded laboratory workup should be considered in selected cases:
  - ASD levels for those with known diagnosis of epilepsy and when an intoxication is suspected.
  - Lumbar puncture and cerebrospinal fluid (CSF) analysis including glucose, cell count, protein, gram stain, and cultures and most common viruses leading to treatable encephalitis such as VZV and HSV. Expanded CSF analysis is often performed to include viral encephalitis panels, IgG index, flow cytometry, cytology, paraneoplastic panel (including NMDA receptor antibodies), and autoimmune epilepsy panel. Table 2.2 includes the main autoantibodies that should be tested in patients with SE.

Table 2.2 Autoantibodies associated with non-infectious inflammatory epilepticus [15]

NMDA	CASPR2	GAD65	Ach receptor binding
AMPA	DPPX	CRMP-5	Amphiphysin
GABAA	LGI-1	Anti-glial nuclear	Anti-neuronal nuclear types 1, 2, and 3
GABAB	Neuronal (V-G) K+ channel	N-type calcium channel	
Purkinje cell cytoplasmic type 2 and type Tr	P/Q-type calcium channel	Ach receptor ganglionic neuronal	

Listed are auto-antibodies which have been associated with SE including those tested for with the Mayo Epilepsy, Autoimmune Evaluation, Serum panel (EPS1), though other autoantibodies may also be linked to SE

NMDA N-methyl-D-aspartate receptor antibody, *AMPA* α-amino-3-hydroxy-5-methyl-4-isoxazolepropionic acid receptor antibody, *GABAA* γ- aminobutyric acid A receptor antibody, *GABAB* γ-aminobutyric acid B receptor antibody, *CASPR2* contactin-associated protein-like2 IgG, *DPPX* dipeptidyl-peptidase-like protein 6 antibody, *LGI-1* leucine-rich glioma-inactivated protein 1 IgG, *neuronal (V-G) K+ channel* voltage-gated potassium channel antibody, *GAD65* glutamic acid decarboxylase antibody, *CRMP-5* collapsing response-mediator protein 5 antibody, *Ach* acetylcholine

Table 2.3 Status epilepticus mimics [17]

Intensive care setting	Ambulatory setting
Chorea-like movements	Psychogenic spells
Semi-purposeful movements	Parasomnias
Tremor-like movements	Syncope
Nonepileptic behavioral spells	
Dystonia	
Myoclonic jerks	

Not all abnormal movements in the ICU setting are caused by SE. Listed are several common mimics which can be seen in both the critically ill and ambulatory patient

- A non-contrast computed tomography of the head is indicated in most cases, particularly in those without clear precipitating factors and when trauma is suspected. A gadolinium-enhanced magnetic resonance imaging (MRI) of the brain can be useful in identifying culprit lesions. Prolonged seizures may cause transient cortical ribboning and thalamic hyperintensities on diffusion-weighted imaging and apparent diffusion coefficient maps, as well as increased T2 signal involving these areas and limbic structures. Mesial temporal sclerosis is commonly found in those with temporal lobe epilepsies, but it may be a late finding in SRSE. Cortical atrophy is commonly seen in SRSE cases and may be reversible [16].
- Continuous EEG (cEEG) is the mainstay of diagnosis and helps guiding therapy in NCSE; thus, it should be promptly initiated in patients who do not return to baseline after prolonged convulsions and in those at risk for nonconvulsive seizures. Centers without cEEG capabilities must be able to repeat 30–60 minutes studies frequently or should transfer patients to centers with increased resources.
- Several conditions may mimic SE. Table 2.3 summarizes common differential diagnoses [17].

Treatment

Prompt termination of SE should be considered a priority given the high morbidity potential associated with prolonged seizures and higher likelihood of treatment failure with delays in therapy.

A tiered approach should be pursued including:

- Adequate doses of benzodiazepine administration as first line of action for seizure termination.
- While benzodiazepines are recommended as first-line therapy for the treatment of SE, up to 40% of patients will not respond to benzodiazepine therapy [18, 19].
- Subsequent loading doses of parenteral ASD (either as second-line therapy in benzodiazepine refractory cases or secondary seizure prophylaxis if SE is successfully treated with benzodiazepines).

- If no response is seen despite adequate doses of first- and second-line therapies, therapeutic coma with intravenous anesthetics should be considered (see Fig. 2.1).
- Rapid progression to anesthesia is definitely justified in patients with refractory generalized convulsive SE and probably in patients with generalized nonconvulsive SE. In cases of focal SE, additional parenteral ASDs may be tried before resorting to induction of anesthesia.

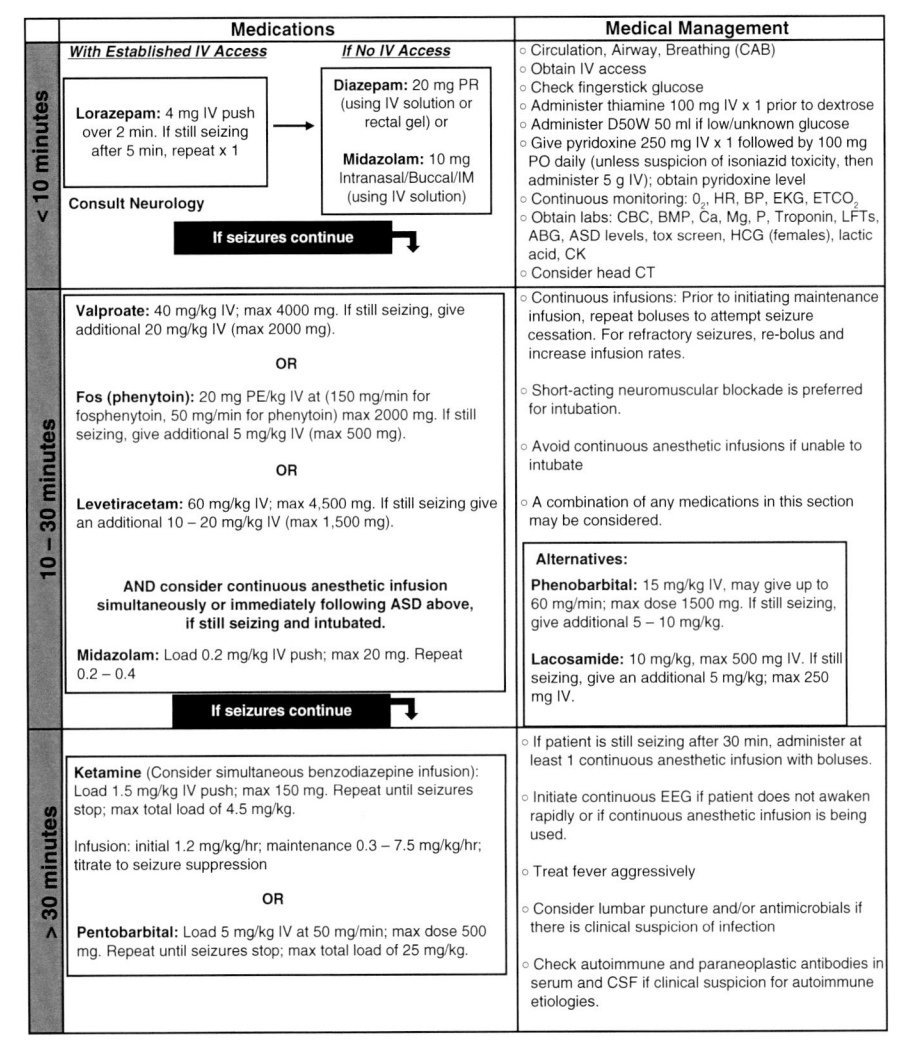

	Medications		Medical Management
< 10 minutes	*With Established IV Access* **Lorazepam:** 4 mg IV push over 2 min. If still seizing after 5 min, repeat x 1 **Consult Neurology**	*If No IV Access* **Diazepam:** 20 mg PR (using IV solution or rectal gel) or **Midazolam:** 10 mg Intranasal/Buccal/IM (using IV solution)	○ Circulation, Airway, Breathing (CAB) ○ Obtain IV access ○ Check fingerstick glucose ○ Administer thiamine 100 mg IV x 1 prior to dextrose ○ Administer D50W 50 ml if low/unknown glucose ○ Give pyridoxine 250 mg IV x 1 followed by 100 mg PO daily (unless suspicion of isoniazid toxicity, then administer 5 g IV); obtain pyridoxine level ○ Continuous monitoring: O_2, HR, BP, EKG, $ETCO_2$ ○ Obtain labs: CBC, BMP, Ca, Mg, P, Troponin, LFTs, ABG, ASD levels, tox screen, HCG (females), lactic acid, CK ○ Consider head CT
	If seizures continue ⬇		
10 – 30 minutes	**Valproate:** 40 mg/kg IV; max 4000 mg. If still seizing, give additional 20 mg/kg IV (max 2000 mg). OR **Fos (phenytoin):** 20 mg PE/kg IV at (150 mg/min for fosphenytoin, 50 mg/min for phenytoin) max 2000 mg. If still seizing, give additional 5 mg/kg IV (max 500 mg). OR **Levetiracetam:** 60 mg/kg IV; max 4,500 mg. If still seizing give an additional 10 – 20 mg/kg IV (max 1,500 mg). AND consider continuous anesthetic infusion simultaneously or immediately following ASD above, if still seizing and intubated. **Midazolam:** Load 0.2 mg/kg IV push; max 20 mg. Repeat 0.2 – 0.4		○ Continuous infusions: Prior to initiating maintenance infusion, repeat boluses to attempt seizure cessation. For refractory seizures, re-bolus and increase infusion rates. ○ Short-acting neuromuscular blockade is preferred for intubation. ○ Avoid continuous anesthetic infusions if unable to intubate ○ A combination of any medications in this section may be considered. **Alternatives:** **Phenobarbital:** 15 mg/kg IV, may give up to 60 mg/min; max dose 1500 mg. If still seizing, give additional 5 – 10 mg/kg. **Lacosamide:** 10 mg/kg, max 500 mg IV. If still seizing, give an additional 5 mg/kg; max 250 mg IV.
	If seizures continue ⬇		
> 30 minutes	**Ketamine** (Consider simultaneous benzodiazepine infusion): Load 1.5 mg/kg IV push; max 150 mg. Repeat until seizures stop; max total load of 4.5 mg/kg. Infusion: initial 1.2 mg/kg/hr; maintenance 0.3 – 7.5 mg/kg/hr; titrate to seizure suppression OR **Pentobarbital:** Load 5 mg/kg IV at 50 mg/min; max dose 500 mg. Repeat until seizures stop; max total load of 25 mg/kg.		○ If patient is still seizing after 30 min, administer at least 1 continuous anesthetic infusion with boluses. ○ Initiate continuous EEG if patient does not awaken rapidly or if continuous anesthetic infusion is being used. ○ Treat fever aggressively ○ Consider lumbar puncture and/or antimicrobials if there is clinical suspicion of infection ○ Check autoimmune and paraneoplastic antibodies in serum and CSF if clinical suspicion for autoimmune etiologies.

Fig. 2.1 Tiered therapeutic approach to status epilepticus. ABG arterial blood gas, ASD antiseizure drug levels, BMP basic metabolic profile, Ca calcium, CBC complete blood count, CK creatine kinase, CSF cerebrospinal fluid, EKG electrocardiogram, ETCO2 end-tidal carbon dioxide, HCG human chorionic gonadotropin, HR heart rate, IV intravenous, IM intramuscular, LFTs liver function tests, Mg magnesium, P phosphorus, PO per oral route, PR per rectum. (Adapted from the Yale New Haven Hospital status epilepticus protocol)

Failure to follow guidelines recommendations (mainly under-dosing and delays in treatment) may lead to worse outcomes.

The pathological foundation of seizures leading to SE plays a paramount role in ASD selection. As such, mechanisms of available ASDs must be considered in selecting an appropriate drug therapy while considering:

- Drug pharmacokinetics
- Tolerability
- Appreciable drug-drug interactions
- Patient specific factors (Table 2.4)

Generally, ASD effects are mediated by increasing the effectiveness of inhibitory transmission via $GABA_A$ receptor or by decreasing the excitatory transmission via inhibition of glutamate release or transmission via ionotropic receptors [19].

Figure 2.2 illustrates ASD targets and classification based on primary mechanisms.

GABAergic Targets

- Benzodiazepines enhance neurotransmission via increasing the frequency of chloride ion channel opening allosterically.
- Barbiturates achieve a similar neurotransmitter effect by prolonging the duration of chloride ion channel opening by binding to the active site of the GABAA receptor [19].
- Among parenteral benzodiazepines:
  - IV lorazepam is the preferred agent in patients with established IV access.
  - IM midazolam is preferred in the absence of established IV access.
  - Diazepam is the preferred agent for rectal administration.
  - Injectable diazepam and lorazepam contain propylene glycol, which can cause hypotension and metabolic acidosis [20].
- Intranasal midazolam recently became an approved therapy to abort seizure clusters/prolonged seizures.
- Clobazam and clonazepam are enteral agents, which have a role as add-on treatment of RSE, though their use is limited by lack of parenteral formulation.
- Clobazam may be associated with less sedation compared to other available benzodiazepines.
- Phenobarbital, a long-acting barbiturate, is an effective alternative in benzodiazepine-resistant SE. It can also be useful to facilitate weaning from continuous infusions of GABAergic anesthetics.
- Other ASDs that target inhibitory synapses include vigabatrin and tiagabine, [19] but their use in SE is limited due to lack of parenteral formulations.

Table 2.4 Suggested dosing, pharmacokinetic data, and considerations of therapeutic agents used in status epilepticus [19, 20]

ASD	Dosing	Approximate half-life (h) in non-critically ill patients	Protein binding	Clinically relevant drug-drug interactions with other ASDs	Considerations for dose adjustment in renal impairment	Considerations for dose adjustment in hepatic impairment	Comments
Injectable anesthetic agents							
Ketamine	LD: 1.5 mg/kg IV push over 3–5 min (max 150 mg); repeat until seizures stop; max total load of 4.5 mg/kg. MD: Initial 1.2 mg/kg/h, range 0.3–7.5 mg/kg/h; titrate to seizure suppression	2.5	45%		None	Consider dose reduction	NMDA antagonist; provides an infusion with a different mechanism of action (non-GABA) May have sympathomimetic properties, but can also cause hypotension when HR/SBP ≥ 0.9
Midazolam	LD: 0.2 mg/kg IV (push over 1–2 min); max 20 mg. Repeat 0.2–0.4 mg/kg boluses (max 40 mg per bolus) q5min until seizures stop; max total load of 2 mg/kg. MD: 0.05–2.9 mg/kg/h; titrate to seizure suppression	7	95%		Consider dose reduction: risk of active metabolite accumulation	Consider dose reduction	Rapid redistribution Active metabolites May be administered via alternate routes: 0.2 mg/kg (up to 10 mg) IM, intranasal, or buccal routes; all well absorbed rapidly

(continued)

Table 2.4 (continued)

ASD	Dosing	Approximate half-life (h) in non-critically ill patients	Protein binding	Clinically relevant drug-drug interactions with other ASDs	Considerations for dose adjustment in renal impairment	Considerations for dose adjustment in hepatic impairment	Comments
Pentobarbital	LD: 5 mg/kg IVP (up to 50 mg/min); max 500 mg. Repeat until seizures stop; max total load of 25 mg/kg. MD: 0.5–10 mg/kg/h; titrate to seizure suppression	22	45–70%		None	Consider dose reduction	Prolonged half-life (up to 50 hours; dose dependent) May cause hypotension, ileus, myocardial suppression, immunosuppression, and thrombocytopenia IV formulation contains 40% propylene glycol; may cause metabolic acidosis
Propofol	LD: 1–2 mg/kg IV over 5 min; max 200 mg. Repeat until seizures stop up to total LD of 10 mg/kg MD: 30–200 mcg/kg/min (1.8–12 mg/kg/h); titrate to seizure suppression	0.6 (Extended with prolonged use) Terminal half-life: 4–7	90%		None	None	May cause respiratory depression, hypotension, hypertriglyceridemia, pancreatitis, and PRIS (metabolic acidosis, bradycardia, cardiac arrest, rhabdomyolysis, renal failure Contraindicated in patients with hypersensitivity to egg or soy products Monitor pH, bicarbonate, triglycerides, creatine kinase, lipase with prolonged therapy (> 48 h) or high doses (> 80 mcg/kg/min or 5 mg/kg/h)

2 Status Epilepticus

Injectable non-anesthetic agents

Drug	Dose	Half-life (hr)	Protein binding	Drug interactions	Renal	Hepatic	Comments
Brivaracetam[a]	LD: 200 mg MD: 200–300 mg/day divided BID to TID	9	<20%	May ↑↑ plasma concentrations of phenytoin and carbamazepine	Not recommended in severe renal impairment	Consider dose reduction	
Carbamazepine	LD: 400–800 mg MD: 400–600 mg/day divided BID	24 8 (with prolonged use due to auto-induction; 2–4 weeks)	75–90%	Major CYP3A4 substrate; major CYP2C19/3A4 inducer. Phenytoin and other CYP3A4 inducers ↓↓levels. Valproic acid and other CYP3A4 inhibitors ↑↑ levels	Consider dose reduction in severe renal impairment (CrCl <10 ml/min): reduce dose by 25%	Consider dose reduction: undergoes extensive hepatic metabolism	Strong association between the risk of developing Stevens-Johnson syndrome/TEN and the presence of HLA-B*1502 allele (documented mostly in Asian descent) Dose-dependent hyponatremia; decreased incidence compared to oxcarbazepine
Diazepam	LD: 0.25 mg/kg IV push over 1–2 min (max 10 mg per dose); repeat every 5 min until seizures stop up to 3 doses or 30 mg. MD: not applicable	40	98%		Not applicable	Not applicable	Rapid redistribution Active metabolite IV formulation contains propylene glycol IV solution may be administered rectally if no IV access. Preferred benzodiazepine for rectal administration

(continued)

Table 2.4 (continued)

ASD	Dosing	Approximate half-life (h) in non-critically ill patients	Protein binding	Clinically relevant drug-drug interactions with other ASDs	Considerations for dose adjustment in renal impairment	Considerations for dose adjustment in hepatic impairment	Comments
Fosphenytoin	LD: 20 mg PE/kg IV (up to 150 mg/min); max 2000 mg. If still seizing, give additional 5 mg/kg IV (max 500 mg) MD: use phenytoin	See phenytoin Conversion half-life to phenytoin ~ 15 to 30 minutes Note: fosphenytoin is dosed in phenytoin equivalents					May be administered IM if no IV access (up to 99% absorption after IM administration) Compatible in saline, dextrose, and lactated ringers solution Nontoxic diluent; ↓cutaneous reactions with extravasation May cause hypotension, arrhythmias Obtain peak phenytoin level 2 hours post IV dose or 4 hours post IM dose
Lacosamide	LD: 10 mg/kg IV over 5–10 min (max 500 mg) If still seizing, give an additional 5 mg/kg over 5 min (max 250 mg IV) MD: 200–600 mg/day divided BID to QID.	13	< 15%		Reduce dose in severe renal impairment (CrCl <30 ml/min); max 300 mg/day HD: 50% removed; lower dose based on CrCl, divide BID and add 50% of AM dose to PM dose post HD CRRT: lower dose based on CrCl, then increase total daily dose by 50% and divide TID	Consider dose reduction	May prolong PR interval or induce tachyarrhythmias, including atrial fibrillation

Levetiracetam	LD: 60 mg/kg over 15 min (max 4500 mg) MD: 1500–4500 mg/day divided TID to QID	6	<10%	Reduce dose based on CrCl <u>HD</u>: 50% removed; lower dose based on CrCl, divide BID, and add 50% of AM dose to PM dose post HD <u>CRRT</u>: lower dose based on CrCl, then increase total daily dose by 50%, and divide QID	May cause behavioral disturbances; consider switch to brivaracetam
Lorazepam	LD: 4 mg IVP over 2 min; repeat every 5 min until seizures stop up to 3 doses or 12 mg MD: not applicable	12	85–90%	Not applicable	Not applicable	Rapid redistribution IV formulation contains 80% propylene glycol; may cause metabolic acidosis. Do not administer IM or SC (IM midazolam preferred if IV access not available)

(continued)

Table 2.4 (continued)

ASD	Dosing	Approximate half-life (h) in non-critically ill patients	Protein binding	Clinically relevant drug-drug interactions with other ASDs	Considerations for dose adjustment in renal impairment	Considerations for dose adjustment in hepatic impairment	Comments
Phenytoin	LD: 20 mg/kg IVP (up to 50 mg/min; 25 mg/min in elderly and patients with preexisting cardiovascular conditions) MD: 200–600 mg/day divided BID or TID	15	90–95%	Induces CYP 1A2, 2B6, 2C, 3A3/4 Generally avoid use with most CYP3A4 substrates Coadministration with valproate displaces phenytoin from protein binding sites. Induces metabolism of valproate	None	Consider dose reduction	May cause rash, fever, hypotension, or arrhythmias IV formulation contains 40% propylene glycol; may cause metabolic acidosis Only compatible in saline (unlike fosphenytoin). Incompatibilities include D5W, potassium, insulin, heparin, norepinephrine, cephalosporins, and dobutamine Severe tissue injury may occur with extravasation, including rare purple glove syndrome
Phenobarbital	LD: 15 mg/kg IV (up to 60 mg/min); max dose 1500 mg. If still seizing, give an additional 5–10 mg/kg. MD: 1–3 mg/kg/day given q day or divided BID or TID	80	50–60%	Strong inducer of UGT, CYP 3A4, 2B6, 2C9, 2A6, 1A2. Dose adjustments of ASDs including phenytoin and valproate might be necessary	Consider dose reduction HD: give full daily dose in evening after hemodialysis	Consider dose reduction	Prolonged half-life (up to 140 hours) May cause hypotension IV formulation contains 70% propylene glycol; may cause metabolic acidosis

Valproate	LD: 40 mg/kg IV (over 5–10 min); max 4000 mg. If still seizing, give additional 20 mg/kg IV (max 2000 mg) over 5 min MD: 2000–6000 mg divided TID to QID	12	90%	Phenytoin and valproate may displace each other from protein binding sites Valproate markedly inhibits lamotrigine metabolism → ↑↑ lamotrigine levels and risk of side effects including rash	None	Caution in hepatic impairment	Highly plasma protein bound (up to 90%) May cause hyperammonemic encephalopathy (treated with L-carnitine supplementation), hepatotoxicity, thrombocytopenia, and platelet dysfunction Concurrent use with carbapenems may result in markedly decreased valproic acid plasma concentrations
Enteral agents							
Clobazam	LD: 20–40 mg MD: 20–60 mg/day divided BID	39	80–90%	Felbamate: ↑plasma concentrations of N-desmethylclobazam	Caution in severe renal impairment (CrCl <30 ml/min)	Consider dose reduction: undergoes extensive hepatic metabolism	Decreased sedation compared to other benzodiazepines
Gabapentin	LD: 1200–3600 mg MD: 2400–4800 mg divided TID to QID	6	<3%		Reduce dose based on CrCl HD: dose based on CrCl, administer supplemental dose post HD	None	

(continued)

Table 2.4 (continued)

ASD	Dosing	Approximate half-life (h) in non-critically ill patients	Protein binding	Clinically relevant drug-drug interactions with other ASDs	Considerations for dose adjustment in renal impairment	Considerations for dose adjustment in hepatic impairment	Comments
Oxcarbazepine	LD: 600–1200 mg MD: 600–2400 mg/day divided BID to QID	5	67%	↑ concentrations of phenobarbital and phenytoin	Consider 50% dose reduction in severe renal impairment HD: IR formulations preferred	ER formulation not recommended	Dose-dependent hyponatremia; more common in elderly
Perampanel	LD: 6–12 mg MD: 12 mg/day	105	95%		Use not recommended in severe renal impairment (CrCl <30 ml/min)	Consider dose reduction in mild to moderate hepatic impairment. Use not recommended in severe hepatic impairment	May cause behavioral issues/agitation
Pregabalin	LD: 150–300 mg MD: 150–600 mg/day divided TID to QID	6	None		Reduce dose HD: dose based on CrCl, administer supplemental dose post HD	None	Occasional peripheral edema

Topiramate	LD: 200–400 mg MD: 200–600 (reports up to 1600) mg/day divided BID to QID	21	15–41%	Use with zonisamide and other carbonic anhydrase inhibitors may worsen metabolic acidosis	Reduce dose by ~50% HD: supplemental dose may be necessary	Consider dose reduction	May cause metabolic acidosis; caution with propofol, acetazolamide, zonisamide and metformin May cause renal stones May be associated with oligohidrosis, with risk of hyperthermia, mainly in pediatric patients
Vigabatrin	LD: 1500 mg. MD: 1000–3000 mg/day divided BID	10 (but sustained effect for several days)	None		Reduce dose based on CrCl	None	Potential progressive permanent peripheral vision loss after months to years of use; regular ophthalmology examinations recommended with prolonged use

Adapted from the Yale New Haven Hospital status epilepticus protocol

ASD antiseizure drug, *CrCl* creatinine clearance, *HD* hemodialysis, *HR* heart rate, *IM* intramuscular, *IV* intravenous, *IVP* intravenous push, *IR* immediate release, *PO* per oral route, *PR* per rectum, *LD* loading dose, *MD* maintenance dose, *PRIS* propofol related infusion syndrome, *SBP* systolic blood pressure

[a]Use in status epilepticus is extrapolated from non-SE data and conversion from levetiracetam to brivaracetam in non-SE

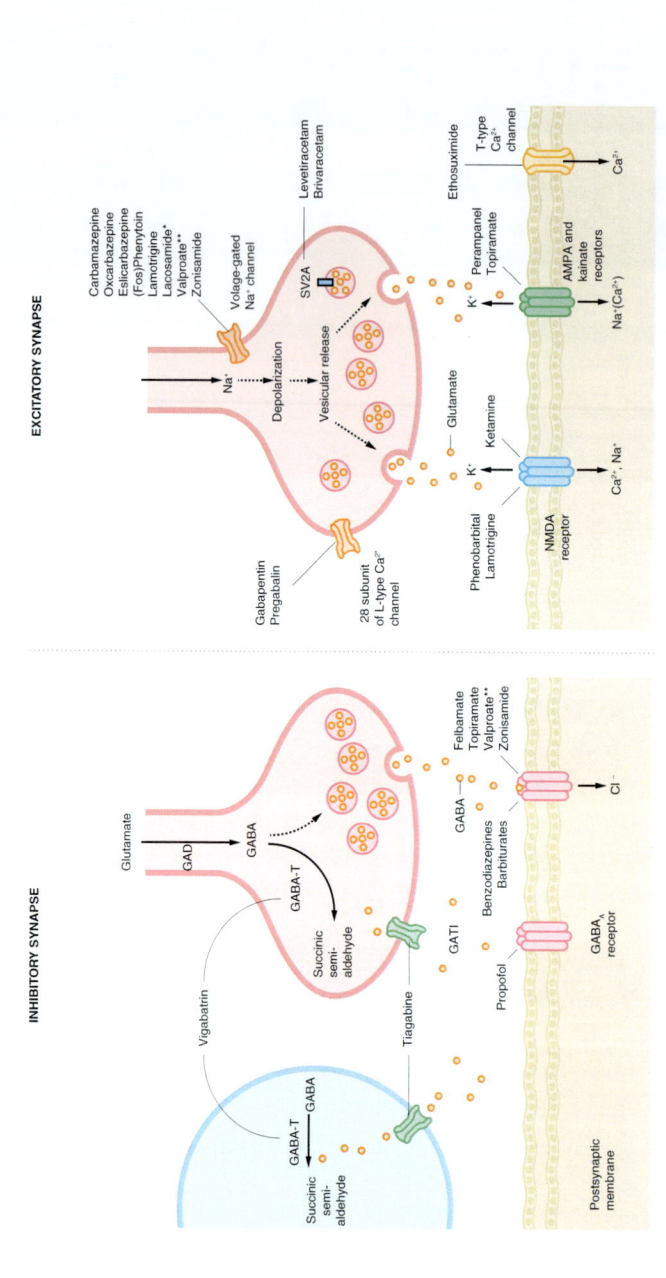

Fig. 2.2 Proposed mechanism of currently available ASDs utilized in SE. ASDs that modulate voltage-gated Na+ channels would be expected to decrease depolarization-induced Ca+ influx and vesicular release of neurotransmitters. *Lacosamide also enhances slow inactivation of voltage-gated Na+ channels unlike the effect seen with other agents in this class, which are thought to enhance fast inactivation. Levetiracetam and brivaracetam bind to SV2A, which might have a role in neurotransmitter release. Gabapentin and pregabalin bind to the α2δ subunit of voltage-gated Ca2+ channels, which is thought to be associated with a decrease in neurotransmitter release. Topiramate acts on AMPA and kainate receptors; and felbamate acts on NMDA receptors leading to inhibition of excitatory neurotransmission at the postsynaptic membrane. GAT1 is inhibited by tiagabine, leading to a decrease in GABA uptake into presynaptic terminals. GABA-T is irreversibly inhibited by vigabatrin which in turn decreases the metabolism of GABA in presynaptic terminals. The benzodiazepines, barbiturates, felbamate, topiramate, and zonisamide enhance inhibitory neurotransmission by modulating GABAA receptor-mediated Cl currents. **Broad spectrum valproic acid with activity at both excitatory and inhibitory synapses. AMPA (α-amino-3-hydroxy-5-methyl-4-isoxazole propionic acid) receptors; GABA, γ-aminobutyric acid; GABA-T, GABA transaminase; GAD, glutamic acid decarboxylase catalyzes the decarboxylation of glutamate to GABA; GAT1, GABA transporter; NMDA (N-methyl-d-aspartate) receptors; SV2A, synaptic vesicle glycoprotein 2A. (Adapted from [18])

Voltage-Dependent Sodium Channel Targets

- ASDs that prolong the inactive state of voltage-dependent sodium channels include carbamazepine, oxcarbazepine, eslicarbazepine, fosphenytoin/phenytoin, lacosamide, and zonisamide [19].
- Phenytoin and fosphenytoin are both recommended for the treatment of benzodiazepine refractory SE [20, 21].
- While the cardiovascular effects of injectable phenytoin may be attributed to the polyethylene glycol and ethanol vehicles used in the parenteral phenytoin formulation, fosphenytoin, a water-soluble phosphate ester prodrug of phenytoin, allows for more rapid administration at a rate of up to 150 mg per minute vs 50 mg per minute for phenytoin.
- Post-loading plasma levels of phenytoin can be checked 1 hour after the completion of infusion. An interval of 2 hours is recommended after fosphenytoin loading to allow for its conversion into phenytoin (mean conversion half-life of approximately 15 minutes).
- The use of lacosamide, a drug that enhances slow-inactivation of voltage-gated sodium channels, in the setting of SE is growing after a few small studies demonstrated similar efficacy and safety profiles to commonly used ASD [22]. The propensity for minimal drug interactions with lacosamide makes it a desirable agent, but it carries a risk of PR interval prolongation.
- Monitoring with frequent EKGs is recommended for all drugs in this class.
- Structural similarities exist between carbamazepine, oxcarbazepine, and eslicarbazepine; the newer drugs appear to have similar efficacy but improved tolerability with fewer drug-drug interactions and less extensive hepatic metabolism. The limited availability of parenteral formulations for carbamazepine-related drugs reserves these agents to an add-on role after other intravenous agents fail, although it is unclear if the recent injectable formulation of carbamazepine (Carnexiv®) may have a role in SE.

Synaptic Vesicle Targets

- Levetiracetam, characterized by its binding to synaptic vesicle protein 2A (SV2A), a protein responsible for glutamate release, is been increasingly used for the treatment of benzodiazepine-refractory SE due to its widespread availability and lack of drug interactions.
- When using levetiracetam for SE, the loading dose of 60 mg/kg should be considered (except in patients with advanced renal failure).
- Brivaracetam, a third-generation ASD with a higher binding affinity to SV2A than levetiracetam, is also thought to have effects on voltage-activated Na+ inflow in cortical neurons and might have a broader anticonvulsant scope than levetiracetam.

Glutamatergic Targets

- Evidence suggests that refractoriness to ASDs during SE is not only due to impaired GABA-mediated inhibition secondary to GABA receptor internalization but also upregulation of a-amino-3-hydroxy-5-methyl-4-isoxazolepropionic acid (AMPA) and NMDA receptors at the synaptic membrane [20].
- Glutamatergic drug targets may have a critical role in the management of RSE, but the lack of parenteral formulations of the majority of agents in this class limits their use in early stages of SE.
- Ketamine, an anti-NMDA receptor drug, can be effective for the treatment of SRSE when used in anesthetic doses [23].

Therapeutic Coma

- Midazolam and propofol infusions are in the frontline of the therapeutic approaches for RSE, but practical approaches utilizing anesthetics as therapeutic coma vary widely [3].
- Recent pre-clinical studies have demonstrated potential benefits of a combined therapeutic strategy to status epilepticus aiming for synergistic mechanisms of action which include the use of lower doses of midazolam and ketamine.
- The prolonged use of anesthetics is associated with higher rates of systemic complications including possible increased mortality and increased length of stay, thus, its use should be carefully balanced in selected cases.
    - Injectable phenobarbital contains propylene glycol and may induce or exacerbate to metabolic acidosis [20].
    - Higher infusion rates of midazolam may lead to hyperchloremic non-anion gap acidosis due its dilution with 0.9% sodium chloride.
    - Ketamine infusions can be diluted in D5W or normal saline, and higher infusion rates are associated with high fluid intake volumes.
    - Propofol infusion syndrome (PRIS) is characterized by refractory bradycardia and metabolic acidosis (lactic acidosis), hyperlipidemia, and rhabdomyolysis. The risk increases with prolonged infusions; therefore, care should be taken when using high infusion rates for more than 48 hours.
        - Younger patients on high-rate propofol infusions for prolonged durations are at highest risk. Additionally, those with inadequate carbohydrate intake are also at increased risk.
        - Routine monitoring includes serial lactic acid, creatine kinase, and triglycerides levels.
        - Propofol infusion should be discontinued upon recognition of PRIS. Supportive treatment is the mainstay of therapy, including renal replacement therapy and cardiac and respiratory support.
- Infusion rates should be titrated with concurrent careful monitoring on EEG. Therapeutic targets remain controversial as not all patients may benefit (or tolerate) burst suppression, and seizure suppression may be as effective and

require less hemodynamic support in some instances. Emerging evidence suggests that the characteristics of bursts of EEG activity during anesthetic infusion and wean may hold prognostic value related to the refractoriness of SE.
- There is no evidence to guide duration of therapeutic coma or anesthetic weaning. The re-emergence of epileptiform patterns during anesthetic weaning is common and may be transient. Whether these EEG findings warrant careful conservative watching or re-introduction of deeper levels of anesthesia remains a matter of debate.
- Inhaled anesthetics such as isoflurane and halothane have been used in super-refractory SE; however, their widespread use is limited by the logistics involved with the utilization of gas anesthesia outside the operating room settings.

Ketogenic Diet

- Ketogenic diet has previously been used for treatment of medically refractory epilepsy in children and adults. It is a diet high in fat with low carbohydrates. As fat metabolism takes place, ketones will be produced [24].
- It has recently been used in the treatment of NORSE, FIRES, SRSE, and anti-NMDA receptor encephalitis-related SE with promising results.
- Adjustment of all concurrently administered medications to formulations that do not include sugar vehicles is necessary in order to allow for establishment of a ketotic state.
- Care should be taken as patients have been noted to experience metabolic acidosis with ketogenic diet, less common effects such as hypoglycemia, hyperlipidemia, poor wound healing, hyponatremia, weight loss, and constipation.

Other Rescue Approaches

- Therapeutic hypothermia added to standard of care has been recently demonstrated to decrease the rate of progression to EEG-confirmed SE in patients with convulsive status epilepticus but was not associated with improved outcomes despite an increase in adverse events [25].
- Empiric surgical approaches such as acute respective surgery in RSE can be viable options in selected cases with focal onset of seizures [26].
- Patients with seizures in the setting of autoimmune encephalitis have been shown to develop freedom from seizures more rapidly and more often when treated with immunotherapeutic agents [27].

Systemic Effects

Systemic complications associated with SE including acid/base disturbances, respiratory compromise, and cardiac injury should always be kept in mind as they can be life-threatening and require urgent or emergent intervention [28].

Table 2.5 Systemic effects of status epilepticus

Cardiac	Pulmonary	Renal and acid-base	Musculoskeletal and tegmentum	Hyperadrenergic	Complications with prolonged hospital course
Arrhythmia	Hypoxia	Acute renal failure due to rhabdomyolysis	Rhabdomyolysis	Hypertension	Infection
Cardiomyopathy	Pulmonary edema	Lactic acidosis	Dislocation	Leukocytosis	Gastrostomy and/or tracheostomy
Cardiac necrosis	Aspiration		Fracture	Tachycardia	Skin breakdown and poor wound healing
Conduction abnormalities	Mucous plugging		Skin breakdown	Hyperglycemia	Critical illness myopathy or neuropathy
	Respiratory acidosis		Poor wound healing		Deep vein thrombosis
					Pulmonary embolism

Systemic complications vary from patient to patient. Listed are many of the more common complications associated with status epilepticus

Additional complications can arise as a result of prolonged hospital course, including deep vein thrombosis, infection, and ARDS. Table 2.5 summarizes many of the systemic complications seen associated with SE.

Medications used as antiseizure therapy can also have a wide range of adverse effects including respiratory depression, platelet and clotting dysfunction, hyperammonemia, sedation, PR prolongation, hypotension, and numerous others. Many of these were previously discussed in the chapter, and consideration of these effects should be taken into account when choosing a therapy.

Prognosis

- Approximately 13% of all patients experience recurrence of SE [11].
- Mortality rates vary significantly depending on age, rates of infectious complications, and, most importantly, etiology of convulsive SE [29].
    - Post-anoxic SE (60–100%)
    - Cerebrovascular disease-related SE (20–60%)
    - Metabolic disorders (10–35%)
    - Acute CNS infection (up to 30%)
- Patients above the age of 50 are particularly at risk for poor outcome [11].
- Multiple scoring systems have been developed to assist the clinician gauging prognosis [30].

The Status Epilepticus Severity Score (STESS) is based on (1) initial level of consciousness, (2) worse seizure type (generalized-convulsive, simple-partial, complex-partial, absence, myoclonic), (3) age, and (4) history of seizure. A score of ≥3 was associated with higher mortality. STESS carries a high negative predictive value (NPV) for survival, particularly with the increased cutoff of 4 points.

The Epidemiology-Based Mortality Score in Status Epilepticus (EMSE) includes (1) etiology, (2) age, (3) comorbidities, and (4) EEG patterns (lateralized periodic discharges, generalized periodic discharges, ictal discharges, and spontaneous burst suppression). A score of ≥64 was associated with higher mortality and a superior performance when compared with STESS-3 and STESS-4 scoring systems. Table 2.6 displays the EMSE score [30, 31].

Table 2.6 Epidemiology-Based Mortality Score in Status Epilepticus (EMSE) [28, 29]

Age	Points	Comorbidity (score each disease)	Points
>80	10	AIDS, metastatic solid tumor	60
71–80	8	Moderate to severe liver disease	30
61–70	7	Moderate to severe renal disease, any tumor (includes lymphoma and leukemia), hemiplegia, diabetes with end-organ damage	20
51–60	5		
41–50	3		
31–40	2	Peripheral vascular disease, connective tissue disease, diabetes, myocardial infarction, cerebrovascular disease, congestive heart failure, dementia, mild liver disease, peptic ulcer disease, chronic pulmonary disease	10
21–30	1		
Score one	____	Score each disease	____
EEG	**Points**	**Etiology**	**Points**
Spontaneous burst suppression	60	Anoxia	65
		Acute central nervous system infection	33
		Acute cerebrovascular disease	26
After status epilepticus ictal discharges (ASIDs)	40	Metabolic disorders	22
		Metabolic, sodium imbalance	17
		Brain tumor	16
Lateralized periodic discharges (LPDs)	40	Cryptogenic	12
		Head trauma	12
		Drug overdose	11
Generalized periodic discharges (GPDs)	40	Alcohol abuse	10
		Hydrocephalus	8
		Remote cerebrovascular event or brain injury	7
No LPDs, GPDs, or ASIDs	0	Multiple sclerosis	5
		Drug withdrawal, reduction, or poor compliance	2
		Central nervous system anomalies	2
Score only worst	____	Score one	____
Total score = sum of above scores			

The scoring system is comprised of four sections with the sum of these scores representing the total EMSE score

The Encephalitis, Nonconvulsive Status Epilepticus, Diazepam Resistance, Image Abnormality, Tracheal Intubation (END-IT) score is superior STESS-3 and STESS-4 scores, but is intended to be used in convulsive SE.

Despite attempts to improve management of SE in recent years, a meta-analysis of adult convulsive SE studies in high-income countries demonstrated no significant improvement in mortality rates over the past 30 years [32].

Special Considerations

SE in pregnancy comprises approximately 5% of all cases. In the majority of cases, it is related to eclampsia; however, other causes, such as posterior reversible encephalopathy, NMDA receptor encephalitis, cortical venous thrombosis, and subarachnoid hemorrhage have been reported. A careful consideration of changes in pharmacokinetics of drugs that occurs during pregnancy is recommended [33].

- Preterm labor is common (35%). Fetal complications can include low birth weight, anoxic brain injury, respiratory distress, and intraventricular hemorrhage.
- Lorazepam and midazolam can be considered as first-line agents for SE in the pregnant patient, with fosphenytoin used as initial ASD.

Post-anoxic patients have an especially high mortality rate when compared with other SE populations, which is largely related to withdrawal of life-sustaining therapies. Seizures are often nonconvulsive and may be further masked by sedation, neuromuscular blockade. Recent evidence suggests that a subset of patients may survive and achieve good outcomes, particularly those with a reactive and continuous EEG background, preserved N20 peaks on somatosensory-evoked potentials and lower levels of neuron-specific enolase [34].

Elderly individuals have a higher incidence of SE than the general population, and they are often at risk of delayed diagnosis of NCSE, as altered mental status may be wrongly attributed to toxic, metabolic, infectious, or dementia as the sole etiology. Using less sedating ASDs is advisable in this population because somnolence due to benzodiazepine use may cloud the clinical picture and mask improvement [35].

Cardinal Points
- Status epilepticus is an emergency requiring prompt initiation of benzodiazepines as first-line therapy.
- EEG remains the mainstay of diagnosis of nonconvulsive SE. Clinicians should have a low threshold to use EEG monitoring because it is also a helpful tool to guide subsequent steps of pharmacologic therapy.
- A stepwise approach should be followed with escalation from benzodiazepines to non-sedating antiseizure medications and finally anesthetic agents.

- It is essential to consider the most common toxicities of the various ASDs and the comorbidities of the patient when selecting second- and third-line agents.
- Despite improvements in diagnosis, mortality from complications of refractory SE remains high, particularly in patients with anoxia, cerebrovascular disease, and metabolic disturbances and in patients older than 50 years.

Disclosures Dr. Carolina B. Maciel reports no disclosures.

Dr. Michael D. Morris reports no disclosures.

Dr. Kent A. Owusu received funding from the Swebilius foundation for a retrospective study comparing different benzodiazepine regimens for seizure termination and seizure cluster prevention in patients admitted to the adult Epilepsy Monitoring Unit.

References

1. Betjemann JP, Josephson SA, Lowenstein DH, Burke JF. Trends in status epilepticus-related hospitalizations and mortality: redefined in US practice over time. JAMA Neurol. 2015;72(6):650–5.
2. Sanchez S, Rincon F. Status epilepticus: epidemiology and public health needs. J Clin Med. 2016;5(8).
3. Alvarez V, Lee JW, Westover MB, Drislane FW, Novy J, Faouzi M, et al. Therapeutic coma for status epilepticus: differing practices in a prospective multicenter study. Neurology. 2016;87(16):1650–9.
4. Trinka E, Cock H, Hesdorffer D, Rossetti AO, Scheffer IE, Shinnar S, et al. A definition and classification of status epilepticus—report of the ILAE task force on classification of status epilepticus. Epilepsia. 2015;56(10):1515–23.
5. Chakraborty T, Hocker S. The clinical spectrum of new-onset status epilepticus. Crit Care Med. 2019;47:970.
6. Hirsch LJ, LaRoche SM, Gaspard N, Gerard E, Svoronos A, Herman ST, et al. American Clinical Neurophysiology Society's standardized critical care EEG terminology: 2012 version. J Clin Neurophysiol. 2013;30(1):1–27.
7. Nagayama M, Yang S, Geocadin RG, Kaplan PW, Hoshiyama E, Shiromaru-Sugimoto A, et al. Novel clinical features of nonconvulsive status epilepticus. F1000Res. 2017;6:1690.
8. Leitinger M, Beniczky S, Rohracher A, Gardella E, Kalss G, Qerama E, et al. Salzburg consensus criteria for non-convulsive status epilepticus—approach to clinical application. Epilepsy Behav. 2015;49:158–63.
9. Hirsch LJ, Gaspard N, van Baalen A, Nabbout R, Demeret S, Loddenkemper T, et al. Proposed consensus definitions for new-onset refractory status epilepticus (NORSE), febrile infection-related epilepsy syndrome (FIRES), and related conditions. Epilepsia. 2018;59(4):739–44.
10. Betjemann JP, Lowenstein DH. Status epilepticus in adults. Lancet Neurol. 2015;14(6):615–24.
11. Dham BS, Hunter K, Rincon F. The epidemiology of status epilepticus in the United States. Neurocrit Care. 2014;20(3):476–83.

12. Delaj L, Novy J, Ryvlin P, Marchi NA, Rossetti AO. Refractory and super-refractory status epilepticus in adults: a 9-year cohort study. Acta Neurol Scand. 2017;135(1):92–9.
13. Kantanen AM, Kalviainen R, Parviainen I, Ala-Peijari M, Backlund T, Koskenkari J, et al. Predictors of hospital and one-year mortality in intensive care patients with refractory status epilepticus: a population-based study. Crit Care. 2017;21(1):71.
14. Ferlisi M, Hocker S, Grade M, Trinka E, Shorvon S. Preliminary results of the global audit of treatment of refractory status epilepticus. Epilepsy Behav. 2015;49:318–24.
15. Spatola M, Novy J, Du Pasquier R, Dalmau J, Rossetti AO. Status epilepticus of inflammatory etiology: a cohort study. Neurology. 2015;85(5):464–70.
16. Hocker S, Nagarajan E, Rabinstein AA, Hanson D, Britton JW. Progressive brain atrophy in super-refractory status epilepticus. JAMA Neurol. 2016;73(10):1201–7.
17. Benbadis SR, Chen S, Melo M. What's shaking in the ICU? The differential diagnosis of seizures in the intensive care setting. Epilepsia. 2010;51(11):2338–40.
18. Treiman DM, Meyers PD, Walton NY, Collins JF, Colling C, Rowan AJ, et al. A comparison of four treatments for generalized convulsive status epilepticus. Veterans Affairs Status Epilepticus Cooperative Study Group. N Engl J Med. 1998;339(12):792–8.
19. Bialer M, White HS. Key factors in the discovery and development of new antiepileptic drugs. Nat Rev Drug Discov. 2010;9(1):68–82.
20. Brophy GM, Bell R, Claassen J, Alldredge B, Bleck TP, Glauser T, et al. Guidelines for the evaluation and management of status epilepticus. Neurocrit Care. 2012;17(1):3–23.
21. Glauser T, Shinnar S, Gloss D, Alldredge B, Arya R, Bainbridge J, et al. Evidence-based guideline: treatment of convulsive status epilepticus in children and adults: report of the Guideline Committee of the American Epilepsy Society. Epilepsy Curr. 2016;16(1):48–61.
22. Strzelczyk A, Zollner JP, Willems LM, Jost J, Paule E, Schubert-Bast S, et al. Lacosamide in status epilepticus: systematic review of current evidence. Epilepsia. 2017;58(6):933–50.
23. Höfler J, Trinka E. Intravenous ketamine in status epilepticus. Epilepsia. 2018;59(Suppl 2):198–206. Epub 2018 Aug 26
24. Cervenka MC, Hocker S, Koenig M, Bar B, Henry-Barron B, Kossoff EH, et al. Phase I/II multicenter ketogenic diet study for adult superrefractory status epilepticus. Neurology. 2017;88(10):938–43.
25. Legriel S, Lemiale V, Schenck M, Chelly J, Laurent V, Daviaud F, et al. Hypothermia for neuroprotection in convulsive status epilepticus. N Engl J Med. 2016;375(25):2457–67.
26. Basha MM, Suchdev K, Dhakar M, Kupsky WJ, Mittal S, Shah AK. Acute resective surgery for the treatment of refractory status epilepticus. Neurocrit Care. 2017;27(3):370–80.
27. Marienke AAM, Bruijn d, van Sonderen A, van Coevorden-Hameete MH, et al. Evaluation of seizure treatment in anti-LGI1, anti-NMDAR, and anti-GABABR encephalitis. Neurology. 2019 May 7;92(19):e2185–96.
28. Hocker S. Systemic complications of status epilepticus—an update. Epilepsy Behav. 2015;49:83–7.
29. Neligan A, Shorvon SD. Frequency and prognosis of convulsive status epilepticus of different causes: a systematic review. Arch Neurol. 2010;67(8):931–40.
30. Giovannini G, Monti G, Tondelli M, Marudi A, Valzania F, Leitinger M, et al. Mortality, morbidity and refractoriness prediction in status epilepticus: comparison of STESS and EMSE scores. Seizure. 2017;46:31–7.
31. Leitinger M, Holler Y, Kalss G, Rohracher A, Novak HF, Hofler J, et al. Epidemiology-based mortality score in status epilepticus (EMSE). Neurocrit Care. 2015;22(2):273–82.
32. Neligan A, Noyce AJ, Gosavi TD, Shorvon SD, Köhler S, Walker MC. Change in mortality of generalized convulsive status epilepticus in high-income countries over time. JAMA Neurol. 2019.

33. Rajiv KR, Radhakrishnan A. Status epilepticus in pregnancy: etiology, management, and clinical outcomes. Epilepsy Behav. 2017;76:114–9.
34. Dragancea I, Backman S, Westhall E, Rundgren M, Friberg H, Cronberg T. Outcome following postanoxic status epilepticus in patients with targeted temperature management after cardiac arrest. Epilepsy Behav. 2015;49:173–7.
35. Canas N, Delgado H, Silva V, Pinto AR, Sousa S, Simoes R, et al. The electroclinical spectrum, etiologies, treatment and outcome of nonconvulsive status epilepticus in the elderly. Epilepsy Behav. 2018;79:53–7.

Chapter 3
Headache Emergencies

Deena M. Nasr and Sherri A. Braksick

Introduction

> **Diagnostic Keys**
> - Obtain a thorough history, examination and identify headache red flags.
> - If there is a high index of suspicion for a secondary cause of headache, pursue a basic serologic testing, CT of head and/or a lumbar puncture as initial diagnostic tests.
> - Further radiographic testing may be determined based on clinical suspicion (i.e., MRI brain, MR/CT angiogram/venogram or catheter angiography).

> **Treatment Priorities**
> - Address emergency treatments prior to aggressive pain management (osmotherapy, neurosurgical consultation, management of hydrocephalus, etc.).
> - Avoid excessive analgesics or sedatives that may confound an examination.

Headache is a common concern in emergency departments and accounts for over 2% of emergency visits [1, 2]. Unfortunately, there is no standard approach to a patient presenting to the emergency department with a headache as this largely depends on the patient and practice demographics at that particular emergency room. There are

D. M. Nasr (✉) · S. A. Braksick
Department of Neurology, Mayo Clinic, Rochester, MN, USA
e-mail: nasr.deena@mayo.edu

> **Prognosis at a Glance**
> - Primary headaches have a benign prognosis although uncontrolled chronic pain may lead to disability.
> - Prognosis of secondary headaches is dependent on etiology, available treatments, and any associated neurologic complications.
> - Early identification of a secondary cause of headache may improve outcomes, particularly in cases of aneurysmal subarachnoid hemorrhage and acute bacterial meningitis.

four questions to consider in the emergency room setting to help guide further management: (1) Is this a thunderclap headache? (2) Does the patient have signs of infection? (3) Are there focal neurologic symptoms associated with the headache? (4) Is this a new and persistent headache? If the answer is yes to any of these questions, one should pursue further testing and rule out secondary etiologies. Red flags in the headache history may also prompt further investigations and are outlined in Table 3.1. Ultimately the goal is to identify which patients would be at risk of secondary etiologies in order to reduce cost and complications from over-testing.

If the headache is concerning for a secondary etiology, initial basic testing should include at a non-contrast CT head and sometimes a lumbar puncture (LP) assuming there are no contraindications, such as an intracranial mass, coagulopathy, or cutaneous infection near the site of LP. Basic cerebrospinal fluid (CSF) analysis should include opening pressure, cell count, protein, glucose, xanthochromia, gram stain and culture. These two tests will exclude most etiologies demanding immediate recognition (subarachnoid hemorrhage, large space-occupying mass, CNS infection, pituitary apoplexy, colloid cyst, and hydrocephalus), though non-contrast CT scan may sometimes be insufficient and clinical suspicion, if strong, should not be dissuaded by a negative CT scan. Further testing with contrast CT or MRI, CT or MRI angiogram/venogram, or conventional angiography is determined based on clinical presentation and suspected etiology.

Thunderclap Headache

A thunderclap headache is defined as a headache that reaches maximum intensity in less than a minute and lasts more than an hour. Although many of these cases have benign or primary etiologies, potential catastrophic and/or lethal etiologies should always be ruled out given the significant morbidity and mortality that can occur if one is missed [3–5]. Table 3.2 presents a list of diagnoses presenting with thunderclap headache.

Table 3.1 Red flags suggesting a secondary etiology

History	Examination
New headache type: Severe at onset or with rapid onset (within seconds) Provocative maneuvers: positional, exertional, Valsalva New headache in age > 55 Awakens patient from sleep (or peak upon awakening) or nausea/vomiting after waking Fixed to one side (aka side-locked headache)	Vitals: Signs of infection: fever, hypotension, tachycardia Cushing syndrome: bradycardia, hypertension, irregular breathing pattern
Review of systems: Systemic symptoms: fever, chills, night sweats, weight loss, rash Neurologic symptoms: syncope, confusion, pulsatile tinnitus, hiccups, blurred vision, diplopia or focal symptoms	Neck: Positive Kernig or Brudzinski signs (Meningismus) Neck bruit
Past medical history: Peripartum Thyroid disease Illicit drug use Recent head trauma Previous venous thrombosis Hypercoagulable state Intracranial aneurysms Immunocompromised (e.g., HIV/AIDS)	Eye[a]: Anisocoria + ptosis (Horner syndrome) Proptosis Ophthalmoparesis/strabismus Visual field cut or tunnel vision Papilledema Glaucoma Vitreous hemorrhage Orbital bruit
Past surgical history: Recent ENT procedure Recent ophthalmologic surgery Recent neurosurgery	Skin: Maculopapular rash Flushing Temporal tenderness
Medications: Immunosuppressants Immunomodulating therapy Steroids Vasoactive medications (SSRI, SNRI, methylphenidate, decongestants, etc.) Estrogen supplementation/birth control	Neuro: Altered mentation Language difficulty Unilateral sensory deficit Unilateral weakness Imbalance/gait disturbance

SSRI selective serotonin reuptake inhibitor, *SNRI* serotonin norepinephrine reuptake inhibitor
[a]Refer to Chap. 5 for a more detailed review of ophthalmologic findings and emergencies

Subarachnoid Hemorrhage

Roughly 25% of patients with thunderclap headache have a subarachnoid hemorrhage (SAH). Thunderclap headache is the most common symptom among patients with SAH, occurring in 50% of these patients, and may be the only symptom [5–7]. Patients with unruptured intracranial aneurysms can develop thunderclap headaches as well. It is controversial whether the unruptured intracranial aneurysm is the culprit; however, it is important not to dismiss this potential sentinel or warning headache because it may signal impending aneurysmal rupture. Other associated symptoms of SAH may

Table 3.2 Thunderclap headache differential diagnosis

Secondary etiologies	Primary headache syndromes
Subarachnoid hemorrhage	Idiopathic/primary thunderclap headache
Reversible cerebral vasoconstriction syndrome	Cluster headache
Posterior reversible encephalopathy syndrome	Coital or orgasmic headache
Giant cell arteritis	Exertional headache
Carotid/vertebral dissection	Cough headache
Cerebral vein thrombosis	Hypnic headache
Pituitary apoplexy	Stabbing headache
Colloid cyst causing intermittent hydrocephalus	Hot-bath-related headache
Spontaneous CSF hypotension	
Hypertensive emergency/crisis	
Pheochromocytoma	
Spontaneous retroclival hematoma	

include nausea, vomiting, altered level of consciousness, seizures, posturing, or neurologic deficits. Head imaging with a CT scan is necessary to evaluate for intracranial hemorrhage or mass lesion. Although a non-contrast CT scan has high sensitivity if performed shortly after the onset of the hemorrhage, it may rarely be falsely negative particularly if performed more than 6 hours after the ictus. Therefore, if the CT scan is negative, a lumbar puncture should subsequently be performed. CSF analysis will typically reveal elevated red blood cells and xanthochromia. Xanthochromia may be detected as early as 2 hours up to 2 weeks after ictus, but sensitivity is suboptimal within the first 4–8 hours and after the first few days. If subarachnoid hemorrhage is found, further testing may include CT angiography (CTA), magnetic resonance angiography (MRA), and/or digital subtraction angiography (DSA). See Chap. 12 for a more in-depth review of the general approach to subarachnoid hemorrhage.

Reversible Cerebral Vasoconstriction Syndrome

Reversible cerebral vasoconstriction syndrome (RCVS) typically presents with recurrent thunderclap headaches with or without a focal neurologic deficit or seizures. There are a number of drugs and comorbid conditions that can predispose to this syndrome (Table 3.3). Typically CT scan is negative unless there is a secondary ischemic infarct or hemorrhage (most often sulcal subarachnoid hemorrhage and rarely intraparenchymal hemorrhage). An angiogram (CTA, MRA, or DSA) may show multifocal intracerebral arterial stenoses mimicking vasculitis that normalizes on subsequent follow-up imaging several months later (Fig. 3.1). Yet, it is important to note that 20% of noninvasive angiograms are falsely negative in RCVS and evidence of vasoconstriction may not be radiologically evident until a week or more from the first thunderclap headache. CSF is typically bland (as compared to vasculitis, which is usually inflammatory), but subtle-mild elevations of white blood cells and protein concentration can be seen. Calcium channel blockers are the treatment

3 Headache Emergencies

Table 3.3 RCVS predisposing triggers

Medical comorbidities	Drugs
Peripartum (preeclampsia, eclampsia)	Alcohol
Neurosurgical procedures (especially carotid endarterectomy)	Illicit drugs (marijuana, cocaine, amphetamine/methamphetamine, ecstasy, LSD)
Head/brain injury	Sympathomimetic nasal decongestants (pseudoephedrine, oxymetazoline)
Intracranial hemorrhage	Serotonergic antidepressants (SSRI, SNRI, TCA)
Pheochromocytoma	Immunosuppressants (tacrolimus, cyclophosphamide)
Carcinoid tumor	Vasoactive abortive medications for migraine (triptans, ergotamines)
	Vasopressors (epinephrine, norepinephrine)
	EPO
	IVIG
	RBC transfusion

SSRI selective serotonin reuptake inhibitor, *SNRI* serotonin norepinephrine reuptake inhibitor, *TCA* tricyclic antidepressant, *EPO* erythropoietin, *IVIG* intravenous immunoglobulin, *RBC* red blood cell

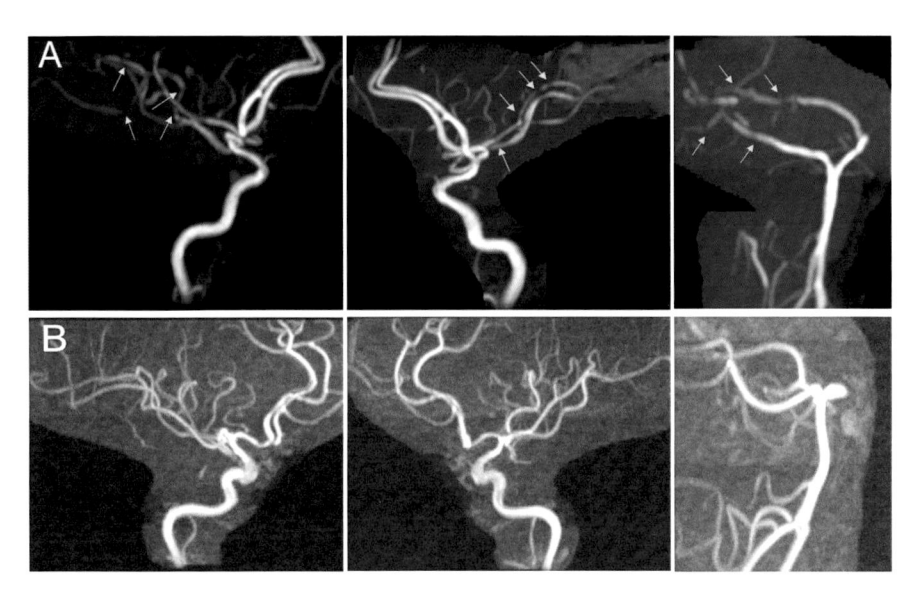

Fig. 3.1 Reversible cerebral vasoconstrictive syndrome. 57-year-old woman with recurrent thunderclap headache. (**A**) 3D time-of-flight MRA demonstrates multifocal vascular narrowing of the distal cerebral vasculature of the bilateral middle and posterior cerebral arteries (yellow arrows). (**B**) Repeat MRA 1 month later following oral verapamil treatment demonstrates reversal of the multifocal intracranial narrowing. Findings were consistent with RCVS

of choice. It is a self-limited and monophasic illness. Prognosis is variable; benign in most cases, but disability can result from brain infarctions or intracerebral hemorrhage and, rarely, fulminant cases can occur, especially during the postpartum period [8–10].

Posterior Reversible Encephalopathy Syndrome

Posterior reversible encephalopathy syndrome (PRES), also known as reversible posterior leukoencephalopathy syndrome (RPLS), is characterized by acute onset of headache, seizures, confusion, and/or visual disturbance [11]. The headache is typically non-distinct and throbbing; however, thunderclap headaches have also been described. This syndrome is most often encountered in the setting of severe hypertension and renal failure, but can also be seen in the setting of pharmacologic agents such as immunosuppressants and chemotherapy. Head imaging demonstrates posterior (parietal and occipital) vasogenic edema seen as hypodensity on CT and T2-FLAIR hyperintensity on MRI. Treatment includes removing or controlling the offending trigger.

Cervical Arterial Dissections

Headache is the most common presenting symptom of cervical arterial dissections (carotid or vertebral) and is acute and fixed ipsilateral to the dissection. There may be associated face and/or neck pain. The headache can be thunderclap or acute and progressive. Cervical arterial dissections occur due to an intimal tear causing an intramural hematoma.

Causes of dissection include neck trauma, prolonged or sudden neck hyperextension, and Valsalva maneuvers (e.g., coughing fits), among others. Chiropractic neck maneuvers have been associated with vertebral artery dissections in young patients [12]. Yet, in up a third of cases, the dissection has no identifiable trigger and these cases are categorized as spontaneous. Dissections are more common in patients with underlying connective tissue disease, and there is some evidence that patients with spontaneous dissections may have abnormal elastin in the vessel walls.

Cervical artery dissection may also manifest with ptosis and miosis due to Horner syndrome. Retinal or cerebral ischemia due to large vessel emboli or occlusion may occur at the time of the dissection or up to 1 month after the dissection. Typical tests include CT and CTA (or MRA) that will show the cervical segment stenosis consistent with an intimal dissection. Neck MRI may show the intramural hematoma at the site of the dissection, particularly on T1 fat-saturated sequences (Fig. 3.2).

There are currently no standard guidelines regarding which antithrombotics to use for stroke prevention (antiplatelet or anticoagulation); a randomized trial (CADISS) showed a low risk of stroke at 1 year (2.5%) which was similar with antiplatelet therapy and with anticoagulation [13]. Yet, some patients will have an acute thrombus at the site of the intramural hematoma with recurrent ischemic infarcts or severe flow limiting stenosis that may require more aggressive intervention such as anticoagulation, angioplasty, and/or stenting.

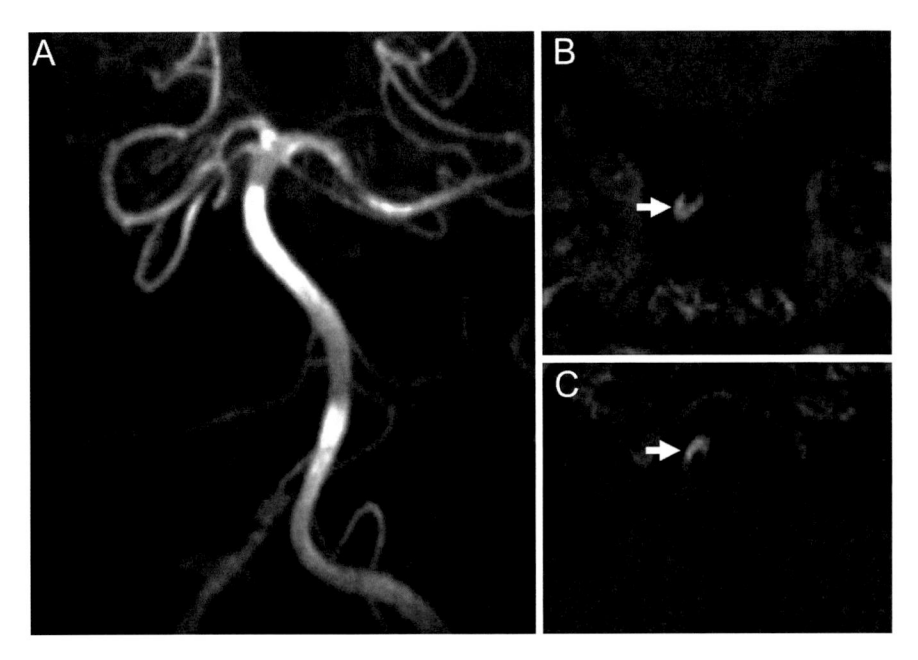

Fig. 3.2 Intradural vertebral artery dissection. 54-year-old man presented with acute onset severe headache but no focal neurological deficit. MRI brain (not shown) was negative for infarction or perfusion deficit. (**A**) 3D time-of-flight MRA demonstrates focal narrowing of the intradural right vertebral artery. There is a "string sign" consistent with flow through the vertebral artery. Shaggy T1 hyperintensity surrounding the artery is consistent with intramural hematoma. (**B**) Axial and (**C**) coronal T1-weighted vessel wall imaging sequences demonstrate T1 hyperintense intramural hematoma, confirming the diagnosis of intracranial dissection (arrows)

Pituitary Apoplexy

A pituitary hemorrhagic infarct can cause thunderclap headache associated with visual disturbances, including bitemporal hemianopia or diplopia due to ophthalmoplegia. Predisposing factors include pituitary adenoma, peripartum period, head trauma, or anticoagulation. MRI of the head will adequately detect this etiology. MRI of the head demonstrates an enlarged pituitary with peripheral enhancement surrounding an infarcted core and possible blood products (Fig. 3.3). CT of the head may show a hyperdense pituitary mass if there is hemorrhage, although it generally has low sensitivity. Treatment includes hormone replacement, hemodynamic monitoring, and possible neurosurgical decompression to restore or preserve vision.

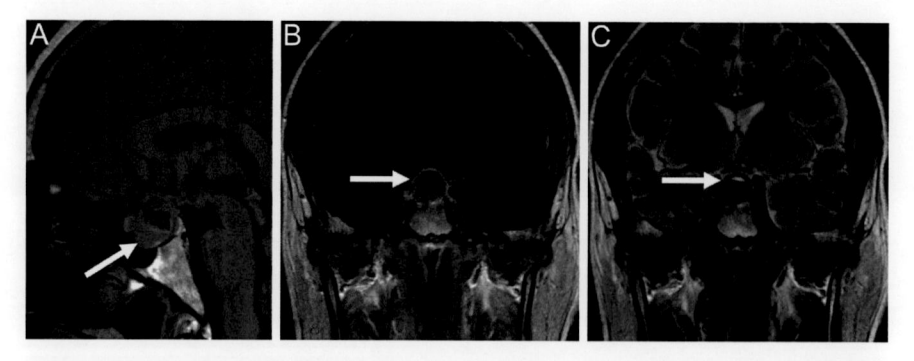

Fig. 3.3 Pituitary apoplexy. 40-year-old man with abrupt onset headache and bitemporal hemianopia during the prior week. (**A**) Sagittal T1-weighted MRI without contrast shows hyperintense subacute blood products in the sella with a fluid-fluid level. (**B**) Post-contrast T1-weighted MRI shows no intra-pituitary enhancement but rather a ring of enhancement surrounding the pituitary gland. (**C**) T2-weighted MRI shows hypointense blood products with a fluid level. Findings were consistent with pituitary apoplexy

Colloid Cyst and Hydrocephalus

A thunderclap headache may be the presenting symptom of a colloid cyst that causes intermittent obstructive hydrocephalus. Typically, this is positional in that it occurs when patient lies down and resolves when they are sitting up due to the dynamic obstruction of the third ventricle causing transient hydrocephalus. A CT or MRI of the brain is sufficient to rule out this diagnosis and treatment is surgical resection (Fig. 3.4).

Retroclival Hematoma

This is an extremely rare cause of intracranial hemorrhage that may either occur due to atlantoaxial dislocation/trauma or spontaneously. There have been a few case reports describing this finding in the setting of an acute onset thunderclap headache [14].

Trigeminal Autonomic Cephalalgias

Trigeminal autonomic cephalalgias are a category of primary headaches characterized by sudden paroxysms of thunderclap-like pain affecting a unilateral trigeminal distribution (often retro-orbital) associated with autonomic features. Different autonomic cephalalgias (e.g., cluster headache, paroxysmal hemicranias, short-lasting unilateral neuralgiform headaches) are primarily classified based on the duration of each headache attack (seconds–hours). Cluster headaches are the most common autonomic cephalalgia.

A cluster headache tends to occur in a cluster period and has a cyclical nature to it. Many patients complain of nighttime awakening due to this type of headache. The

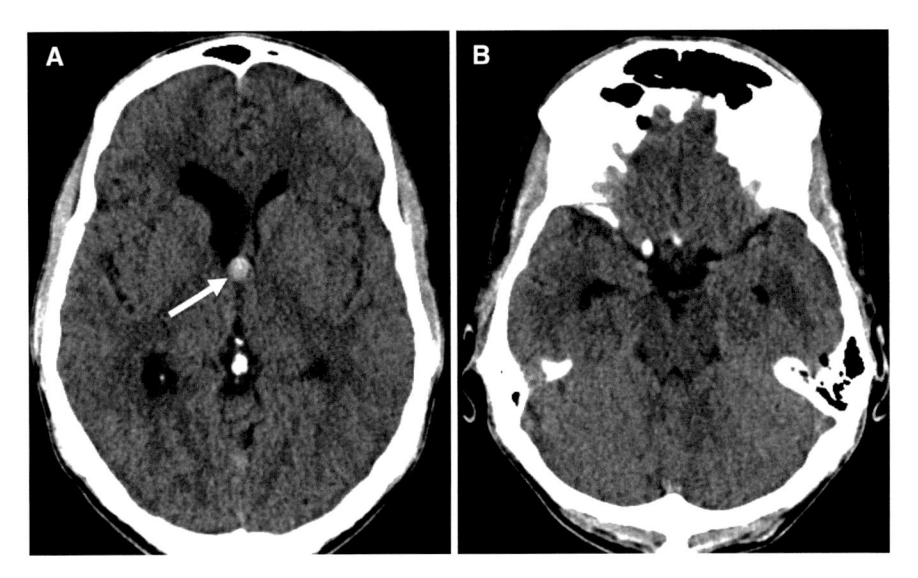

Fig. 3.4 Third ventricular colloid cyst. (**A**) Non-contrast CT demonstrates a hyperdense colloid cyst at the foramen of Monro (arrow). There is associated dilatation of the frontal horn and atrium of the right lateral ventricle as well as dilatation of the temporal horn of the right lateral ventricle consistent with hydrocephalus (**B**)

duration of cluster periods may be weeks to months and then recur after a period of remission. The headache is typically associated with autonomic features, such as tearing, rhinorrhea, ptosis, facial pallor, or flushing. Patients with cluster headache have great difficulty staying still while in pain; they will continually pace or rock. Fortunately, it is a primary headache and is not directly life-threatening although patients who suffer from these headaches have a high risk of suicide due to the disability that occurs from unrelenting acute pain. It is therefore important to diagnose and treat these headaches urgently. Typically the neurologic examination is normal with the exception of pupillary changes and ptosis. CT or MRI is important to rule out mimickers, such as a carotid dissection. Treatment in the emergency or urgency setting should include high flow 100% oxygen delivered through a face mask at a minimum rate of 12 L per minute. Other acute treatments include injectable triptans or dihydroergotamine (DHE). Additional treatments that can be pursued in the outpatient setting include occipital nerve block, intranasal lidocaine, or oral steroids. Long-term preventive treatments include calcium channel blockers or lithium.

A New Acute or Subacute Headache with Focal Neurologic Features

A subacute progressive headache is a headache that worsens over the course of days to weeks. This is typically due to a benign etiology, but if it represents a new headache type or is associated with abnormal neurologic symptoms and signs, the patient should be studied with head imaging to rule out a mass lesion, vascular etiology, hydrocephalus, infection, or inflammatory disease. Further testing depends on the specific clinical scenario. Common emergencies presenting with subacute, progressive headaches are briefly discussed below.

Ischemic Stroke

Acute ischemic strokes can occasionally be associated with a headache at onset, particularly if it is in the posterior circulation [15, 16]. The characteristics of these headaches can be deceivingly benign and similar to those of a migraine or tension headache. Furthermore, these patients often have a preexisting history of migraines. It is also thought that patients with a history of migraine with aura are at increased risk of stroke, but this is uncommon. See Chap. 9 for a more in-depth information on a practical approach to ischemic stroke evaluation and management.

Cerebral Vein Thrombosis (CVT)

CVT typically presents with a subacute insidious headache, but can rarely present as an acute thunderclap headache [14]. It may be accompanied with other symptoms, such as seizures, blurry vision, or focal neurological deficits, and it may worsen when the patient is lying recumbent. The patient may have a history of recent head trauma or hypercoagulable state (pregnancy, oral contraceptive use, cancer, Crohn's disease, antiphospholipid antibody syndrome, etc.). Physical examination findings may include papilledema due to intracranial hypertension or focal neurologic deficits if there is associated venous infarct or intracerebral hemorrhage. Along with the standard non-contrast CT scan, a CT venogram (CTV) or MR venogram (MRV) is needed to confirm the diagnosis. Lumbar puncture may reveal elevated opening pressure and CSF may have increased protein concentration without concomitant pleocytosis.

Once the diagnosis is confirmed, treatment usually includes anticoagulation, even in the presence of intracerebral hemorrhage. Rarely, intra-sinus infusion of thrombolytic or mechanical venous thrombectomy can be pursued, but data on the value of these interventions are limited, and they should be reserved for cases refractory to anticoagulation. See Chap. 10 for a more in-depth overview on acute cerebral venous thrombosis.

Brain Tumor Headache

Many patients with brain tumors may experience headache as one of their symptoms, but headache rarely occurs in isolation [17]. It is often described as a subacute headache that worsens over days to weeks and may be associated with features suggestive of increased intracranial pressure (i.e., worsened with Valsalva or exertion, worse when patient is lying supine or awakening the patient from sleep). Headache from brain tumor can also be associated with other manifestations depending on location of the tumor, such as papilledema, weakness, sensory disturbance, or subacute mood/personality change. A history of malignancy raises suspicion for metastasis and a history of HIV/AIDS or immunosuppressive medications may suggest opportunistic conditions, such as CNS lymphoma. Further evaluation usually includes searching for a primary systemic cancer with CT chest/abdomen or pelvis or a PET scan in the case of suspected metastasis and a biopsy for tissue diagnosis. In some cases, direct resection may be undertaken immediately in lieu of a biopsy.

Initial treatment may include steroids to reduce vasogenic edema and assist with pain control. Depending on the number, size, and type of tumor, tumor resection, chemotherapy, and/or radiation may be employed for targeted treatment.

Subdural Hematoma Headache

These headaches are similar to the brain tumor headaches described above. It is important to ask about a history of head trauma and anticoagulation, but spontaneous subdural hemorrhage may occur in elderly patients in the absence of trauma. Treatment involves cessation of any antithrombotic agents until resolution and hematoma evacuation (via craniotomy or trephination) depending on the size, acuity of the collection and the severity of the brain compression.

Stroke-Like Migraine Attacks After Radiation Therapy (SMART) Syndrome

SMART syndrome is a rare and delayed complication of cranial irradiation for intracranial tumors [18, 19] where patients experience subacute stroke-like deficits (unilateral weakness, sensory loss, ataxia, aphasia, visual field defect, etc.) associated with a migrainous headache. Other symptoms may include seizures or encephalopathy. These symptoms often resolve over the course of several weeks, although a minority of patients may have residual deficits [20]. Onset occurs several years after whole-brain or lesion-targeted radiation. In the setting of a headache associated with focal neurologic deficits, a thorough workup with head (MRI or CT) and sometimes vascular imaging (MRA or CTA) must be pursued to rule out stroke or tumor recurrence, as SMART syndrome is a diagnosis of exclusion. MRI of the head showing gyriform enhancement and T2 hyperintensity and thickening near the area of prior radiation is suggestive of this syndrome (Fig. 3.5).

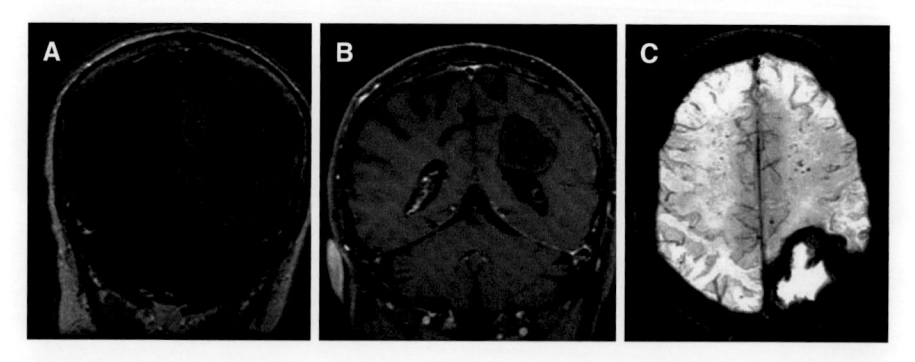

Fig. 3.5 SMART syndrome. 61-year-old man with a history of left parieto-occipital grade 2 oligodendroglioma treated with surgical resection and radiation therapy 13 years before presented for evaluation of new neurologic symptoms, most notably aphasia as well as right arm paresthesias and dysmetria. He did not have any impairment of consciousness or seizure activity. (**A**) Post-contrast MRI demonstrates gyral enhancement in the left temporal, parietal, occipital, and posterior frontal lobes around the resection cavity. (**B**) In addition, there is clear gyral swelling. (**C**) Susceptibility-weighted imaging sequence demonstrates multiple foci of T2* hypointensity in the bilateral deep cerebral white matter consistent with radiation related microhemorrhages

Hemiplegic Migraine

Hemiplegic migraine presents with subacute progressive headache associated with lateralizing neurologic deficits. The headache is described as unilateral and throbbing and associated with a combination of photophobia, phonophobia, or nausea and vomiting as per migraine criteria [21]. This rare form of migraine also includes transient focal neurologic deficits as one of the manifestations of an aura (e.g., unilateral numbness, scotomas, diplopia, aphasia, etc.) and can be hereditary or sporadic. It is often difficult to clinically discriminate from a stroke, particularly on initial presentation. It is prudent to pursue and evaluations to exclude stroke or seizure at the time of initial presentation, or if the character of the symptoms changes over time. This is a challenging group of patients but a thorough history may aid in guiding the diagnostic and therapeutic approach. Fortunately, this is a primary headache disorder and therefore not life-threatening, although it may cause transient disability. Treatment usually includes acute symptom management with analgesics and antiemetics. Vasoactive agents such as triptans and ergotamine are generally contraindicated due to the hypothetical risk of vasospasm in these patients. A small study actually supported triptan use [22], but most experts prefer to avoid the potential risk. Long-term preventative therapies are typically pursued in the outpatient setting and acetazolamide and verapamil are most commonly prescribed.

Subacute-Chronic Progressive Headache with Signs of Infection

Most often headaches accompanied by fevers are benign and likely secondary to systemic infections such as the common cold, flu, or sinusitis, particularly in the outpatient setting. Yet, one must have a low suspicion for meningitis, particularly in urgent and emergent setting. Although aseptic or viral meningitis commonly is self-limited and it has a good prognosis, late intervention with antibiotics for acute bacterial meningitis can be fatal. For in-depth review of CNS infections, please refer to Chap. 7.

Bacterial Meningitis

Meningitis can present with a subacute headache associated with photophobia and phonophobia, nuchal rigidity and other signs of meningismus, encephalopathy, and signs of sepsis (such as tachycardia, hypotension, and fever). Advanced age, immunocompromised status, and recent neurosurgical or ENT procedures increase risk for CNS infection. Evaluation should include blood cultures, head imaging with contrast (ideally an MRI but a CT scan is sufficient to exclude space occupying lesion), and a lumbar puncture. Most often meningitis is aseptic or viral and self-limited; however, it is crucial to initiate antibiotic therapy as soon as possible and to continue them until bacterial meningitis is ruled out. Concomitant initiation of steroids is recommended when community-acquired acute bacterial meningitis is suspected. If there is a purpuric rash, meningococcal meningitis should be considered and the type of antibiotics tailored accordingly. Antibiotic choice depends on the suspected or confirmed organism and individual patient characteristics (including age, history of alcohol use, neurosurgical or ENT procedures, immunocompromised state, etc.). Prognosis is often good with early treatment. However, fulminant meningitis with rapid progression to coma has a much poorer prognosis.

Intracranial Abscess/Empyema

This presents as a subacute headache that worsens over days to weeks. It can be associated with fever and vomiting in half of the cases [23], focal neurologic symptoms, and signs of increased intracranial pressure. It is important to ask about a history of recent ENT or neurosurgical procedures, dental procedures, and conditions associated with immunocompromised state (such as immunosuppressant therapy or AIDS). Brain imaging is diagnostic. Treatment involves drainage and broad-spectrum antibiotics.

New Persistent Headache

Temporal Arteritis

Temporal arteritis (also known as giant cell arteritis) should always be considered in patients over 50 years old with new-onset and persistent headache because prompt diagnosis and treatment can prevent vision loss and strokes. Vision loss is most commonly associated with anterior ischemic optic neuropathy (see also Chap. 5). However, posterior ischemic optic neuropathy, central retinal or cilio-retinal artery occlusion, and occipital lobe infarct can also be seen. This vasculitis can also cause brain infarctions and rarely intracerebral hemorrhages. The headache is variable but usually affects the temporal/occipital head region and is somewhat nonspecific; it tends to be pervasive. It can be associated with temporal scalp tenderness, jaw claudication, fatigue, and arthralgia (as seen with polymyalgia rheumatica). Angiography will demonstrate multi-vessel narrowing described as "beading" in appearance and a lumbar puncture will yield inflammatory CSF. Further diagnostic testing should include a temporal artery biopsy, which typically shows mononuclear cell infiltration or granulomatous inflammation of the arterial wall. Treatment includes steroids and possibly other immunomodulatory therapy.

Idiopathic Intracranial Hypertension

Although intracranial hypertension is most often due to mass lesion, it can also occur without a structural lesion. Idiopathic intracranial hypertension (IIH) typically presents with a subacute headache and tends to be more common among young obese females, who may have a history of other headache types (such as migraines). Other associated features include blurred vision, visual obscurations, and visual field abnormalities from an enlarged blind spot due to papilledema, diplopia due to ophthalmoplegia, and pulsatile tinnitus. MRI/V should be performed to rule out mass lesion and cerebral vein thrombosis, which can present similarly. MRI brain in IIH is usually normal but may show an empty sella, flattening of the posterior globes, and optic nerve tortuosity and kinking (Fig. 3.6). A lumbar puncture will show elevated opening pressures (above 22 cmH_2O). Medical management includes weight loss and acetazolamide or other second-line diuretics like furosemide. Surgical options include optic sheath fenestration if there is vision loss. In patients who are refractory to medical therapy, CSF shunting can be considered. There is limited data on the value of transvenous dural stenting in the setting of dural venous stenosis.

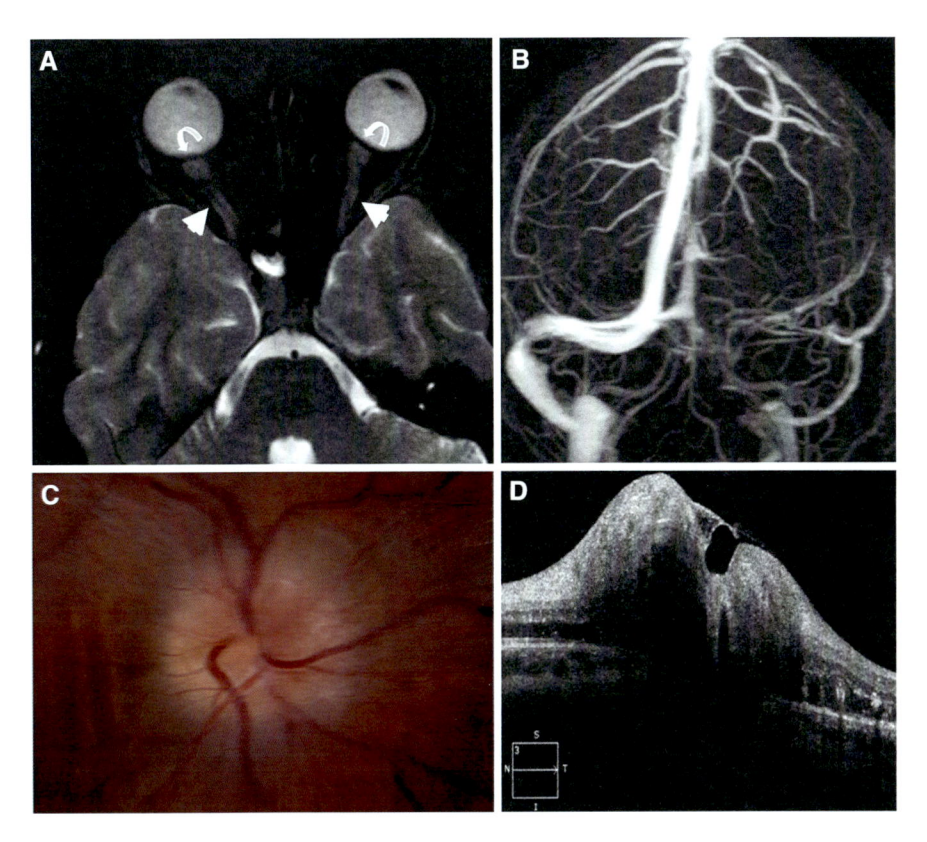

Fig. 3.6 Idiopathic intracranial hypertension. 31-year-old woman with a body mass index of 41.3 who presented with an acute visual deterioration in the setting of chronic severe headaches. Opening CSF pressure of 46 cmH$_2$O. (**A**) T2-weighted MRI demonstrates dilatation of the optic nerve sheaths (short arrows) as well as flattening of the optic discs (arrow heads). (**B**) MR venogram demonstrates congenital absence of the left transverse sinus and a stenosis of the right transverse sinus. (**C**) Funduscopic examination demonstrates papilledema. (**D**) Optical coherence tomography demonstrates macular exudates, which are typical of IIH

Intracranial Hypotension

An orthostatic headache that occurs upon sitting up or standing and resolves with laying supine is characteristic of intracranial hypotension. Typically these headaches are dull or pulsatile in nature, but may rarely have a thunderclap onset. This disorder is most commonly caused by a CSF leak from a dural tear. Lumbar puncture is the most common etiology; trauma, ENT, or neurosurgical procedures, severe cough/Valsalva, meningeal diverticula, or connective tissue diseases can also cause this problem. MRI findings

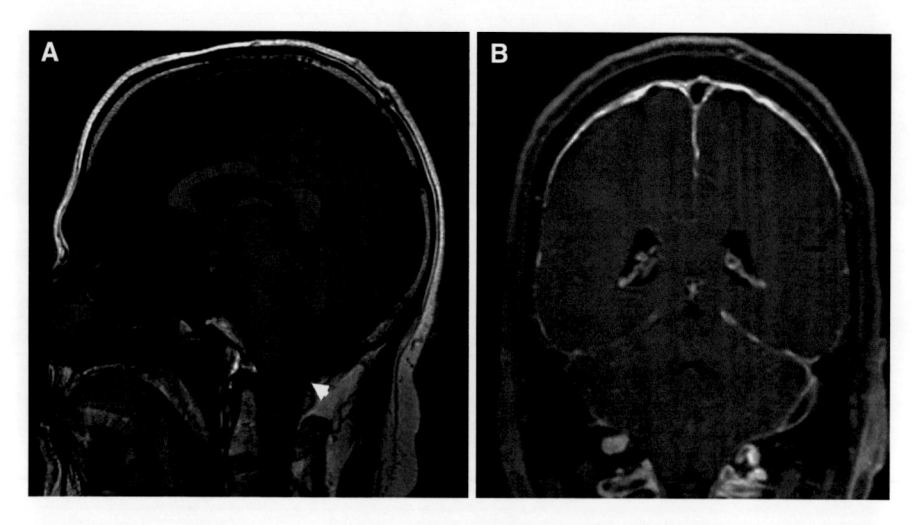

Fig. 3.7 Intracranial hypotension. 55/M with multiple symptoms including chronic severe headache which improved when the patient was in a dependent position. The patient was improperly diagnosed with chronic meningitis. Opening CSF pressure was 3 cm H_2O. (**A**) Sagittal T1-weighted MRI demonstrates brain sag with flattening of the pons, downward shift of the cerebellar tonsils (arrow) and enlargement of the pituitary. (**B**) Post-contrast MRI demonstrates prominent diffuse dural thickening and enhancement, typical imaging findings of CSF hypotension

usually show pachymeningeal enhancement, low-lying cerebellar tonsils, a flattened pons, pituitary enlargement, and spinal epidural venous plexus prominence (Fig. 3.8). If rhinorrhea is present, a sample can be used to detect beta-2 transferrin, which is only present in CSF. Other diagnostic tests may include CT myelography or indium nuclear cisternography. Medical treatment for headache includes caffeine and fluids. Often an epidural blood patch over the area of suspected leak is needed. In the case of an identified source and an epidural blood patch failure, a direct surgical repair may be necessary. If no source is found, a blind blood patch may still be beneficial (Fig. 3.7).

Status Migrainosus

A new headache in a patient with migraines should be evaluated for possible secondary etiologies. However, a typical migraine headache that has been unrelenting is a reassuring sign and suggestive of status migrainosus. Although this is not a life-threatening problem, it can be disabling and may lead to an ED evaluation for IV hydration and parenteral analgesics in the setting of vomiting. There is no standard or universal approach to status migrainosus, and therapies are usually chosen based on the patient's comorbidities and medication history. Treatment may include ergotamines; triptans; antiemetics, such as metoclopramide and prochlorperazine; IV non-steroidal anti-inflammatory agents such as ketorolac; intravenous magnesium; steroids; or valproic acid.

Cardinal Messages
- A thunderclap headache is an abrupt, severe headache with peak intensity occurring in less than a minute and may herald an emergent medical condition. Urgent investigations for secondary etiologies are necessary.
- Any headache with red flags requires urgent evaluation with CT head and possibly lumbar puncture with further testing (MRI, angiogram, and venogram) chosen on a case-by-case basis.
- Angiographic testing (i.e., CTA, MRA, digital subtraction angiography) should be highly considered in the setting of a thunderclap headache or an acute headache with focal neurologic features.
- CT head (and possibly MRI) with serologic and CSF infectious workup should be highly considered in the setting of a new headache with any signs of infection.
- Although status migrainosus, cluster headache, and hemiplegic migraine are not life-threatening, they should not be disregarded in the ED as these can cause significant morbidity and disability. The rate of suicide is increased in cluster headache due to unrelenting pain if left untreated.

References

1. Goldstein JN, Camargo CAJ, Pelletier AJ, Edlow JA. Headache in United States emergency departments: demographics, work-up and frequency of pathological diagnoses. Cephalalgia. 2006;26(6):684–90.
2. Lucado J, Paez K, Elixhauser A. Headaches in U.S. hospitals and emergency departments, 2008: statistical brief #111. Healthcare Cost and Utilization Project (HCUP) Statistical Briefs. Rockville; 2006.
3. Devenney E, Neale H, Forbes RB. A systematic review of causes of sudden and severe headache (Thunderclap Headache): should lists be evidence based? J Headache Pain . [Research Support, Non-US Gov't Review]. 2014;15:49.
4. Wijdicks EF, Kerkhoff H, van Gijn J. Long-term follow-up of 71 patients with thunderclap headache mimicking subarachnoid haemorrhage. Lancet. 1988;2(8602): 68–70.
5. Landtblom AM, Fridriksson S, Boivie J, Hillman J, Johansson G, Johansson I. Sudden onset headache: a prospective study of features, incidence and causes. Cephalalgia. [Research Support, Non-U.S. Gov't]. 2002;22(5):354–60.
6. Linn FH, Wijdicks EF, van der Graaf Y, Weerdesteyn-van Vliet FA, Bartelds AI, van Gijn J. Prospective study of sentinel headache in aneurysmal subarachnoid haemorrhage. Lancet. [Research Support, Non-U.S. Gov't]. 1994;344(8922):590–3.
7. Ducros A, Bousser MG. Thunderclap headache. BMJ. [Review]. 2013;346:e8557.
8. Katz BS, Fugate JE, Ameriso SF, Pujol-Lereis VA, Mandrekar J, Flemming KD, et al. Clinical worsening in reversible cerebral vasoconstriction syndrome. JAMA Neurol. [Case Reports Multicenter Study]. 2014;71(1):68–73.
9. Suchdev K, Norris G, Zak I, Mohamed W, Ibrahim M. Fulminant reversible cerebral vasoconstriction syndrome. Neurohospitalist. 2018;8(1):NP5–8.
10. Fugate JE, Ameriso SF, Ortiz G, Schottlaender LV, Wijdicks EF, Flemming KD, et al. Variable presentations of postpartum angiopathy. Stroke. 2012;43(3):670–6.

11. Fugate JE, Rabinstein AA. Posterior reversible encephalopathy syndrome: clinical and radiological manifestations, pathophysiology, and outstanding questions. Lancet Neurol. 2015;14(9):914–25. Epub 2015 Jul 13
12. Biller J, Sacco RL, Albuquerque FC, Demaerschalk BM, Fayad P, Long PH, Noorollah LD, Panagos PD, Schievink WI, Schwartz NE, Shuaib A, Thaler DE, Tirschwell DL, American Heart Association Stroke Council. Cervical arterial dissections and association with cervical manipulative therapy: a statement for healthcare professionals from the American Heart Association/American Stroke Association. Stroke. 2014;45(10):3155–74. Epub 2014 Aug 7
13. Markus HS, Levi C, King A, Madigan J, Norris J, Cervical Artery Dissection in Stroke Study (CADISS) Investigators. Antiplatelet therapy vs anticoagulation therapy in cervical artery dissection: the Cervical Artery Dissection in Stroke Study (CADISS) Randomized Clinical Trial Final Results. JAMA Neurol. 2019;76:657–64.
14. Narvid J, Amans MR, Cooke DL, Hetts SW, Dillon WP, Higashida RT, et al. Spontaneous retroclival hematoma: a case series. J Neurosurg. [Case Reports]. 2016;124(3):716–9.
15. Wolf ME, Szabo K, Griebe M, Forster A, Gass A, Hennerici MG, et al. Clinical and MRI characteristics of acute migrainous infarction. Neurology. 2011;76(22):1911–7.
16. Mitsias P, Ramadan NM. Headache in ischemic cerebrovascular disease. Part I: clinical features. Cephalalgia. [Review]. 1992;12(5):269–74.
17. Weingarten S, Kleinman M, Elperin L, Larson EB. The effectiveness of cerebral imaging in the diagnosis of chronic headache. Arch Intern Med. 1992;152(12):2457–62.
18. Black DF, Bartleson JD, Bell ML, Lachance DH. SMART: stroke-like migraine attacks after radiation therapy. Cephalalgia. [Case Reports]. 2006;26(9):1137–42.
19. Zheng Q, Yang L, Tan LM, Qin LX, Wang CY, Zhang HN. Stroke-like migraine attacks after radiation therapy syndrome. Chin Med J (Engl). [Review]. 2015;128(15):2097–101.
20. Black DF, Morris JM, Lindell EP, Krecke KN, Worrell GA, Bartleson JD, et al. Stroke-like migraine attacks after radiation therapy (SMART) syndrome is not always completely reversible: a case series. AJNR Am J Neuroradiol. [Case Reports]. 2013;34(12):2298–303.
21. The International Classification of Headache Disorders, 3rd edition (beta version). Cephalalgia. 2013;33(9):629–808.
22. Artto V, Nissila M, Wessman M, Palotie A, Farkkila M, Kallela M. Treatment of hemiplegic migraine with triptans. Eur J Neurol. [Evaluation Studies Research Support, N.I.H., Extramural Research Support, Non-U.S. Gov't]. 2007;14(9):1053–6.
23. Hakan T, Ceran N, Erdem I, Berkman MZ, Goktas P. Bacterial brain abscesses: an evaluation of 96 cases. J Infect. 2006;52(5):359–66.

Chapter 4
Neuro-otologic Emergencies: A Practical Approach

Kiersten L. Gurley and Jonathan A. Edlow

> **Diagnostic Keys**
> - Stroke is an important cause of acute dizziness in the emergency setting.
> - Small posterior strokes can present with an isolated acute vestibular syndrome.
> - Physical exam findings often allow for a confident and specific diagnosis and reliably discriminate between peripheral and central disorders.
> - Early (<48 hours of onset) neuroimaging even with DW-MRI may miss up to 15–20% of posterior circulation strokes presenting as isolated dizziness.
> - Sudden sensorineural hearing loss (SSNHL) can be diagnosed with careful physical examination.

> **Treatment Priorities**
> - Benign paroxysmal positional vertigo can be treated at the bedside with simple maneuvers.
> - Posterior circulatory ischemia requires prompt recognition and treatment to prevent recurrent stroke and decrease short-term complications.
> - Large cerebellar strokes may require surgical decompression.
> - Early glucocorticoids are the mainstay of treatment in SSNHL.

K. L. Gurley (✉) ·
Department of Emergency Medicine, Beth Israel Deaconess Medical Center/Harvard University School of Medicine, Boston, MA, USA
e-mail: kgurley@bidmc.harvard.edu

J. A. Edlow
Department of Emergency Medicine, Beth Israel Deaconess Medical Center and Harvard Medical School, Boston, MA, USA

© Springer Nature Switzerland AG 2020
A. A. Rabinstein (ed.), *Neurological Emergencies*,
https://doi.org/10.1007/978-3-030-28072-7_4

> **Prognosis at a Glance**
> - Prognosis of posterior circulation strokes depends on the location and extension of the infarction.
> - Approximately two-thirds of patients with idiopathic SSNHL will experience a partial recovery.
> - Acute vestibular disorders, even if recurrent, are usually not severely disabling.

Introduction

Dizziness is a common chief complaint with multiple possible causes and high risk of misdiagnosis. Physicians must distinguish between the large majority of dizzy patients with self-limiting or easily treatable conditions and the minority with life- or brain-threatening problems. In 2013, total health-care-related costs for patients with dizziness in the USA were estimated to exceed $10 billion [1, 2]. Additional "costs" include adverse events such as patient anxiety, injuries from falls or other dizziness-related trauma, and preventable major strokes following misdiagnosed minor cerebrovascular events [3].

Taking a history from a dizzy patient should be no different than taking a history in other patients. The timing, triggers and evolution over time, associated symptoms, and context (and *not* the descriptor used) best inform the differential diagnosis. Bedside examination can frequently establish a specific diagnosis [4]. A confident diagnosis of a peripheral vestibular problem obviates the need for specialty consultation, imaging, and hospitalization. When the evaluation suggests a central problem, especially stroke, steps can be taken to prevent harm by early initiation of secondary stroke prevention (milder presentations) or thrombolysis or surgical interventions (more severe presentations) [5]. In this chapter, we use the general term, "dizziness," to encompass various words patients use to describe disturbed balance or spatial orientation, such as "lightheaded," "spinning," "rocking," "vertigo," "off balance," and others.

Sudden sensorineural hearing loss (SSNHL) is an otologic emergency requiring a careful physical examination, early treatment, and specialist referral. Early glucocorticoid therapy is the mainstay of treatment. It is important to rule out central nervous system (CNS) causes in all cases.

Dizziness

Differential Diagnosis

Numerous conditions cause acute dizziness. Of 9472 patients in a study from a national database, dizziness was caused by general medical (including non-stroke cardiovascular) diagnoses in approximately 50%, oto-vestibular diagnoses in 33%, and neurologic (including stroke) diagnoses in 11% and a "symptom only" dizziness without otherwise specific diagnosis in 22% [6]. Prospectively defined "dangerous" diagnoses were found in 15% of patients and were more common in those who were 50 years or older. The most common serious diagnoses were fluid and electrolyte disturbances (5.6%), cerebrovascular diseases (4.0%), cardiac arrhythmias (3.2%), acute coronary syndromes (1.7%), anemia (1.6%), and hypoglycemia (1.4%). The overall incidence of important CNS disease in adult patients evaluated in the Emergency Department with acute dizziness is approximately 5%, mostly posterior circulation strokes. Risk factors for CNS causes of dizziness include older age, history of vascular disease or previous stroke, complaint of "instability," abnormal gait, and focal neurological findings [7].

Use of the word "vertigo" is not associated with a stroke diagnosis [8]. Patients with a cardiovascular cause of dizziness describe "vertigo" in almost 40% of cases, more than the fraction that described presyncope [9]. Patients with benign paroxysmal positional vertigo (BPPV) often describe non-vertiginous dizziness, especially elderly patients [10]. Eliciting timing and triggers, evolution of symptoms, and related symptoms when taking the history can help the clinician develop a rank-ordered differential diagnosis.

Diagnostic Pitfalls

In a study of 475 consecutive acutely dizzy patients seen by neurologists (who routinely performed a detailed ocular motor exam using Frenzel lenses), the neurologists diagnosed benign conditions in 73% of cases and serious (mostly cerebrovascular and inflammatory CNS disease) in 27% of cases [11]. A neurologist masked to the initial Emergency Department visit changed the diagnosis at follow-up in 44% of those reevaluated within 30 days. Benign vestibular diagnoses were deemed wrong in 58% ($n = 21/36$), including 17% ($n = 6/36$) with missed cerebrovascular diagnoses. The most common reason for misdiagnosis was an evolution of the clinical course over time, which factored in 70% of misdiagnoses. This study illustrates that correct diagnosis at initial presentation can be difficult even for specialists.

Posterior circulation strokes mimic peripheral causes of dizziness. In one study from an ENT clinic, almost 3% of patients referred for vertigo had a missed cerebellar stroke [12]. Stroke misdiagnosis is important because the underlying vascular pathology goes untreated (leaving the patient vulnerable to another stroke) and because patients can develop posterior fossa edema, which can be fatal [13]. Lost opportunity for thrombolysis or mechanical thrombectomy is another potential negative consequence in some cases.

Younger age and vertebral dissection as the cause for the acute dizziness are risk factors for missed cerebellar stroke [14]. Posterior circulation location is a risk factor for stroke misdiagnosis in general [15]. Knowledge gaps regarding eye movement findings contribute to misdiagnosis [16]. In a study of 1091 dizzy patients in

US Emergency Departments, physicians used templates to document the presence or absence of nystagmus in 887 (80%) cases. Nystagmus was said to be present in 185 (21%). However, the nystagmus was adequately described in only 10 (5.4%). Of patients given a peripheral vestibular diagnosis, the nystagmus description conflicted with the final diagnosis in 81%. Misdiagnosis of common peripheral vestibular problems, such as BPPV and vestibular neuritis, leads to ineffective treatments and resource over-utilization [17].

Misdiagnosis of patients with dizziness results from five common pitfalls: over-reliance on symptom quality, under-use of a timing and triggers approach, unfamiliarity with key physical examination findings, over-weighting traditional factors such as age and vascular risk factors to screen patients, and over-reliance on CT scan [13, 14].

Acute Vestibular Syndrome (AVS)

Spontaneous AVS is defined as the acute onset of persistent dizziness associated with nausea or vomiting, gait instability, nystagmus, and head-motion intolerance lasting days to weeks [18, 19]. Patients are usually symptomatic at presentation and focused physical examination is often diagnostic. The most common cause is vestibular neuritis (dizziness only) or labyrinthitis (dizziness plus hearing loss or tinnitus). The most frequent dangerous cause is posterior circulation ischemic stroke, generally in the cerebellum or brainstem. A small minority are due to multiple sclerosis [20]. Rare causes of an isolated AVS include cerebellar hemorrhage [21], thiamine deficiency [22], and various autoimmune, infectious, or other metabolic conditions [20]. Importantly, although nystagmus is implicit in the classic definition of AVS, some patients with AVS will present without nystagmus, especially those with a stroke etiology. This concept is important when interpreting the physical examination.

Another key concept is understanding the distinction between symptoms that are *exacerbated* (dizzy at baseline, worse with movement) versus *triggered* (not dizzy at baseline, dizziness develops with movement). Patients with an AVS typically experience worse dizziness with head movement (exacerbation), such as when performing the Dix-Hallpike maneuver, but this is *not* a sign of BPPV. Confusion on this point contributes to difficulty differentiating BPPV from vestibular neuritis or stroke [16, 18]. Occasionally, BPPV patients may endorse mild, persistent symptoms of malaise or unsteadiness between triggered, brief bouts of dizziness; this may be due to repeated symptoms triggered by small, inadvertent head movements or anticipatory anxiety about moving and is more common among older patients. This can usually be teased out by careful history taking. When such patients lack obvious features of vestibular neuritis or stroke, the Dix-Hallpike and supine roll tests can be performed to assess for an atypical, AVS-like presentation of BPPV [23].

Vestibular neuritis (the most common cause of AVS) is a benign, self-limited, presumed viral or post-viral inflammatory condition affecting the vestibular nerve.

Diagnosis is clinical. Most cases are idiopathic, possibly linked to herpes simplex infections [24]. Ramsay Hunt syndrome from herpes zoster presents with AVS, usually in conjunction with hearing loss, facial palsy, and a vesicular eruption in the external ear or palate [25]. Brain MRI is usually normal in these cases [26].

Posterior fossa strokes can mimic vestibular neuritis or labyrinthitis [27]. The prevalence of cerebrovascular disease in patients presenting to the Emergency Department with dizziness is as high as 3–5% [18], but it can be as high as 25% among those with AVS. Almost all (96%) of these strokes are ischemic [19, 21]. Sensitivity of CT scan for acute posterior circulation ischemic stroke is as low as 7–16% in the first 24 hours [28]. Therefore, CT *cannot* "rule out" ischemic stroke in AVS [13, 16]. Importantly, even MRI with diffusion-weighted imaging misses 15–20% of strokes presenting with an AVS within the first 48 hours after onset, mostly small strokes affecting the lower portions of the brainstem [29, 30]. Delayed MRI (3–7 days post symptom onset) may be required to confirm the presence of a new infarct in such cases [19, 29].

Fortunately, the physical examination can make the distinction between vestibular neuritis and posterior circulation stroke with greater sensitivity than early MRI [29–31]. The studies reaching this conclusion were conducted by neuro-otologists performing a targeted three-component ocular motor exam—the head impulse test (HIT), gaze testing for nystagmus, and alternate cover test for skew deviation (HINTS—head impulse, nystagmus, test of skew). Trained general neurologists may achieve similar accuracy; however, because this approach has not been validated, we suggest performing two additional components for the basic evaluation of patients with AVS—a targeted neurological examination and gait testing [32].

We perform these tests in the following sequence: (1) nystagmus testing; (2) alternate cover test for skew deviation; (3) HIT; (4) targeted neurological exam, focusing on cranial nerves, cerebellar testing, and long-tract signs; and (5) gait testing (Table 4.1). Nystagmus testing is the least "intrusive" part of the examination, and it informs the interpretation of the HIT. Thus, nystagmus helps to anchor and inform the rest of the process. Nearly all patients with an AVS due to a vestibular cause will have nystagmus if examined within the first days, so its absence makes the diagnosis of vestibular neuritis unlikely.

Nystagmus is usually visible with the naked eye. Subspecialists often use Frenzel lenses to block visual fixation and magnify the view, thus improving detection. Other bedside alternatives to block visual fixation may be used, including lightweight plastic lenses or a penlight. If nystagmus is truly absent, acute vestibular neuritis is very unlikely and the HIT can yield misleading information. Bedside examination for nystagmus is straightforward and the details are diagnostically important [33]. Table 4.2 shows the nystagmus findings for patients with the AVS. Two patterns suggest stroke: (1) dominantly vertical or torsional nystagmus in any gaze position and (2) dominantly horizontal nystagmus that changes direction in different gaze positions.

Skew deviation is a vertical misalignment of the eyes due to imbalance in gravity-sensing vestibular pathways [34]. Skew deviation is elicited using the "alternate

Table 4.1 Sensitivity of various components of the physical examination for central mechanism in patients with the acute vestibular syndrome

Component of exam	Sensitivity for central cause[a]	Comments
Nystagmus	50–60%	See Table 4.2
Skew deviation	25%	This finding is not very sensitive but it is specific for a central etiology, usually in the brainstem. See Table 4.2
Head impulse test[b] (see description below)	85–90%	Extremely important to *only* use this test in patients with the AVS with nystagmus. All other patients will have a "negative" test, which is "worrisome" for a stroke
Focused neurological exam	65%	In addition to obvious neurological findings, it is important to look for subtle findings that can be easily missed
Gait and/or truncal ataxia	65%	This is an essential test in patients with dizziness. Some patients without the first four findings may unable to sit up or stand and walk unaided. Apart from obvious disposition issues, many of these patients will have a stroke causing this finding

Abbreviation: AVS acute vestibular syndrome

Head impulse test: This maneuver tests the vestibulo-ocular reflex (VOR). Standing in front of the patient, the examiner holds the patient's head by each side and instructs the patient to focus on the examiner's nose and to keep their head and neck loose. The examiner gently displaces the patient's head about 10–15° from the midline to one side; from there, a flick of the wrists brings the head back towards the center position rapidly (>120°/sec) where it stops "dead" at the midline, while the examiner observes the eyes carefully. Both sides should be tested several times each. The normal response (normal VOR) is that the patient's gaze remains locked on the examiner's nose. The presence of a corrective saccade (the eyes move with the head, then snap back in a fast corrective movement back to the examiner's nose) is a "positive" test (abnormal VOR), which generally indicates a peripheral process, usually vestibular neuritis. Somewhat counterintuitively, it is the "positive" test which is reassuring as it suggests a peripheral vestibular problem and a "negative" test that is worrisome (in patients with the AVS because it suggests a stroke)

[a]Approximate numbers based on pooled data from multiple studies in some cases

[b]For AVS patients with nystagmus, the combined sensitivity of the first three elements (HINTS) approaches 100%

cover" test (Table 4.2). A normal response is no vertical correction, and an abnormal response suggests brainstem localization.

Next, use the HIT to test of the vestibulo-ocular reflex (VOR) (Table 4.1). The absence of a corrective saccade on both sides suggests a central cause for the AVS. It may seem counterintuitive that a normal finding predicts a dangerous disease. This is why the HIT is *only useful* in patients with the AVS with nystagmus. A HIT done in a patient without nystagmus (e.g., a dizzy patient with urosepsis or dehydration) will be normal (i.e., worrisome for stroke) and therefore misleading.

Because the circuit of the VOR does not loop through the cerebellum, cerebellar stroke patients typically have a negative (normal) HIT [35]. However, it does loop through the lateral pons, so some patients with brainstem strokes have a falsely "positive" (abnormal) HIT, from anterior inferior cerebellar artery (AICA) strokes affecting the pons or the labyrinth itself [34]. Bedside hearing testing ("HINTS plus") helps diagnose these patients [31]. The traditional teaching that coincident

Table 4.2 Nystagmus and skew deviation interpretation in patients with the acute vestibular syndrome

Finding	Significance	Comments
No nystagmus	Normal finding	Essentially rules out vestibular neuritis but is consistent with a cerebellar stroke. Rare patients with BPPV will endorse continuous dizziness and not have nystagmus at rest
Spontaneous horizontal nystagmus in primary gaze[a]	Does not distinguish between central and peripheral causes	Seen more commonly with peripheral causes of AVS, but is not diagnostic
Gaze evoked horizontal nystagmus that beats in only one direction	Does not distinguish between central and peripheral causes	Suggests a peripheral cause of AVS, but is not diagnostic. Note that in neuritis, there is often a slight torsional component
Direction-changing gaze evoked horizontal nystagmus	Central	This is central but can be a benign central cause (e.g., acute alcohol intoxication or anticonvulsant use)
Pure vertical nystagmus	Central	This should always be considered a central finding
Torsional nystagmus	Central	Torsional nystagmus is the expected finding in posterior canal BPPV, but these patients do not present with the AVS but rather a triggered episodic vestibular syndrome. There is often a slight torsional component in neuritis
Skew deviation[b]	Normally absent; its presence means a central cause	Not very sensitive, but if present it signals a central cause of the AVS

Abbreviations: *AVS* acute vestibular syndrome, *ED* emergency department, *BPPV* benign paroxysmal positional vertigo

[a]Nystagmus is nearly always present in vestibular neuritis (at least in the first few days) but only seen in 50% of cerebellar stroke patients and variably in other brainstem strokes. It is the quality of the nystagmus that is diagnostically important, not the mere presence or absence. The absence of nystagmus, after a careful examination to eliminate fixation, essentially excludes a diagnosis of acute vestibular neuritis or "labyrinthitis" in patients presenting during the first few days of the process

[b]Test skew deviation by using the alternate cover test. With the patient's eyes focused on a target (the examiner's nose), the examiner alternately covers and then uncovers each of the patient's eyes, every 2–3 seconds. It is important for the examiner to focus just on one eye (it does not matter which one) in order to see the small amplitude vertical corrections that occur when one eye is uncovered (one eye will go up and the other down, so either one will have a vertical correction, which is why either eye can be observed). Horizontal eye corrections are not meaningful for recognition of skew deviation

hearing loss and dizziness is always peripheral (a problem in the labyrinth) is wrong. Combined audio-vestibular loss is often a sign of stroke [36]. The relative frequency of labyrinthitis (inflammation of both components of the eighth nerve) versus AICA stroke is unknown.

Patients with the AVS who have worrisome nystagmus, skew deviation, or a bilaterally normal HIT have a presumed stroke. If all three tests are reassuring, the clinician should perform a targeted neurological examination [4] to identify anisocoria, facial weakness or sensory asymmetry, dysarthria/dysphonia, or limb ataxia. Lateral medullary stroke (Wallenberg syndrome) merits special attention. In addition to acute dizziness, patients may complain of dysarthria, dysphagia, or hoarseness due to lower cranial neuropathy. They may have Horner syndrome with subtle ptosis and anisocoria only evident in dim light (the normal larger pupil fully dilates, accentuating the difference in pupil size) [37]. The physical finding of decreased pain and temperature sensation on one side of the face may be missed if one only tests light touch (Table 4.3).

Finally, if these four exam components (nystagmus, skew deviation, HIT, and targeted neurological exam) are reassuring, the clinician should still test the gait. Ideally have the patient walk unassisted, but for severely nauseated patients who are

Table 4.3 Important components of the focused exam for posterior circulation stroke in patients presenting with the acute vestibular syndrome

Finding	Significance	Comments
Hearing by finger rub in each ear	Can be central or peripheral	The classic teaching that dizziness plus decreased hearing is nearly always peripheral is wrong. Infarcts of the labyrinth or eighth nerve root entry one (AICA distribution) can also cause this combination of findings
Abnormal extraocular movements	If diplopia is present, this should be considered central	The nuclei of these three cranial nerves (III and IV, midbrain; IV and VI, upper pons) suggest a brainstem localization
Ptosis	Suggests a lateral medullary infarct	Part of Horner syndrome
Anisocoria	Suggests a lateral medullary infarct	Seen best in a dark room to accentuate the difference in pupillary size. Part of Horner syndrome
Facial weakness	Suggests a lesion in the internal auditory canal or brainstem	Standard seventh nerve testing
Decreased facial pain and temperature sensation	Suggests a lateral medullary infarct	Light touch is preserved so one must test pain or temperature
Hoarseness (listening to the patient speak)	Suggests a lateral medullary infarct	Be careful about administering oral medications in this setting
Limb ataxia (finger-to-nose and heel-to-shin)	Suggests a cerebellar stroke	In the dizzy patient, these findings should be tested, but may be absent in some patients with cerebellar strokes
Truncal ataxia	Cerebellar or brainstem stroke	Test the ability of the patient maintain the seated position unassisted in the stretcher without holding on to the guard rails for support
Gait ataxia	Cerebellar or brainstem stroke	Test the ability of the patient to stand and walk unassisted. Patients with neuritis may have some unsteadiness but usually can stand and walk, whereas many patients with stroke cannot

Abbreviation: *AICA* anterior inferior cerebellar artery

too symptomatic to walk, test for truncal ataxia by asking the patient to sit upright with arms crossed. Patients who cannot walk or sit up unassisted are unsafe for discharge and are more likely to have a stroke (or other CNS pathology) rather than vestibular neuritis [38].

Although bedside examination trumps brain imaging in the early diagnosis of patients with the AVS, CT or MR angiography is required for stroke patients to define large vessel occlusions or vertebral dissections. For those patients with AVS who have clinical signs concerning for stroke and are candidates for intravenous thrombolysis, a non-contrast CT head is sufficient to exclude hemorrhage. For patients with a HINTS plus exam suggesting stroke who are not eligible for thrombolysis, neither CT nor MRI in the first 48 hours excludes stroke.

Management of Patients with Acute Posterior Circulation Stroke

Treatment should follow other guidelines for acute stroke in general. Close monitoring for deterioration is important. Acute reperfusion therapy should be pursued whenever possible. Intravenous thrombolysis is recommended within 4.5 hours of symptom onset in patients with disabling deficits. Mechanical thrombectomy is a valuable therapeutic alternative in patients with vertebral artery or basilar artery occlusions; success rates are greater with embolic occlusions as compared to thrombosis in situ [39]. Should a patient deteriorate, one must distinguish between primary continuing brainstem ischemia vs secondary brainstem compression or hydrocephalus. Imaging can help make this distinction. Clinical monitoring should ideally be done in a Neurocritical Care unit with access to neurosurgeons.

Medical Treatments Fluids and electrolytes need to be monitored and corrected, and vomiting can be controlled pharmacologically. Vestibular suppressants and restrictions in head movement can be prescribed initially but should be rapidly tapered, and vestibular rehabilitation should be started as soon as feasible. Isolated dizziness is usually not considered an indication for thrombolysis due to the low risk of disability. Prevention of future events should be promoted via risk factor modification and use of antithrombotics.

Surgical Treatments Subacute edema from large cerebellar infarctions may require decompression and/or external ventricular drainage to prevent brainstem compression. Placement of stents or surgery can be considered in patients with severe symptomatic vertebral artery stenosis, subclavian steal, or rotational vertebral artery syndrome refractory to medical treatments. Rarely, carotid endarterectomy/stenting can be used in carefully selected patients such as those with vascular anatomic variants placing them at higher risk for recurrence (e.g., persistent trigeminal or persistent hypoglossal artery connecting the carotid system to the post circulation directly) [40].

Rehabilitation Rehabilitation is often necessary, and most return of function is seen within the first few months. Vestibular rehabilitation is useful for reducing symptoms and improving patient function. The goal of rehabilitation is to promote CNS compensation through exercise.

Spontaneous Episodic Vestibular Syndrome (s-EVS)

The s-EVS is marked by recurrent, spontaneous episodes of dizziness that range in duration from seconds to days, the majority lasting minutes to hours. If patients are still symptomatic at presentation, one should use the approach to AVS described in the previous section. However, most patients are asymptomatic at the time of clinical assessment, the dizziness cannot be triggered at the bedside, and the examination is normal; in such cases the evaluation usually relies entirely on the history.

The most common benign cause of s-EVS is vestibular migraine [41]. The most frequent dangerous cause is posterior circulation TIA [42]. Ménière's disease also presents with the s-EVS but is less common [41]. Other causes include reflex (e.g., vasovagal) syncope and panic attacks [43]. Uncommon dangerous causes of s-EVS include cardiovascular (cardiac arrhythmia, unstable angina pectoris, pulmonary embolus), endocrine (hypoglycemia, neuro-humoral neoplasms), and toxic (intermittent carbon monoxide exposure) disorders.

Vestibular migraine presentations are variable [44] (Table 4.4). Attack duration ranges from seconds to days [41]. Nystagmus, if present, can be of peripheral, central, or mixed type. Headache, often absent during the attack, may begin before, during, or after the dizziness and may differ from the patient's "typical" migraine headaches. Nausea, vomiting, photophobia, phonophobia, and visual auras may accompany vestibular migraine, but these features are often absent. Hearing loss or tinnitus sometimes occurs, mimicking Ménière's disease. Since there are no pathognomonic signs or biomarkers, the diagnosis is clinical [41].

Ménière's disease classically presents with the triad of episodic vertigo with unilateral tinnitus and/or aural fullness and reversible sensorineural hearing loss. Episodes typically last minutes to hours. Only one in four patients initially present with the complete triad [45], and non-vertiginous dizziness is common [46]. Usually patients will have ipsiversive horizontal nystagmus and later contraversive paretic nystagmus. Patients with suspected Ménière's disease should be referred to an otolaryngologist; care should be taken not to miss TIA with audiovestibular symptoms that can mimic Ménière's disease.

Table 4.4 Diagnostic criteria for vestibular migraine

At least five episodes with vestibular symptoms (spontaneous, positional, or visually induced vertigo, head-motion-induced dizziness with nausea) of moderate or severe intensity lasting between 5 minutes and 72 hours
Presence of migraine or history of migraine with or without aura
One or more migraine features with at least 50% of the vestibular episodes
Headache with at least two of the following characteristics: unilateral location, pulsatile quality, moderate or severe pain, or aggravation by routine physical activity
Photophobia or phonophobia
Visual aura
No other vestibular explanation

Reflex (or neurocardiogenic) syncope includes vasovagal syncope, carotid sinus hypersensitivity, and situational syncope (e.g., micturition, defecation, cough) [47]. Presyncopal episodes (i.e., without loss of consciousness) outnumber spells with full syncope [48]. Dizziness is the most common presyncopal symptom and it may be of any type, including vertigo. Diagnosis is based on clinical history, excluding dangerous mimics (especially arrhythmia), and can be confirmed by formal head-up tilt table testing [49].

Episodic dizziness from panic attacks (with or without hyperventilation) begins rapidly, peaks within 10 minutes, and, by definition, is accompanied by at least three other symptoms [50]. Although a situational precipitant (e.g., claustrophobia) may be present, spells often occur without obvious reasons and classical symptoms are absent in 30% of cases. Ictal panic attacks from temporal lobe epilepsy generally last only seconds, and they typically exhibit altered mental status [43]. Hypoglycemia, cardiac arrhythmias, pheochromocytoma, and basilar TIA can also mimic panic attacks by producing a combination of neurologic and autonomic features.

The principal dangerous diagnosis presenting as s-EVS is TIA [51]. Traditionally, isolated vertigo was not considered a TIA symptom, but epidemiological evidence shows that isolated attacks of spontaneous dizziness are the most common symptom in vertebrobasilar TIAs [42]. Although TIAs can last seconds to hours, in one prospective series the highest risk was observed with symptoms lasting minutes [52]. Focal neurological symptoms and head or neck pain were associated with stroke and TIA. Of the 27 patients diagnosed with a cerebrovascular cause, DWI was only 58% sensitive, presumably because these patients with transient symptoms had either smaller lesions or ischemia without infarction [52]. Perfusion weighted MRI (MR-PWI) was able to nearly double the proportion of patients in whom they could make a definite diagnosis. However, despite the intensive investigations these patients underwent, the authors could not determine a cause in 56% [52].

TIA causing dizziness or vertigo is easily missed; in a population-based study of transient symptoms preceding vertebrobasilar stroke, 9 of 10 who sought medical attention were initially missed [42]. Dizziness is a common symptom in basilar artery occlusion. Dizziness is the most common presenting symptom of vertebral artery dissection, which affects younger patients, mimics migraine, and is easily misdiagnosed [13]. Because 5% of TIA patients suffer a stroke within 48 hours, prompt diagnosis and treatment are critical [53].

Cardiac arrhythmias should also be considered in patients with s-EVS, particularly when true syncope occurs [54]. Although some clinical features may increase or decrease the odds of a cardiac cause [47], additional testing (e.g., cardiac loop recording) is often required to confirm the final diagnosis [49].

Triggered Episodic Vestibular Syndrome (t-EVS)

Patients with t-EVS have brief episodes of dizziness lasting seconds to minutes, depending on the underlying etiology. There is an "obligate" trigger; a specific movement or action that consistently causes dizziness. Common triggers are changes in head position or body posture. Patients with nausea and vomiting may overestimate episode duration. Again, clinicians must distinguish *exacerbating* features (worsens preexisting baseline dizziness) from *triggers* (provokes new dizziness not present at baseline). The most common etiologies of t-EVS are BPPV and orthostatic hypotension. Dangerous causes include central (neurologic) mimics of BPPV and serious causes of orthostatic hypotension. By definition, physicians should be able to reproduce the dizziness at the bedside.

BPPV, the most common vestibular cause of dizziness (with a lifetime prevalence of 2%) [55], is caused by mobile crystalline debris in one or more semicircular canals ("canaliths") of the vestibular labyrinth. Classical symptoms are repetitive, brief, triggered episodes of rotational vertigo lasting less than a minute, though nonvertiginous dizziness is also frequent. The diagnosis is confirmed by reproducing symptoms using canal-specific positional testing maneuvers and identifying a canal-specific nystagmus.

While BPPV can be easily diagnosed and treated, it is not an emergency; however central mimics of BPPV (*central* paroxysmal positional vertigo—CPPV) caused by posterior fossa neoplasm, infarction, hemorrhage, and demyelination may be. BPPV nystagmus usually begins after a delay (latency) of a few seconds, peaks in intensity rapidly, and then rapidly decays as long as the head is held stationary. Instead, CPPV may begin immediately or after a delay, may decay or persist, and may or may not change direction during testing [44, 56] (Table 4.5).

Orthostatic hypotension accounts for 24% of acute syncopal presentations. The classical symptom is lightheadedness or presyncope on arising, but vertigo is common [9]. Because BPPV produces dizziness on arising in 58% [55], it can mimic the

Table 4.5 Central paroxysmal positional vertigo (CPPV) clues in patients with a triggered episodic vestibular syndrome

Presence of symptoms or signs that are not observed in BPPV
Headache
Diplopia
Abnormal cranial nerve or cerebellar function
Atypical nystagmus characteristics or symptoms during positional tests
Downward-beating nystagmus[a]
Nystagmus that starts instantaneously, persists for longer than 90 s, or lacks a crescendo-decrescendo pattern of intensity
Prominent nystagmus with mild or absent associated dizziness or vertigo
Poor response to therapeutic maneuvers
Repetitive vomiting during positional maneuvers
Unable to cure patient with canal-specific canalith repositioning maneuver (modified Epley or equivalent for posterior canal BPPV, Lempert's barbecue maneuver for horizontal canal BPPV)
Frequent recurrent symptoms

[a]Downward-beating nystagmus can be observed with superior canal BPPV; however this is uncommon and is usually seen with central structural lesions

postural lightheadedness of orthostatic hypotension and often goes undiagnosed in the elderly [10]. Orthostatic hypotension may be incidental, especially in older patients taking antihypertensive medications [57]. Positional triggers, such as rolling over in bed, are common in BPPV, but should not occur with orthostatic hypotension. Orthostatic dizziness without systemic orthostatic hypotension has been reported with hemodynamic TIA (due to low flow across a vascular stenosis) [58] and in patients with intracranial hypotension [59].

Sudden Sensorineural Hearing Loss (SSNHL)

SSNHL is an acute, unexplained hearing loss, nearly always unilateral, that develops over days. Most cases are idiopathic, with an annual incidence from 2 to 20 per 100,000 people, usually middle-aged. It is considered a medical emergency [60]. Patients with older age, diet low in fresh vegetables, low folate, and chronic otitis media and those with metabolic syndrome may be at increased risk. Several known etiologies for SSNHL are listed in Table 4.6.

Table 4.6 Identifiable causes of sudden sensorineural hearing loss (SSNHL)

Infectious	Bacterial meningitis	Toxic	Aminoglycosides
	Cryptococcal meningitis		Chemotherapeutic agents
	Lyme disease		Non-steroidal anti-inflammatory drugs
	HIV		Salicylates
	Herpes virus	Traumatic	Inner ear concussion
	Mumps		Iatrogenic trauma/surgery
	Mycoplasma		Perilymphatic fistula
	Otosyphilis		Temporal bone fracture
	Lassa fever		Barotrauma
	Toxoplasmosis	Autoimmune	Autoimmune inner ear disease
Neurologic	Migraine		Systemic lupus erythematosus
	Multiple sclerosis		Behcet's disease
	Pontine ischemia		Cogan's syndrome
Vascular	Cardiovascular bypass	Otologic	Fluctuating hearing loss
	Sickle cell disease		Ménière's disease
	Cerebrovascular accident/stroke		Otosclerosis
Functional	Conversion disorder		Enlarged vestibular aqueduct
	Malingering		Hereditary/congenital hearing loss
Neoplastic	Vestibular schwannoma	Metabolic	Diabetes mellitus
	Myeloma		Hypothyroidism
	Meningiomas, petrous apex metastases		Thyrotoxicosis

Adapted from Kuhn et al. [63]

The majority of patients report hearing loss upon awakening and often do not recognize they have lost hearing. Instead, patients may complain of having the sensation of a blocked ear; thus, increasing the risk of initial misdiagnosis. More than 90% of patients also report tinnitus, increasing the psychological burden for patients [60]. Some have vertigo, ear pain, and paresthesia, but there is no neck pain.

History gathering should include questions about trauma, ear pain or drainage, fever or focal neurologic symptoms, headache, diplopia, and history of similar symptoms. Should the hearing loss fluctuate over time, Ménière's disease should be considered.

Physical examination should include a full otoscopic exam during which any cerumen should be removed. The external canal and tympanic membrane should be unremarkable. The classical Weber and Rinne tests can help distinguish between sensorineural and conductive hearing loss. A full neurologic examination should be performed to exclude the presence of an ipsilateral Horner syndrome, diplopia, nystagmus, facial weakness, limb incoordination, gait ataxia, and contralateral loss of pain and temperature. Lyme titers can be checked in endemic areas. MRI with gadolinium should be performed with close ENT follow-up for formal audiometric evaluation.

Treatment Glucocorticoids are the usual first-line therapy and may be given orally or locally via intratympanic installation by otolaryngologists (usually when oral treatment has failed or in patients for whom oral steroids may cause serious side effects). The benefit of oral glucocorticoids is unclear but may be more beneficial in those with severe hearing loss [61]. It is recommended to start treatment within 2 weeks of onset of hearing loss using prednisone 1 mg/kg/day (up to 60 mg) for 10–14 days [60]. Antiviral agents are sometimes prescribed because HSV-1 is presumed to be a common etiology for SSNHL; however there is a lack of evidence that antiviral treatment is helpful and its use is controversial. Should one choose to add an antiviral, valacyclovir 1 g three times daily or famciclovir 500 mg three times daily may be used.

Prognosis Approximately two-thirds of patients with idiopathic SSNHL will experience a partial recovery. Patients having low-frequency hearing loss are more likely to experience complete recovery; however, the prognosis is poor for patients with profound hearing loss across all frequencies. Most patients improve within 10 days and almost all within 3 months of symptom onset [62].

Conclusions

Dizziness, vertigo, and unsteadiness are common complaints caused by numerous diseases, including otological, neurological, and systemic disorders. Diagnosis can be difficult. Misconceptions, resource over-utilization, and misdiagnosis are common. History taking guided by the timing and triggers approach along with a focused physical examination is more accurate than early neuroimaging (even with MRI) and more likely to result in a specific diagnosis. Sudden sensorineural hearing loss requires a careful physical examination to rule out central processes, early treatment, and otolaryngology referral.

> **Cardinal Messages**
> - One in five acute ischemic strokes affect the posterior circulation.
> - Posterior circulation strokes are more likely to be misdiagnosed.
> - Understanding neuroanatomy is essential to adequately interpret posterior circulation symptoms and brain and vascular imaging findings.
> - Most patients with posterior circulation stroke or TIA will have associated symptoms and focal deficits on examination. However, dizziness can be the sole manifestation of posterior circulation ischemia.
> - Brain imaging—both CT and MRI—has important limitations in the early diagnosis of posterior circulation ischemic stroke. In fact, among acutely dizzy patients, the physical examination can be more sensitive than early MRI in differentiating acute ischemia from a peripheral vestibular disorder.
> - Sudden sensorineural hearing loss requires a careful physical examination, early treatment, and prompt specialist referral.

References

1. Saber Tehrani AS, Coughlan D, Hsieh YH, et al. Rising annual costs of dizziness presentations to U.S. emergency departments. Acad Emerg Med. 2013;20:689–96.
2. Newman-Toker DE. Missed stroke in acute vertigo and dizziness: it is time for action, not debate. Ann Neurol. 2016;79:27–31.
3. Newman-Toker DE, McDonald KM, Meltzer DO. How much diagnostic safety can we afford, and how should we decide? A health economics perspective. BMJ Qual Saf. 2013;22(Suppl 2):ii11–20.
4. Newman-Toker DE. Symptoms and signs of neuro-otologic disorders. Continuum (Minneap Minn). 2012;18:1016–40.
5. Edlow JA, Newman-Toker DE, Savitz SI. Diagnosis and initial management of cerebellar infarction. Lancet Neurol. 2008;7:951–64.
6. Newman-Toker DE, Hsieh YH, Camargo CA Jr, Pelletier AJ, Butchy GT, Edlow JA. Spectrum of dizziness visits to US emergency departments: cross-sectional analysis from a nationally representative sample. Mayo Clin Proc. 2008;83:765–75.
7. Kerber KA, Meurer WJ, Brown DL, et al. Stroke risk stratification in acute dizziness presentations: a prospective imaging-based study. Neurology. 2015;85(21):1869–78.
8. Kerber KA, Brown DL, Lisabeth LD, Smith MA, Morgenstern LB. Stroke among patients with dizziness, vertigo, and imbalance in the emergency department: a population-based study. Stroke. 2006;37:2484–7.
9. Newman-Toker DE, Dy FJ, Stanton VA, Zee DS, Calkins H, Robinson KA. How often is dizziness from primary cardiovascular disease true vertigo? A systematic review. J Gen Intern Med. 2008;23:2087–94.

10. Lawson J, Johnson I, Bamiou DE, Newton JL. Benign paroxysmal positional vertigo: clinical characteristics of dizzy patients referred to a Falls and Syncope Unit. QJM. 2005;98:357–64.
11. Royl G, Ploner CJ, Leithner C. Dizziness in the emergency room: diagnoses and misdiagnoses. Eur Neurol. 2011;66:256–63.
12. Casani AP, Dallan I, Cerchiai N, Lenzi R, Cosottini M, Sellari-Franceschini S. Cerebellar infarctions mimicking acute peripheral vertigo: how to avoid misdiagnosis? Otolaryngol Head Neck Surg. 2013;148:475–81.
13. Savitz SI, Caplan LR, Edlow JA. Pitfalls in the diagnosis of cerebellar infarction. Acad Emerg Med. 2007;14:63–8.
14. Newman-Toker DE, Moy E, Valente E, Coffey R, Hines AL. Missed diagnosis of stroke in the ED: a cross-sectional analysis of a large population based sample. Diagnosi. 2014;2:29–40.
15. Kuruvilla A, Bhattacharya P, Rajamani K, Chaturvedi S. Factors associated with misdiagnosis of acute stroke in young adults. J Stroke Cerebrovasc Dis. 2011;20:523–7.
16. Kerber KA, Newman-Toker DE. Misdiagnosing dizzy patients: common pitfalls in clinical practice. Neurol Clin. 2015;33:565–75.
17. Newman-Toker DE, Camargo CA Jr, Hsieh YH, Pelletier AJ, Edlow JA. Disconnect between charted vestibular diagnoses and emergency department management decisions: a cross-sectional analysis from a nationally representative sample. Acad Emerg Med. 2009;16:970–7.
18. Newman-Toker DE, Edlow JA. TiTrATE: a novel, evidence-based approach to diagnosing acute dizziness and vertigo. Neurol Clin. 2015;33:577–99.
19. Tarnutzer AA, Berkowitz AL, Robinson KA, Hsieh YH, Newman-Toker DE. Acute vestibular syndrome: does my patient have a stroke? A systematic and critical review of bedside diagnostic predictors. Can Med Assoc J 2011;Jun 14;183(9):E571–92.
20. Edlow JA, Newman-Toker DE. Medical and nonstroke neurologic causes of acute, continuous vestibular symptoms. Neurol Clin. 2015;33:699–716.
21. Kerber KA, Burke JF, Brown DL, et al. Does intracerebral haemorrhage mimic benign dizziness presentations? A population based study. Emerg Med J. 2012;29(1):43–6.
22. Kattah JC, Dhanani SS, Pula JH, Mantokoudis G, Saber Tehrani AS, Newman-Toker D. Vestibular signs of thiamine deficiency during the early phase of suspected Wernicke encephalopathy. Neurol Clin Pract. 2013;3:260–468.
23. Cutfield NJ, Seemungal BM, Millington H, Bronstein AM. Diagnosis of acute vertigo in the emergency department. Emerg Med J. 2011;28(6):538–9.
24. Arbusow V, Theil D, Strupp M, Mascolo A, Brandt T. HSV-1 not only in human vestibular ganglia but also in the vestibular labyrinth. Audiol Neurootol. 2001;6:259–62.
25. Lu YC, Young YH. Vertigo from herpes zoster oticus: superior or inferior vestibular nerve origin? Laryngoscope. 2003;113:307–11.
26. Strupp M, Jager L, Muller-Lisse U, Arbusow V, Reiser M, Brandt T. High resolution Gd-DTPA MR imaging of the inner ear in 60 patients with idiopathic vestibular neuritis: no evidence for contrast enhancement of the labyrinth or vestibular nerve. J Vestib Res. 1998;8:427–33.
27. Baloh RW. Clinical practice. Vestibular neuritis. N Engl J Med. 2003;348:1027–32.
28. Newman-Toker DE, Della Santina CC, Blitz AM. Vertigo and hearing loss. Handb Clin Neurol. 2016;136:905–21.
29. Kattah JC, Talkad AV, Wang DZ, Hsieh YH, Newman-Toker DE. HINTS to diagnose stroke in the acute vestibular syndrome: three-step bedside oculomotor examination more sensitive than early MRI diffusion-weighted imaging. Stroke. 2009;40:3504–10.
30. Saber Tehrani AS, Kattah JC, Mantokoudis G, et al. Small strokes causing severe vertigo: frequency of false-negative MRIs and nonlacunar mechanisms. Neurology. 2014;83:169–73.
31. Newman-Toker DE, Kerber KA, Hsieh YH, et al. HINTS outperforms ABCD2 to screen for stroke in acute continuous vertigo and dizziness. Acad Emerg Med. 2013;20:986–96.
32. Chen L, Lee W, Chambers BR, Dewey HM. Diagnostic accuracy of acute vestibular syndrome at the bedside in a stroke unit. J Neurol. 2010;May;258(5):855–61
33. Edlow J, Newman-Toker D. Using the physical examination to diagnose patients with acute dizziness and vertigo. J Emerg Med. 2016;50(4):617–28.

34. Newman-Toker DE, Curthoys IS, Halmagyi GM. Diagnosing stroke in acute vertigo: the HINTS family of eye movement tests and the future of the "eye ECG". Semin Neurol. 2015;35:506–21.
35. Newman-Toker DE, Kattah JC, Alvernia JE, Wang DZ. Normal head impulse test differentiates acute cerebellar strokes from vestibular neuritis. Neurology. 2008;70:2378–85.
36. Lee SH, Kim JS. Acute diagnosis and management of stroke presenting dizziness or vertigo. Neurol Clin. 2015;33:687–98, xi.
37. Kim JS. Pure lateral medullary infarction: clinical-radiological correlation of 130 acute, consecutive patients. Brain. 2003;126:1864–72.
38. Carmona S, Martinez C, Zalazar G, et al. The diagnostic accuracy of truncal ataxia and HINTS as cardinal signs for acute vestibular syndrome. Front Neurol. 2016;7:125.
39. Baik SH, Park HJ, Kim JH, Jang CK, Kim BM, Kim DJ. Mechanical thrombectomy in subtypes of basilar artery occlusion: relationship to recanalization rate and clinical outcome. Radiology. 2019;291:730–7.
40. Kim DU, Han MK, Kim JS. Isolated recurrent vertigo from stenotic posterior inferior cerebellar artery. Otol Neurotol. 2011;32:180–2.
41. Seemungal B, Kaski D, Lopez-Escamez JA. Early diagnosis and management of acute vertigo from vestibular migraine and Meniere's disease. Neurol Clin. 2015;33:619–28, ix.
42. Paul NL, Simoni M, Rothwell PM, Oxford Vascular S. Transient isolated brainstem symptoms preceding posterior circulation stroke: a population-based study. Lancet Neurol. 2013;12:65–71.
43. Kanner AM. Ictal panic and interictal panic attacks: diagnostic and therapeutic principles. Neurol Clin. 2011;29:163–75.
44. Jonathan EA. Diagnosing patients with acute-onset persistent dizziness. Ann Emerg Med. 2018;71:625–31.
45. Mancini F, Catalani M, Carru M, Monti B. History of Meniere's disease and its clinical presentation. Otolaryngol Clin North Am. 2002;35:565–80.
46. Faag C, Bergenius J, Forsberg C, Langius-Eklof A. Symptoms experienced by patients with peripheral vestibular disorders: evaluation of the Vertigo Symptom Scale for clinical application. Clin Otolaryngol. 2007;32:440–6.
47. van Dijk JG, Thijs RD, Benditt DG, Wieling W. A guide to disorders causing transient loss of consciousness: focus on syncope. Nat Rev Neurol. 2009;5:438–48.
48. Romme JJ, van Dijk N, Boer KR, et al. Influence of age and gender on the occurrence and presentation of reflex syncope. Clin Auton Res. 2008;18:127–33.
49. Moya A, Sutton R, Ammirati F, et al. Guidelines for the diagnosis and management of syncope (version 2009). Eur Heart J. 2009;30:2631–71.
50. Katon WJ. Clinical practice. Panic disorder. N Engl J Med. 2006;354:2360–7.
51. Blum CA, Kasner SE. Transient ischemic attacks presenting with dizziness or vertigo. Neurol Clin. 2015;33:629–42, ix.
52. Choi JH, Park MG, Choi SY, et al. Acute transient vestibular syndrome: prevalence of stroke and efficacy of bedside evaluation. Stroke. 2017;48(3):556–62.
53. Shah KH, Kleckner K, Edlow JA. Short-term prognosis of stroke among patients diagnosed in the emergency department with a transient ischemic attack. Ann Emerg Med. 2008;51:316–23.
54. Newman-Toker DE, Camargo CA Jr. 'Cardiogenic vertigo'—true vertigo as the presenting manifestation of primary cardiac disease. Nat Clin Pract Neurol. 2006;2:167–72.
55. von Brevern M, Radtke A, Lezius F, et al. Epidemiology of benign paroxysmal positional vertigo: a population based study. J Neurol Neurosurg Psychiatry. 2007;78:710–5.
56. Soto-Varela A, Rossi-Izquierdo M, Sanchez-Sellero I, Santos-Perez S. Revised criteria for suspicion of non-benign positional vertigo. QJM. 2013;106:317–21.
57. Poon IO, Braun U. High prevalence of orthostatic hypotension and its correlation with potentially causative medications among elderly veterans. J Clin Pharm Ther. 2005;30:173–8.
58. Stark RJ, Wodak J. Primary orthostatic cerebral ischaemia. J Neurol Neurosurg Psychiatry. 1983;46:883–91.

59. Blank SC, Shakir RA, Bindoff LA, Bradey N. Spontaneous intracranial hypotension: clinical and magnetic resonance imaging characteristics. Clin Neurol Neurosurg. 1997;99:199–204.
60. Stachler RJ, Chandrasekhar SS, Archer SM, et al. Clinical Practice Guideline: sudden hearing loss. Otolaryngol Head Neck Surg. 2012;146:S1–35.
61. Nosrati-Zarenoe R, Hultcrantz E. Corticosteriod treatment of idiopathic sudden sensorineural hearing loss: randomized triple-blind study. Otol Neurotol. 2012;33:523.
62. Yeo SW, Lee DH, Jun BC. Hearing outcome of sudden sensorineural hearing loss: long term follow-up. Otolaryngol Head Neck Surg. 2007;136:221.
63. Kuhn M, Heman-Ackah SE, Shaikh JA, Roehm PC. Sudden sensorineural hearing loss: a review of diagnosis, treatment, and prognosis. Trends Amplif. 2011;15(3):91–105.

Chapter 5
Neuro-ophthalmologic Urgencies and Emergencies

Devon A. Cohen and John J. Chen

Vision Loss

> **Diagnostic Keys**
> - Timing and associated symptoms are important in determining the urgency of evaluation in a patient presenting with visual loss.
> - Pain is a harbinger of danger in acute vision loss, with pituitary apoplexy, mucormycosis, and giant cell arteritis among the main possible causes.
> - Giant cell arteritis should be suspected in any patient over 50 with vision loss in conjunction with systemic symptoms until proven otherwise.
> - Checking for a relative afferent pupillary defect (RAPD) is one of the most important exam techniques because, if present, it indicates unilateral or asymmetric bilateral optic nerve or retinal disease.
> - Patients with acute central or branch retinal artery occlusion require urgent embolic workup, especially imaging for carotid disease.

D. A. Cohen
Department of Neurology, Mayo Clinic, Rochester, MN, USA

J. J. Chen (✉)
Department of Neurology, Mayo Clinic, Rochester, MN, USA

Department of Ophthalmology, Mayo Clinic, Rochester, MN, USA
e-mail: chen.john@mayo.edu

© Springer Nature Switzerland AG 2020
A. A. Rabinstein (ed.), *Neurological Emergencies*,
https://doi.org/10.1007/978-3-030-28072-7_5

> **Treatment Priorities**
> - Giant cell arteritis with acute vision loss demands immediate treatment with corticosteroids (even before definite pathological confirmation).
> - The value of intravenous or selective intra-arterial thrombolysis for acute central or branch retinal artery occlusion is not well established.
> - Pituitary apoplexy may require emergency surgical decompression and should be treated with stress-dose corticosteroids.

> **Prognosis at a Glance**
> - Unless promptly treated, giant cell arteritis can cause permanent visual loss.
> - Patients with acute central or branch retinal artery occlusion have substantially increased short-term risk of brain infarction.
> - Vision recovery over time is the rule among survivors of pituitary apoplexy.

Introduction

Visual loss is among the most common neuro-ophthalmologic presenting symptoms in emergency departments. A few simple questions and exam techniques can help guide the next steps in workup and management.

The first step should be lesion localization. History aids in this process. It is important to determine if the deficit is monocular or binocular as it localizes the pathology to anterior versus posterior to the chiasm, respectively. A monocular deficit indicates a unilateral eye or optic nerve disorder. Examining visual fields will further refine location of the pathology. A bitemporal hemianopia points to a chiasmal lesion. A homonymous hemianopia indicates a retro-chiasmal lesion involving the optic tract, optic radiations, or occipital lobe.

Loss of central visual acuity points toward a primary ophthalmologic disorder, which can have various etiologies, some of which can be neurologically dangerous and involve the retina or optic nerve, while others can be as benign as refractive error or cataracts. Presence of a relative afferent pupillary defect (RAPD) with the swinging flashlight test indicates unilateral or asymmetric bilateral optic nerve or retinal disease; it manifests as pupillary dilatation with direct illumination of the affected eye and constriction when the contralateral eye is illuminated. Other causes of vision loss, including cataract, amblyopia, refractive error, or media opacity will not cause a frank RAPD. Similarly, bilateral symmetric retinal or optic nerve pathology will not cause a RAPD.

Other exam techniques and pieces of history can help localize the pathology. Visual acuity improved with pinhole indicates that the vision loss is from refractive error and can be corrected with glasses. Delayed visual acuity recovery following bright light shone on each eye for 10 seconds (photostress test) suggests retinal pathology. Image distortion (metamorphopsia) or size distortion (micropsia) points to a maculopathy, such as an epiretinal membrane or macular degeneration.

Timing and associated symptoms are important in determining the urgency of an evaluation. When patients present with pain and acute vision loss, urgent evaluation is necessary.

Arteritic Anterior Ischemic Optic Neuropathy from Giant Cell Arteritis

Giant cell arteritis (GCA) should be suspected in any patient older than 50 years with vision loss in conjunction with systemic symptoms. The systemic symptoms are classically headache, scalp tenderness, and jaw claudication, but may also include weight loss, anorexia, malaise, and myalgias. The average annual incidence rate of GCA is 17.8 cases per 100,000 persons older than 50 years, according to a population study in Olmsted County, Minnesota [1]. Approximately 8–20% of patients with GCA can develop severe irreversible vision loss and become a neuro-ophthalmic emergency [2]. Arteritic anterior ischemic optic neuropathy (AAION) is responsible for the vision loss in about 90% of cases, but other causes such as posterior ischemic optic neuropathy and central retinal artery occlusion can also cause vision loss in GCA [2]. AAION tends to present with pallid disc edema and usually causes severe vision loss with the majority of patients having a visual acuity of 20/400 or worse (Fig. 5.1). It is important to note that up to 20% of patients with vision loss from GCA can have "occult" GCA without noticeable systemic symptoms [2].

Though vision loss is the most commonly reported visual symptom, patients can present with diplopia. Less common symptoms include eye pain, anisocoria, and ptosis secondary to cranial neuropathies. Patients may even present with stroke symptoms; around 3% of patients with GCA have cerebrovascular events.

Fig. 5.1 Pallid disc edema from arteritic anterior ischemic optic neuropathy due to giant cell arteritis

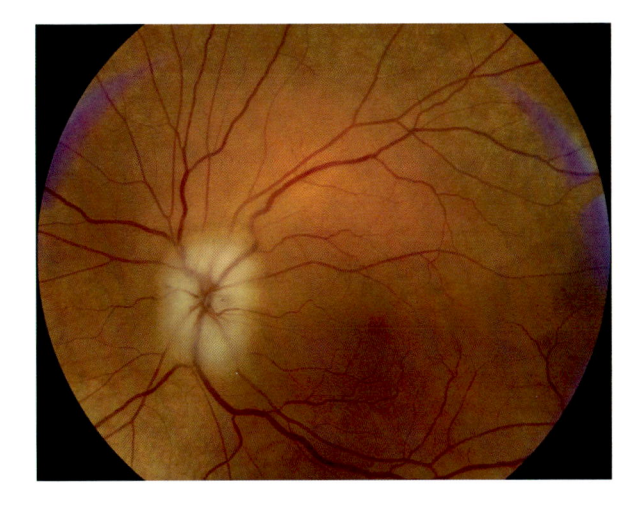

Laboratory workup should include CBC, ESR, and CRP; CRP is more sensitive than ESR [3]. Patients also often have an increase in platelet count. If the suspicion is high, steroids should be initiated immediately without waiting for temporal artery biopsies to be performed.

Patients with vision loss should be treated with high-dose IV steroids (methylprednisolone 1 g per day for 3–5 days). Steroid treatment will generally not reverse the vision loss already present, but is imperative to attempt to prevent worsening vision loss or bilateral involvement. Patient will typically be continued on a slow oral prednisone taper over 6–12 months based on the evolution of symptoms and inflammatory markers. Steroid-sparing agents have recently gained traction, particularly with the 2017 FDA approval of tocilizumab (humanized monoclonal antibody against the interleukin-6 receptor) for the specific indication of GCA, although these medications should not be used without concomitant steroids.

Retinal Artery Occlusion and Stroke

Patients with a central (CRAO) or branch (BRAO) retinal artery occlusion present with sudden unilateral painless vision loss. Patients may report prior episodes of amaurosis fugax with transient vision loss lasting 5–15 minutes, which is classically described as a shade coming over the eye. Patients with CRAO typically present with severe vision loss and classically have retinal whitening with a macular cherry red spot (Fig. 5.2). A calcified plaque is visible (white arrow). A BRAO will lead to a scotoma or segmental field loss depending on the extension of retinal ischemia. Both CRAO and BRAO may show box car segmentation and cotton wool spots. The presence of a CRAO or BRAO is a neuro-ophthalmic emergency because the majority of

Fig. 5.2 Central retinal artery occlusion causing retinal whitening with a cherry red spot (red arrow). A calcified plaque is visible (white arrow)

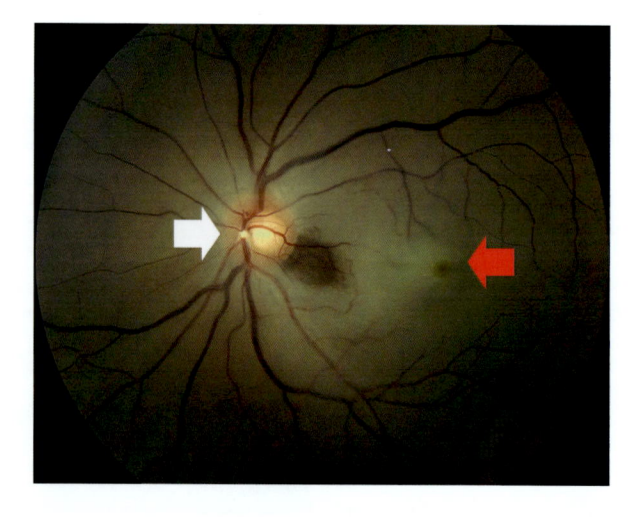

these cases are caused by embolism. Recent studies indicate that up to 5% of patients have a symptomatic brain infarction within a month of the retinal artery occlusion and 20–25% have evidence of an asymptomatic infarct on MRI. Therefore, patients with acute BRAO or CRAO require urgent workup to exclude embolic sources, starting from excluding vulnerable carotid plaques. The value of intravenous or selective intra-arterial thrombolysis for CRAO is not well established.

Homonymous visual field deficits indicate a retrochiasmal lesion; however, patients might only report unilateral field loss as they assume they are only missing vision in the eye with the temporal defect. Therefore, assessment of visual fields by confrontation is very helpful in differentiating a monocular process versus a bilateral homonymous process. An acute homonymous quadrantanopia or hemianopia may be indicative of a posterior circulation stroke. An isolated dense homonymous hemianopia points to a posterior cerebral artery occlusion causing an occipital stroke, while strokes affecting the parietal and temporal lobe often have accompanying neurologic symptoms. In these cases, the evaluation should include imaging of the cervical arteries, Holter monitor, and transesophageal echocardiogram. The differential includes hemorrhage, tumor, demyelination, and infection—all of which will be seen on brain MRI. Visual aura from migraine tends to cause a scintillating scotoma with gradual onset and resolution lasting 15–60 minutes, which can help differentiate this diagnosis from a stroke or transient ischemic attack that are characterized by sudden onset and absence of positive visual phenomena.

Pituitary Apoplexy

Pituitary apoplexy typically presents with acute onset headache often associated with sudden vision loss or diplopia, and it is an important diagnosis to be considered for patients presenting with a thunderclap headache in the emergency department. Differential diagnoses include subarachnoid hemorrhage and reversible cerebral vasoconstriction syndrome. Pituitary apoplexy occurs with sudden enlargement of the pituitary gland secondary to infarction or hemorrhage of a tumor (or rarely from ischemic necrosis of the pituitary gland due to hypovolemic shock during or after childbirth—a clinical entity known as Sheehan's syndrome). An inciting factor might be found in up to a third of patients, such as anticoagulant use, dopaminergic agents, malignant hypertension, or hypotension. Resultant mass effect on the optic chiasm causes patients to present most commonly with bitemporal field loss or potentially a junctional scotoma, as well as ophthalmoplegia in the setting of cavernous sinus involvement. Given the poor sensitivity of CT scan for this diagnosis, brain MRI should be performed if pituitary apoplexy is suspected. The disease can be fatal. Acute management includes high-dose corticosteroids and surgical intervention for decompression of the sella. Ophthalmological complications include vision loss and diplopia, though visual improvement over time is the rule [4].

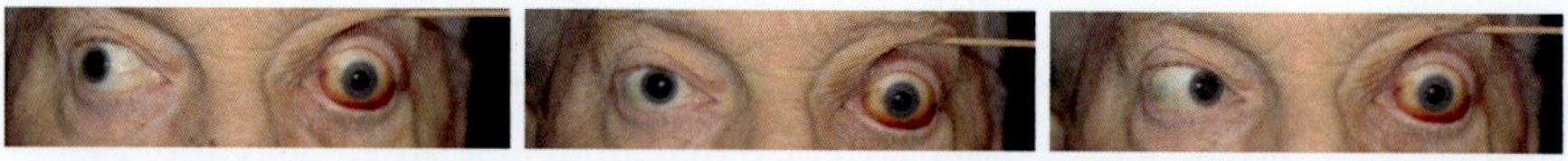

Fig. 5.3 Severe left-sided proptosis and complete ophthalmoplegia from mucormycosis causing an orbital apex syndrome. This patient had no light perception in the left eye

Mucormycosis

Mucormycosis, an invasive fungal infection, can present with painful orbital apex syndrome with subacute vision loss and ophthalmoplegia often in the setting of fever, periorbital swelling and facial pain, as well as sinusitis (Fig. 5.3). The pathognomonic black eschar involving the nasal mucosa occurs much less commonly and is seen in only approximately 20% of patients [5]. Mucormycosis is typically found in diabetic and immunocompromised patients. If there is a high clinical index of suspicion for this diagnosis, even if neuroimaging does not reveal bone erosion or extra sinus extension, paranasal sinus biopsy should be performed, and empiric antifungal treatment initiated. Surgical consultation for debridement is imperative. Retrobulbar amphotericin B has also shown promise. Early diagnosis and aggressive management is necessary because invasive fungal sinusitis from mucormycosis carries a 30% mortality rate.

Toxic Optic Neuropathy

The differential diagnosis for bilateral vision loss should include toxic optic neuropathy, though this will typically occur more progressively and non-emergently except for methanol toxicity.

Methanol is an optic nerve toxin that can cause sudden onset vision loss associated with optic disc swelling in the setting of an underlying metabolic acidosis. Patients will initially develop bilateral visual blurring—that may be transient—occurring within 18–48 hours of methanol ingestion. Patients will typically have systemic symptoms such as nausea and emesis, headache, and abdominal pain and may ultimately become comatose. Recognizing the diagnosis is fundamental to emergent intervention with IV ethyl alcohol and potentially dialysis to interfere with methanol metabolism. Visual recovery is often poor. Poison Control should be notified if there is no protocol in place when patients present with these toxicities.

Non-emergent Differentials

Less emergent causes of vision loss include idiopathic intracranial hypertension, nutritional and other optic toxic neuropathies, as well as optic neuritis. These all require appropriate semi-urgent workups, but not immediate interventions.

Papilledema

Introduction

Papilledema is optic disc swelling from increased intracranial pressure. Patients presenting with papilledema often have symptoms of increased intracranial pressure, including headache, transient visual obscurations, and pulse synchronous tinnitus, and may have diplopia from 6th nerve palsies. If the raised intracranial pressure is acute, nausea and emesis is also often present. Patients with papilledema will typically have bilateral optic disc edema and preserved central vision, unlike other optic neuropathies associated with disc edema, such as ischemic optic neuropathy, which typically causes loss of central visual acuity.

A sudden rise in intracranial pressure secondary to acute subarachnoid or intraparenchymal hemorrhage may cause acute onset papilledema, though these changes typically occur after 1–5 days of elevated intracranial pressure. Papilledema can have associated peripapillary retinal hemorrhages and cotton wool spots representing nerve fiber layer ischemia. Venous pulsations will disappear secondary to compression of the central retinal vein resulting in retinal venous engorgement and tortuosity. Severe disc swelling can cause subretinal fluid extension to the macula that will result in reduction in visual acuity and metamorphopsia. Patients may also be noted to have retinal or choroidal folds.

Papilledema typically causes blind spot enlargement. Papilledema can lead to visual field defects, most commonly inferior nasal defects, but severe or persistent papilledema can cause significant field loss and even blindness if left untreated.

The most common acute causes of papilledema in the emergency department include hydrocephalus, venous sinus thrombosis, meningitis, intracranial hemorrhage, and idiopathic intracranial hypertension. Malignant hypertension should be on the differential. History and the remainder of the neurologic exam should help identify the correct etiology.

Intracranial Hypertension

Intracranial hypertension can either be chronic, as with idiopathic intracranial hypertension (pseudotumor cerebri), or acute, often occurring secondary to a tumor, obstructive hydrocephalus, traumatic brain injury, intracranial hemorrhage, or venous sinus thrombosis (Fig. 5.4). Head CT scan may demonstrate small ventricles and cistern and sulcal effacement. Brain MRI and MR venogram will provide more detail and help eliminate secondary causes of raised intracranial pressure. A patient with focal neurological deficits in association with signs of meningismus and/or fevers should be worked up for meningitis, encephalitis, and abscess. Since papilledema indicates increased intracranial pressure, neuroimaging should be performed prior to lumbar puncture to rule out a mass lesion that could increase the risk of iatrogenic herniation.

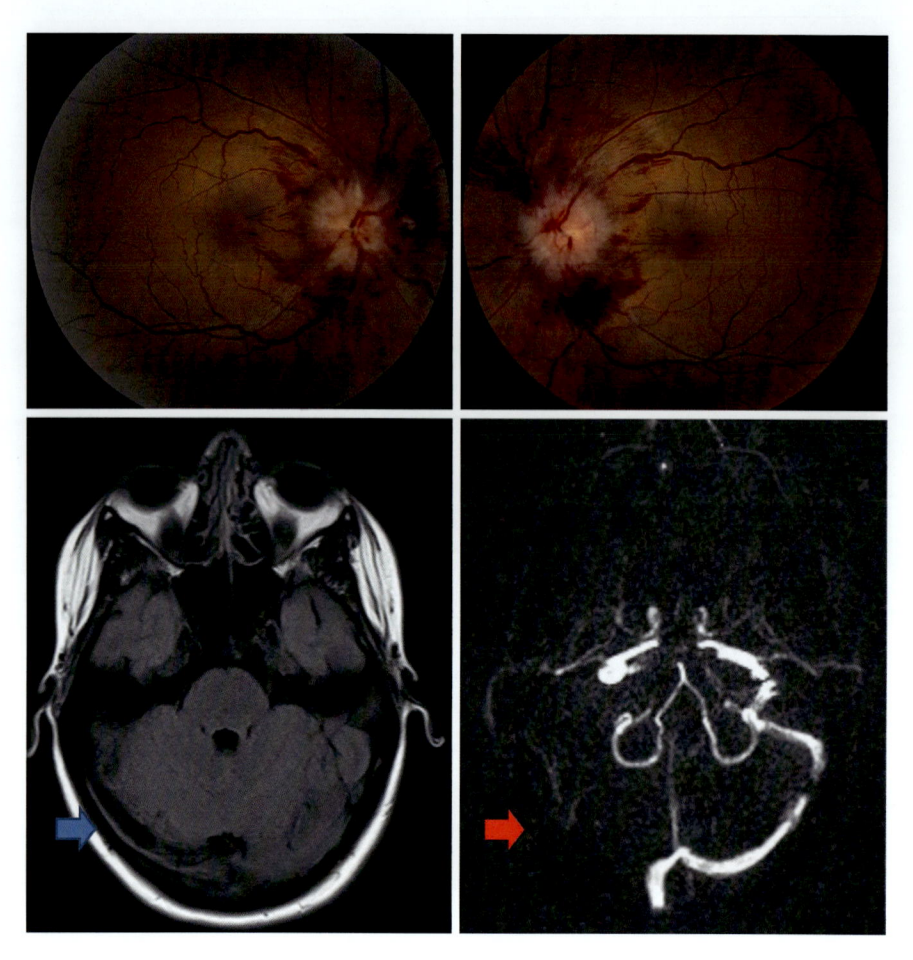

Fig. 5.4 Bilateral severe papilledema from cavernous sinus thrombosis. MRI shows poor signal of the right transverse sinus (blue arrow). MRV confirms lack of flow through the right transverse sinus indicative of a cavernous sinus thrombosis (red arrow)

If a patient is at risk of herniation, the intracranial pressure can be acutely reduced with head of the bed elevation, intravenous mannitol 20% (1–1.5 g/kg), as well as hyperventilation (PCO2 of 26 to 30 mmHg). Emergency neurosurgical consultation for decompression should be considered for severe cases.

Hypertensive Optic Neuropathy and Retinopathy

Patients with malignant hypertension can develop disc edema, often occurring with retinal hemorrhages, exudates, cotton wool spots, and arteriolar narrowing (Fig. 5.5) [3]. The disc edema can mimic papilledema, and therefore malignant hypertension

Fig. 5.5 Disc edema, retinal hemorrhages, cotton wool spots, and exudates from malignant hypertension

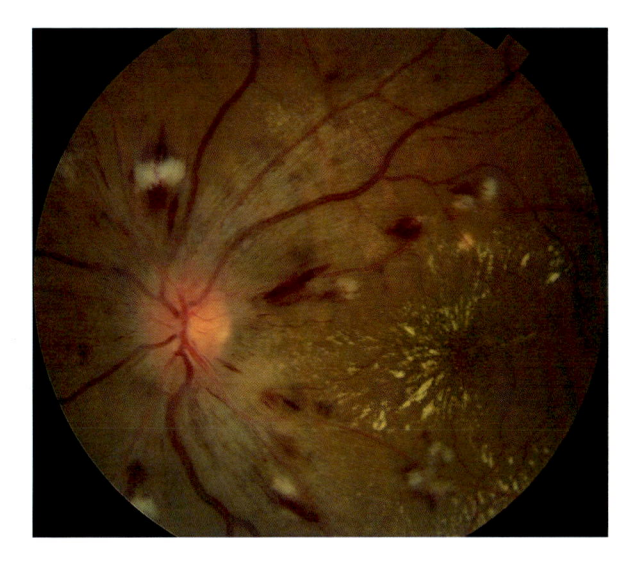

needs to be on the differential diagnosis list of patients presenting with bilateral disc edema. Disrupted autoregulation of the cerebral vasculature results from sudden or extreme elevations in blood pressure, causing increased vascular permeability and vasogenic cerebral edema. Disc edema is unlikely to occur in isolation and patients typically present with headache and/or confusion. If malignant hypertension is left untreated, it can lead to seizures, focal deficits, and progression to coma, in addition to serious damage to other organs.

Blood pressure reduction is indispensable, but abrupt drops in blood pressure should be strictly avoided because they can produce severe ischemia to the optic nerves, brain, myocardium, kidneys, and other organs. Steady blood pressure reduction over 1–2 days is ideal, usually in an ICU setting for patients with encephalopathy, cardiac ischemia, pulmonary edema, or renal insufficiency [3].

Non-emergency Differential Diagnoses

Chronic Papilledema

Chronic papilledema is most commonly caused by idiopathic intracranial hypertension, but mass lesions and other causes of papilledema need to be ruled out. The onset and severity of symptoms will guide the urgency of the evaluation. While the majority of cases of idiopathic intracranial hypertension can be evaluated in an outpatient setting, there are rare cases of fulminant idiopathic intracranial hypertension that can lead to rapid blindness and require urgent surgical intervention, such as optic nerve sheath fenestration or ventriculoperitoneal shunting.

Pseudopapilledema

Pseudopapilledema, which is an elevated-appearing optic nerve without true edema, is an important mimicker of papilledema. History and examination usually suffice to differentiate between these two diagnoses, but some cases require ancillary ophthalmologic testing. Pseudopapilledema is often caused by optic nerve head drusen or congenital anomalies, such as tilted optic disc or crowded hyperopic disc, which usually require confirmation by an ophthalmologist or neuro-ophthalmologist. Findings suggestive of pseudopapilledema include absence of a central cup and abnormal branching of the retinal vasculature with preserved venous pulsations.

Diagnostic Keys
- Papilledema typically causes blind spot enlargement and can lead to visual field defects, most commonly inferior nasal defects.
- Optic disc swelling in a patient with severe acute onset headache and focal neurologic deficits warrants immediate CT scan to rule out intracranial hemorrhage.
- The most common acute causes of papilledema in the ED include hydrocephalus, venous thrombosis, meningitis, intracranial hemorrhage, and idiopathic intracranial hypertension.
- Disc edema from malignant hypertension can mimic papilledema and therefore needs to be on the differential of patients presenting with bilateral disc edema.

Treatment Priorities
- In patients with disc edema from hypertensive encephalopathy, blood pressure reduction should start immediately but should be gradual to avoid inducing ischemia.
- Acute papilledema from intracranial hypertension related to an intracranial process represents a medical emergency that demands immediate intervention, brief hyperventilation, osmotic agents, and, in some cases, surgery which are possible therapeutic options.

Prognosis at a Glance
- Prognosis depends on the underlying cause of the papilledema.
- Severe or persistent papilledema can cause significant field loss and even blindness if left untreated.

Anisocoria

Introduction

Obtaining a detailed history is fundamental in the evaluation of anisocoria (i.e., pupillary asymmetry). Of particular importance is the acuity and the determination of which pupil is abnormal (the smaller or the larger pupil). Dangerous causes of anisocoria typically produce other signs or symptoms that will lead to the correct diagnosis, as is the case with Horner syndrome (mild ptosis on the side with the smaller pupil) or a third nerve palsy (ptosis and ipsilateral ophthalmoplegia association with the larger pupil). Thus, careful evaluation of the lids and ocular motility is imperative when evaluating patients with anisocoria because isolated anisocoria is rarely neurologically dangerous.

Light reactivity should be assessed to determine which one is the abnormal pupil. A pathologically larger pupil will have decreased reactivity to light stimulation. Assessing asymmetry with the room lights on and off can help decipher which eye is abnormal: larger asymmetry in light indicates the larger pupil is the abnormal due to poor constriction of the larger pupil relative to the normal pupil while larger asymmetry in the dark indicates the smaller pupil is the abnormal due to poor dilation in the dark of the smaller pupil relative to the normal pupil.

Horner Syndrome

Oculosympathetic disruption from a Horner syndrome will cause ipsilateral miosis, ptosis, and sometimes anhidrosis (Fig. 5.6). The anisocoria will be more prominent in dim conditions because of the impaired sympathetic tone in the smaller pupil. Of note, the small pupil of Horner syndrome will constrict normally with near vision and on direct light stimulation.

Acute Horner syndrome can be a neurologic emergency because it can be caused by carotid or vertebral artery dissection—especially if associated with ipsilateral neck or facial pain or other signs of brainstem stroke. Evaluating for accompanying signs or symptoms can help determine the underlying etiology of the Horner syndrome.

Carotid Dissection: Post-ganglionic Horner Syndrome

The differential for thunderclap headache includes carotid dissection, which typically commences with an ipsilateral neck pain or headache. In more than half of patients, this will be followed by a partial Horner syndrome manifested by ptosis and miosis, but without anhidrosis (post-ganglionic, third-order neuron lesion). Sometimes the pain can be mild so carotid dissection is on the differential for any Horner syndrome. Patients less often present with monocular vision loss from central retinal artery occlusion or ocular motor nerve palsies. These neuro-ophthalmologic

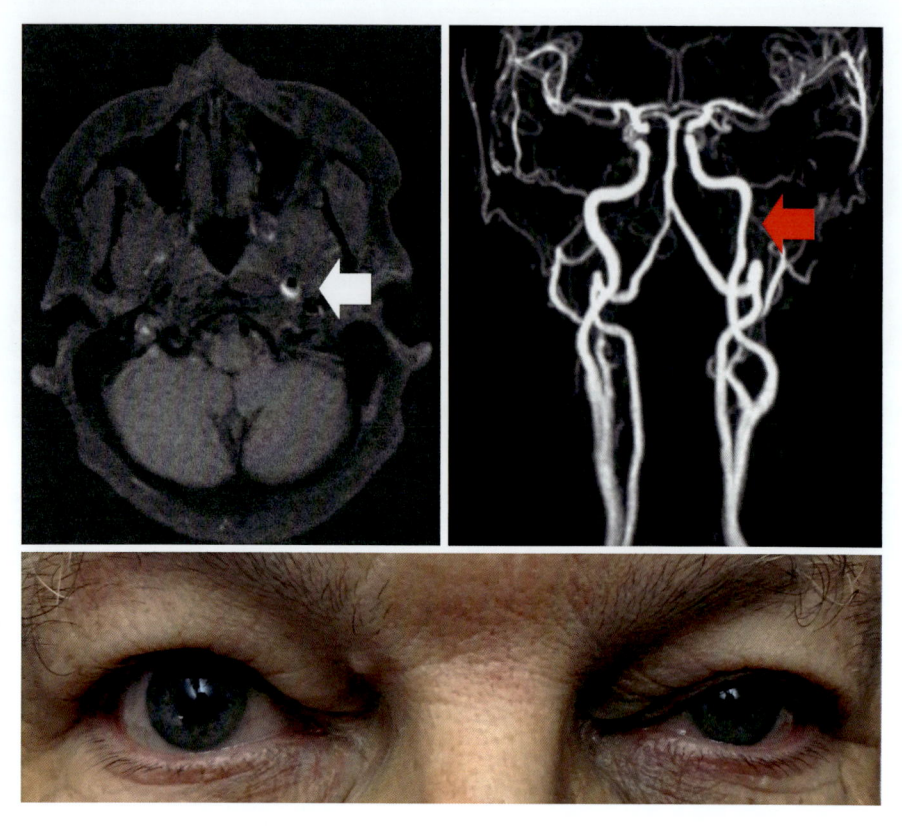

Fig. 5.6 Carotid dissection causing a left Horner syndrome. MRI axial shows a left internal carotid dissection with a classic crescent sign (white arrow) and MRA showed narrowing of the left internal carotid artery (red arrow). The patient had the classic ipsilateral ptosis and miosis of a Horner syndrome

manifestations of a carotid dissection can represent a warning sign for an impending hemispheric stroke that may occur within the following week [6].

Acute painful Horner syndrome necessitates emergent neuroimaging to rule out a carotid artery dissection, which is a significant cause of stroke in younger patients [7]. Preference to perform either MRI/MRA or CTA varies by institution [8]. Patients found to have a dissection need immediate anticoagulation and/or antiplatelet therapy to avoid subsequent strokes. There is currently insufficient evidence to support anticoagulation over antiplatelet therapy [9].

Lateral Medullary Infarction: Central Horner Syndrome

Ipsilateral Horner syndrome is present in at least three quarters of lateral medullary strokes as part of the classical Wallenberg syndrome. Patients with lateral medullary infractions can also present with ipsilateral corneal and facial anesthesia, ipsilateral appendicular and gait ataxia, contralateral hemi-body anesthesia, vertigo, nausea and vomiting, dysphagia, and dysarthria. They may additionally have oculomotor abnormalities including skew deviation, torsional or horizontal nystagmus, or ocular lateropulsion (tendency for the eye to deviate toward the side of the lesion).

Third Nerve Compression

When a clinician is asked to see a patient with an acutely fixed and dilated pupil, the first concern is often transtentorial (uncal) herniation. However, uncal herniation causing a dilated pupil from compression of the third nerve will be accompanied by severe neurologic deficits and often coma. Therefore, if a patient has a large poorly reactive pupil but is not at a minimum obtunded, uncal herniation should not be of concern, and more common causes of isolated mydriasis should be considered such as a tonic pupil or pharmacologic mydriasis.

Yet, acute pupillary dilatation may also occur because of compression of the third nerve by an enlarging aneurysm (typically arising from the posterior communicating artery). These patients may have preserved level of alertness and also preserved ocular motility because the compression may affect the parasympathetic (pupillary constricting) fibers overlying the third nerve without compromising the function of the motor fibers controlling extraocular movements.

Non-emergency Differential Diagnoses

Physiologic Anisocoria

The differential diagnosis of anisocoria should include physiologic anisocoria, a normal asymmetry of the pupils that can be seen in approximately 20% of the normal population. Physiologic anisocoria can fluctuate and thus a patient may first notice the pupillary asymmetry when experiencing other visual symptoms, such as eye pain or retro-orbital headache; in these cases, old photos or a driver's license can help uncover a chronic, less obvious asymmetry. When testing light reaction, these patients will commonly have an equal degree of asymmetry in light and dark, though it may be more obvious in the dark; in such cases additional investigation may be justified to rule out a Horner syndrome.

Pharmacologic Exposure

This commonly occurs due to inadvertent eye contact with drugs containing mydriatic properties, such a scopolamine patch, ipratropium inhaler, or sprays with adrenergic agents.

Tonic Pupil

A tonic pupil is caused by postganglionic disruption of the parasympathetic fibers innervating the pupil that results in mydriasis, which is often asymptomatic, but can cause photophobia or impede accommodation, making it difficult to read with the affected eye. It is more common in women and usually idiopathic. When it occurs in conjunction with areflexia, it is termed Holmes-Adie syndrome.

Diplopia/Ocular Motility Disorders

Diagnostic Keys and Treatment Priorities
- A comatose or stuporous patient with an acutely fixed and dilated pupil should be considered to have transtentorial brain herniation, which constitutes a medical/surgical emergency.
- A fixed or poorly light-responsive, dilated pupil in a patient who is awake should not be caused by brain herniation, but could be caused by local compression from an enlarging intracranial aneurysm thus representing a medical/surgical urgency.
- Anisocoria due to Horner syndrome will be more prominent in dim light conditions.

Prognosis at a Glance
- Horner syndrome can be caused by carotid dissection or medullary stroke and therefore be associated with increased risk of subsequent brain ischemia.

Diagnostic Keys
- The first step in the evaluation of diplopia is to determine if it is monocular or binocular: monocular diplopia is an expression of ocular disease, while binocular diplopia is often caused by a neurological disorder producing ophthalmoparesis.
- Signs of danger in patients with eye movement disorders include the presence of severe pain or accompanying neurologic symptoms suggestive of a systemic etiology.
- Acute ophthalmoparesis associated with proptosis and severe congestion of conjunctival vessels should prompt evaluation for a carotid cavernous fistula.
- Vertical gaze paralysis localizes to the dorsal midbrain.

> **Treatment Priorities**
> - Encephalopathic patients with ophthalmoparesis should immediately receive intravenous thiamine supplementation.
> - Patients with encephalopathy and vertical gaze paralysis or skew deviation of the eyes must undergo emergency evaluation for possible top of the basilar occlusion and undergo acute recanalization therapy (intravenous thrombolysis and/or mechanical thrombectomy) if the occlusion is present.
> - Cavernous sinus thrombosis should be treated with anticoagulation. Antibiotics should be added whenever septic thrombophlebitis is suspected.
> - Carotid cavernous fistulas, when symptoms are severe, may require endovascular closure.

> **Prognosis at a Glance**
> - Embolic occlusion of the top of the basilar artery is often fatal unless rapid recanalization is achieved.
> - Wernicke encephalopathy can cause major permanent disability when diagnosis and treatment are delayed.
> - Diplopia from compression of cranial nerves responsible for extraocular movements often improve over time when the compression is relieved promptly.

Introduction

History is fundamental to localizing the lesion in ocular motility disorders. When a patient presents with diplopia, the first step is to determine if it is monocular or binocular. If it does not resolve when closing one eye, it is monocular. Monocular diplopia is caused by an ocular problem, such as dry eye or astigmatism and is not neurologically dangerous.

Binocular diplopia will be the focus of this section given the potential for neurologic causes. Further localization is facilitated by determining image orientation and the gaze direction of diplopia exacerbation. Harbingers of danger include the presence of severe pain or accompanying neurologic symptoms suggestive of a systemic etiology. Some causes of binocular diplopia, such as pituitary apoplexy and mucormycosis have been previously mentioned in this chapter.

Aneurysmal Third Nerve Palsy

A third nerve palsy causes impaired ipsilateral elevation, adduction, and depression and classically presents with a "down and out" eye in association with ptosis and mydriasis. It is important to note that third nerve palsies may be partial (i.e., only

Fig. 5.7 MRA showing a left posterior communicating artery aneurysm (red arrow) that caused a complete pupil involving left third nerve palsy

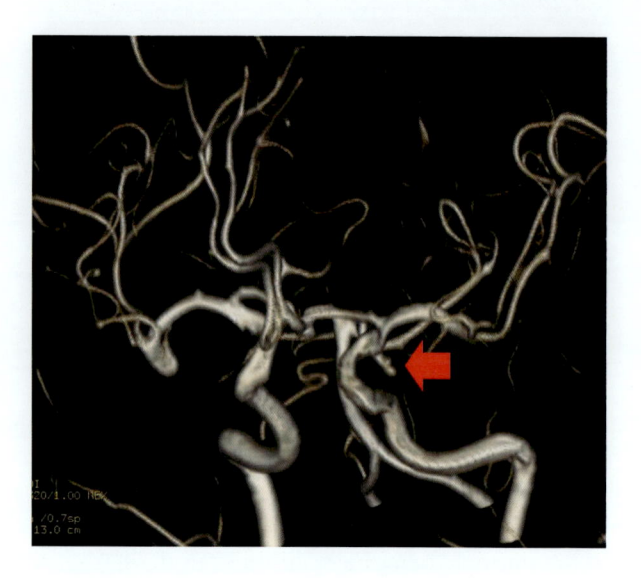

have some of the third nerve functions impaired). Because third nerve palsies can be the first sign of an enlarging intracranial aneurysm, third nerve palsies are neuro-ophthalmic emergencies. This is especially true if there is a large degree of anisocoria (>1 mm) because this typically indicates a compressive lesion as opposed to a microvascular ischemic third nerve palsy that tends to spare the pupil. However, there are reports of compressive lesions causing third nerve palsies while sparing the pupil, and therefore all suspected third nerve palsies should prompt neuroimaging.

The aneurysms affecting the third nerve are classically located at the junction of the posterior communicating and the internal carotid arteries (Fig. 5.7), though aneurysms affecting the third nerve can also occur at the top of the basilar artery and the junction of the basilar and superior cerebellar arteries. Cavernous sinus aneurysmal third nerve palsies will often have accompanying signs, such as other cranial neuropathies (fourth cranial nerve, sixth cranial nerve, V1 and V2 branches of the trigeminal nerve) and Horner syndrome (from the compromise of sympathetic fibers) because of the close proximity of these structures within the cavernous sinus.

Cerebral angiography is indicated in patients with acute mydriasis, particularly if associated with acute headache or retroocular pain, to exclude an intracranial aneurysm. Noninvasive angiographic studies (MRI/MRA or CT/CTA) are more frequently utilized [10]. Three-dimensional time-of-flight (3D TOF) magnetic resonance angiography has a sensitivity of approximately 98% for detecting aneurysm causing third nerve palsies. Though CT/CTA is often the preferred initial test in the emergency department for aneurysm exclusion due to its speed and availability, MRI/MRA will better determine alternative etiologies underlying a third nerve palsy [11]. If an aneurysm is found, open surgical or endovascular intervention becomes necessary and should not be delayed. If the suspicion remains high for aneurysmal isolated third nerve palsy despite a negative CTA or MRA, then cerebral angiogram may be warranted.

Increased risk of aneurysmal rupture has been found to occur with increased age (most notably in the sixth decade), female gender, tobacco smoking, hypertension, alcohol use, pertinent family history, genetic predisposition (adult polycystic kidney disease), aneurysm size ≥10 mm, and aneurysm location (posterior communicating and basilar tip locations have higher cumulative rupture risk at 5 years) [12].

Cavernous Sinus Thrombosis

Cavernous sinus thrombosis classically causes a cavernous sinus syndrome with potential involvement of cranial nerves III, IV, V1, V2, VI, and Horner syndrome, which can be accompanied by proptosis, chemosis, and ptosis secondary to impaired venous drainage. Diminished visual acuity secondary to ischemic optic neuropathy or retinal artery or vein occlusion is noted in up to half of the cases. Cavernous sinus thromboses can either be septic or aseptic. Early neuroimaging and treatment of the underlying cause is necessary because cavernous sinus thrombosis can carry a mortality rate of at least 6–10%. In fact, septic thrombosis of the cavernous sinuses has a mortality rate of about 20–30% even with treatment [3].

Carotid Cavernous Fistula (CCF)

Patients with a carotid cavernous fistula (CCF) will classically present with headache and tortuous (corkscrew-appearing) congested blood vessels of the conjunctiva (Fig. 5.8), often associated with diplopia and/or elevated intra-ocular pressure [13]. CCF is either classified as direct or dural. Direct CCFs, which present more acutely and dramatically, typically occur secondary to trauma or iatrogenically following surgical intervention, though they can occur spontaneously from an aneurysm, with resultant tear in the branch artery from the internal carotid artery within the cavernous sinus [14]. Patients may report pulse synchronous tinnitus and a bruit may be audible. Dural CCFs involve anomalous communication between the cavernous sinus and a branch of the internal and/or external carotid arteries. Dural CCFs have a lower flow rate than direct CCFs. They are presumed to drain posteriorly at first and ocular symptoms ensue when drainage shifts anteriorly via superior and inferior ophthalmic veins.

CCF can cause glaucoma, serous retinal hemorrhages, retinal detachment, vitreous hemorrhage, and papilledema. Up to 30% of patients with CCF can develop vision loss secondary to uncontrolled glaucoma or ischemic optic neuropathy [14]. A direct CCF can become a life-threatening problem if it results in intracranial hemorrhage (due to acutely increased intracranial venous hypertension) or even from massive epistaxis.

Fig. 5.8 Classic conjunctival corkscrew vessels of a carotid-cavernous sinus fistula

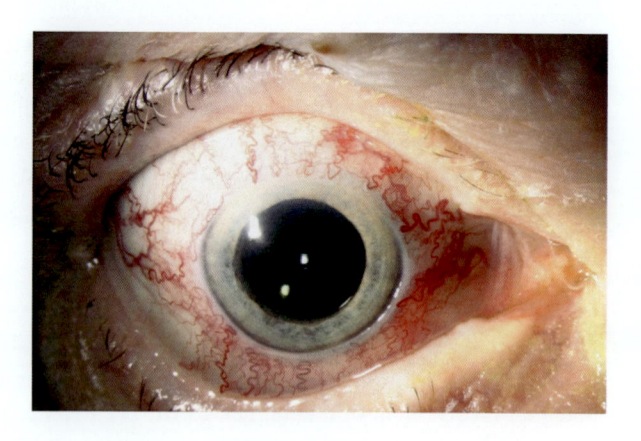

While CT angiography or MR angiography can often confirm the diagnosis, the gold standard is catheter angiography. Up to half of CCFs spontaneously close; thus, patients with mild symptoms can undergo conservative management with regular monitoring of visual function, intra-ocular pressure, and ophthalmologic examination. Severely increased intra-ocular pressure or neurologic deficits warrant neurosurgical consultation for endovascular treatment.

Top of the Basilar Syndrome (Conjugate Gaze Abnormality)

"Top of the basilar syndrome" presents with acute encephalopathy associated with homonymous visual field defects and vertical eye movement abnormalities (upgaze or downgaze palsy or both, vertical "one-and-a-half" syndrome, Parinaud/dorsal midbrain syndrome, skew deviation) [15]. The syndrome is caused by injury to areas supplied by the rostral basilar artery, most frequently due to an embolic event. Emergency CT head and CTA head and neck should be performed, and intravenous thrombolysis plus endovascular therapy must be pursued without delay because of the extreme severity of the prognosis without recanalization [16].

Dorsal Midbrain Syndrome (Parinaud Syndrome)

Lesions of the dorsal midbrain will cause supranuclear vertical gaze palsy, pupillary light/near dissociation, convergence–retraction nystagmus, lid retraction, and convergence and accommodation deficits [17]. Typically, not all features of dorsal midbrain syndrome will be present and any of these components should raise the suspicion of dorsal midbrain injury. Dorsal midbrain syndrome is seen with pineal gland tumors, midbrain stroke, multiple sclerosis, mesencephalic hemorrhage, and obstructive hydrocephalus. In patients with a ventriculo-peritoneal shunt, the emergence of dorsal midbrain features could signal shunt malfunction.

Skew Deviation

Patients presenting with the chief complaint of binocular vertical diplopia should be examined for skew deviation. Skew deviation results from vertical misalignment of the eyes. When it occurs in association with ataxia, it should raise suspicion for an acute cerebellar or brainstem lesion, such as a stroke involving pre-nuclear vestibular pathways to the third and fourth nerve nuclei, though a skew deviation can rarely be seen in peripheral vestibular lesions.

Botulism

Patients with botulism initially develop external ophthalmoplegia and ptosis, followed by poorly reactive dilated pupils and accommodation paralysis. This is soon followed by dysphagia, dysarthria, dysphonia, and symmetric descending paralysis [18]. Nausea and vomiting are typically present. Botulism is a clinical diagnosis and patients suspected to have botulism require close observation because they can suddenly develop cardiorespiratory collapse. Treatment with botulism antitoxin should be initiated while the serum toxin result is pending. The Health Department should be notified, particularly if there is concern for a foodborne outbreak.

Wernicke Encephalopathy

B1 - thiamine Deficiency Along B-6, B12

Wernicke encephalopathy causes the classic triad of encephalopathy, gait ataxia, and ophthalmoplegia due to thiamine deficiency, although not all features of the triad are consistently present. It is most commonly seen in individuals with chronic alcoholism, malnutrition or gastric resection or bypass.

Patients will often have upbeat nystagmus, horizontal and/or vertical gaze palsy, and bilateral abduction deficits, but any pattern of ophthalmoplegia can be seen. MRI brain often reveals symmetric lesions in the periaqueductal area, midbrain tegmentum, mammillary bodies, and dorsomedial thalamus, but the absence of these lesions does not preclude the diagnosis of Wernicke encephalopathy [19].

Wernicke encephalopathy can be confirmed by measuring erythrocyte transketolase activity, though the result is not available emergently. Treatment with 100 mg thiamine IV every 8 hours must be initiated as soon as the diagnosis is suspected because treatment delays can have devastating consequences for the patient.

Non-emergency Differential Diagnoses

Myasthenia Gravis

Myasthenia gravis must be considered in the differential diagnosis of painless ocular motility disorders without pupillary involvement. Fluctuating weakness of non-ocular muscles is often present, but may be absent in pure ocular myasthenia.

Monocular Diplopia

This suggests an optical problem, including cataracts, corneal scars, irregular astigmatism, and abnormal tear film (dry eye). A refractive etiology can be corrected with monocular pinhole testing. Monocular diplopia can also occur secondary to a macular problem, including epiretinal membranes and retinal or choroidal folds.

> **Cardinal Messages**
> - Pain is a red flag when it occurs with a neuro-ophthalmologic complaint.
> - Giant cell arteritis (GCA) should be suspected in any patient over 50 with vision loss in conjunction with systemic symptoms.
> - Patients with acute central or branch retinal artery occlusion require urgent embolic workup, especially imaging for carotid disease.
> - Determining which pupil is abnormal is the first step in evaluating patients with anisocoria.
> - Isolated anisocoria without eyelid or eye motility abnormalities is almost never neurologically dangerous.
> - Acute third nerve palsies are a neuro-ophthalmologic emergency, particularly if there is a large degree of anisocoria, because they may be the first sign of an enlarging intracranial aneurysm.
> - Acute proptosis and chemosis associated with impaired extraocular movements should raise suspicion for a cavernous sinus process (such as thrombosis or fistula).
> - Always consider brainstem ischemia and Wernicke encephalopathy in patients presenting to the emergency department with depressed alertness and ophthalmoparesis.

References

1. Chandran AK, et al. The incidence of giant cell arteritis in Olmsted County, Minnesota, over a 60-year period 1950–2009. Scand J Rheumatol. 2015;44(3):215–8.
2. Chen JJ, et al. Evaluating the incidence of arteritic ischemic optic neuropathy and other causes of vision loss from giant cell arteritis. Ophthalmology. 2016;123(9):1999–2003.
3. Purvin V, Kawasaki A. Neuro-ophthalmic emergencies for the neurologist. Neurologist. 2005;11(4):195–233.
4. Singh TD, Valizadeh N, Meyer FB, Atkinson JL, Erickson D, Rabinstein AA. Management and outcomes of pituitary apoplexy. J Neurosurg. 2015;122(6):1450–7. Epub 2015 Apr 10.
5. Ferry AP, Abedi S. Diagnosis and management of rhino-orbitocerebral mucormycosis (phycomycosis): a report of 16 personally observed cases. Ophthalmology. 1983;90(9):1096–104.
6. Biousse V, et al. Ophthalmologic manifestations of internal carotid artery dissection. Am J Ophthalmol. 1998;126(4):565–77.
7. Lemos J, Eggenberger E. Neuro-ophthalmological emergencies. Neurohospitalist. 2015;5(4):223–33.
8. Provenzale JM, Sarikaya B. Comparison of test performance characteristics of MRI, MR angiography, and CT angiography in the diagnosis of carotid and vertebral artery dissection: a review of the medical literature. AJR Am J Roentgenol. 2009;193(4):1167–74.
9. Chowdhury MM, et al. Antithrombotic treatment for acute extracranial carotid artery dissections: a meta-analysis. Eur J Vasc Endovasc Surg. 2015;50(2):148–56.
10. Heiserman JE, et al. Neurologic complications of cerebral angiography. AJNR Am J Neuroradiol. 1994;15(8):1401–7; discussion 1408–11
11. Jacobson DM, Trobe JD. The emerging role of magnetic resonance angiography in the management of patients with third cranial nerve palsy. Am J Ophthalmol. 1999;128(1):94–6.
12. Wiebers DO, et al. Unruptured intracranial aneurysms: natural history, clinical outcome, and risks of surgical and endovascular treatment. Lancet. 2003;362(9378):103–10.
13. Miller NR. Dural carotid-cavernous fistulas: epidemiology, clinical presentation, and management. Neurosurg Clin. 2012;23(1):179–92.
14. Liu GT, Volpe NJ, Galetta SL. Neuro-ophthalmology diagnosis and management. 3rd ed. Philadelphia: Elsevier; 2019.
15. Mehler MF. The neuro-ophthalmologic spectrum of the rostral basilar artery syndrome. Arch Neurol. 1988;45(9):966–71.
16. Kaneko J, Ota T, Tagami T, Unemoto K, Shigeta K, Amano T, Ueda M, Matsumaru Y, Shiokawa Y, Hirano T, TREAT Study Group. Endovascular treatment of acute basilar artery occlusion: Tama-REgistry of Acute Thrombectomy (TREAT) study. J Neurol Sci. 2019 Jun 15;401:29–33. [Epub ahead of print]
17. Keane JR. The pretectal syndrome: 206 patients. Neurology. 1990;40(4):684–90.
18. Chatham-Stephens K, et al. Clinical features of foodborne and wound botulism: a systematic review of the literature, 1932–2015. Clin Infect Dis. 2017;66(suppl_1):S11–s16.
19. Antunez E, et al. Usefulness of CT and MR imaging in the diagnosis of acute Wernicke's encephalopathy. AJR Am J Roentgenol. 1998;171(4):1131–7.

Chapter 6
Neuro-Oncologic Emergencies

Michael W. Ruff and Alyx B. Porter

Diagnostic Keys
- New-onset neurologic symptoms in a patient with a known cancer diagnosis should prompt urgent neuroimaging with and without contrast.
- Altered mental status in a patient with cancer should trigger encephalopathy workup, including imaging, EEG, electrolyte and drug levels if appropriate, and consideration for CSF analysis.
- Imaging findings consistent with posterior reversible encephalopathy syndrome (PRES) in a patient with cancer can be related to systemic therapy.

Treatment Priorities
- Dexamethasone is frequently used in neuro-oncologic emergencies to treat the tumor-associated vasogenic edema and the resulting mass effect.
- Neurosurgery and Radiation Oncology consultations should be obtained urgently when concern arises for epidural spinal cord compression.
- Neurologic symptoms appearing after chemotherapy should be managed by holding and then either reducing or potentially discontinuing treatment based on degree of toxicity.

M. W. Ruff
Department of Neurology, Mayo Clinic, Rochester, MN, USA

A. B. Porter (✉)
Department of Neurology, Mayo Clinic Arizona, Phoenix, AZ, USA
e-mail: Porter.alyx@mayo.edu

Prognosis at a Glance
- Neurologic symptoms related to mass effect that persist >48 hours after initiation of dexamethasone are less likely to be reversible.
- Inability to walk at the time of diagnosis of epidural cord compression is associated with worse prognosis for recovery of independent ambulation.
- Overall survival varies related to primary tumor type and performance status.

In this chapter, we will describe the most common occurring neurological emergencies directly and indirectly related to neoplastic disease. While some neuro-oncologic emergencies require urgent neurosurgical intervention, others require early recognition and implementation of appropriate medical management. Identification of herniation syndromes as well as management of status epilepticus, reviewed in greater detail elsewhere within this book, are applicable to neuro-oncologic disease. As cancer treatment evolves, specific syndromes related to radiation and chemotherapy are becoming more frequent. This chapter not only includes neurologic symptoms that may be emergently related to radiation, but also includes updated understanding of the spectrum of neurologic disease resulting from traditional chemotherapy as well as some of the newer targeted immunotherapies.

Neurologic Emergencies Directly Related to the Tumor

Mass Effect

Brain tumors cause neurologic symptoms based on the size and location of the tumor in addition to the surrounding edema caused by its presence. Based on the degree of mass effect and cerebral edema, patients may have varied symptoms ranging from focal deficits to a more generalized brain dysfunction. Progressive headache followed by an altered level of consciousness raises immediate concern for a herniation syndrome [1]. Tumors may cause obstructive hydrocephalus, resulting in positional headache, eye movement abnormalities, and pupillary changes. New-onset focal weakness, sensory changes, seizure, or exacerbation of an underlying seizure disorder may also be presenting symptoms.

CT scan without contrast can reveal low attenuation changes of vasogenic edema and may be the first indication of an underlying mass. MRI shows vasogenic edema as hyperintense signal on T2/FLAIR sequences and hypointense signal on T1-weighted images. Brain imaging can also demonstrate the degree of mass effect and tissue shift in different planes (lateral subfalcine herniation and craniocaudal transtentorial and transforaminal herniation).

Neurosurgical intervention may be required for resection of the mass, which can be both diagnostic and therapeutic. The placement of an external ventricular device

Fig. 6.1 MRI of the brain (FLAIR sequence, axial view) showing a necrotic brain tumor consistent with glioblastoma multiforme

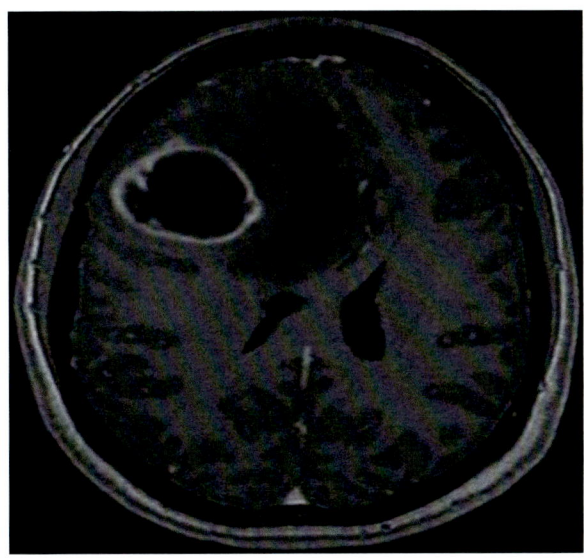

(EVD) or a ventricular shunt in the case of obstruction may also be indicated. Treatment of the vasogenic edema depends on the degree to which the clinician feels it is causative of the patient's symptoms. Dexamethasone can be given 10 mg IV or PO once followed by 4 mg PO or IV q6 hourly. Larger bolus doses of dexamethasone (50–100 mg) are justified in emergency situations. Reversal of the symptoms within 24 hours of initiating treatment with dexamethasone is frequently seen as a positive prognostic sign [2]. Hyperventilation and osmotic diuretics such as mannitol or hypertonic saline can also be used in an ICU setting to reduce mass effect from an underlying tumor.

Although effective during emergency circumstances, corticosteroid usage can be associated with significant morbidity both acutely and especially over time. Side effects including psychosis, steroid-induced hyperglycemia, myopathy, osteopenia, avascular hip necrosis, gastritis, and gastric intestinal bleeding can be a result of long-term use. Thus, as soon as clinically feasible, weaning of dexamethasone is advised (Fig. 6.1).

Epidural Spinal Cord Compression

Epidural spinal cord compression (ESCC) is typically a late emergency complication of metastatic cancer [3]. Lung, breast, and prostate cancers are the most common solid tumors that cause this complication while non-Hodgkin lymphoma is the hematologic malignancy most frequently associated with ESCC. There are two main mechanisms implicated in the occurrence of ESCC. The first is through direct extension of the tumor into the spinal canal. The second is through hematogenous spread via either arterial emboli, or through Batson's plexus, the lumbosacral vasculature that drains the blood volume from the abdomen and pelvis.

Back pain is the most common presenting symptom, with the thoracic spine being the most frequent location of pain complaint and ESCC occurrence. Other symptoms may also occur including gait changes or difficulty with ambulation, changes in bowel/bladder function, focal weakness, and sensory changes. In a patient with cancer and new-onset neurologic symptoms, MRI with and without contrast is considered the gold standard for radiographic diagnosis. An extradural enhancing mass with the compression of the spinal cord is the anticipated finding with or without FLAIR or T2 signal changes seen within the cord. CT scan with contrast may be performed in instances where MRI is contraindicated. Suggestive changes can be seen on plain X-ray, bone scan, and PET imaging as well.

Once detected, treatment is palliative. Dexamethasone should be started immediately. Urgent consultations with Neurosurgery and Radiation Oncology should be obtained. Based on ambulation and duration of symptoms, urgent neurosurgical intervention with a goal of tumor excision and spine stabilization may be preferred prior to radiation therapy. Similarly, if radiation is initiated first, Neurosurgery may choose to intervene if the patient's neurologic function decompensates during treatment.

Factors that may impact survival include ambulatory status at the time of presentation and the underlying tumor type. For example, ESCC related to breast or prostate cancer is typically associated with a longer overall survival than ESCC resulting from metastatic lung cancer. Despite aggressive intervention, the median survival is roughly 6 months, 8–10 months if the patient is still ambulatory. If the patient is non-ambulatory at the time of presentation, the median survival is reduced to 2–4 months (Fig. 6.2).

Fig. 6.2 Sagittal view of the spine MRI showing epidural spinal cord compression from metastatic brain cancer

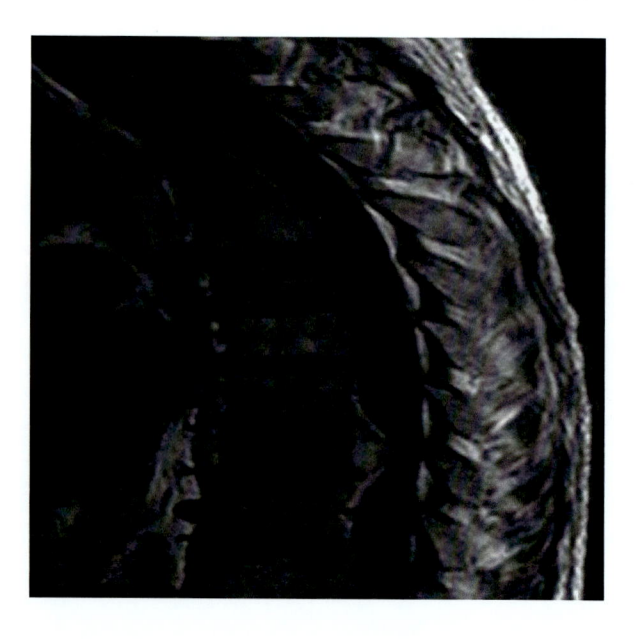

Tumor-Related Epilepsy

New-onset seizure in an adult should always prompt neuroimaging, preferably MRI with and without contrast. When no causative lesion is identified, additional workup with lumbar puncture should be obtained to rule out infectious, inflammatory, and paraneoplastic causes. Anti-N-methyl-D-aspartate (NMDA)-receptor antibody encephalitis (ovarian teratoma) and voltage-gated potassium channel (VGCC) associated limbic encephalitis (lung and breast cancer) are the most common paraneoplastic syndromes that can lead to this neurologic complication. Standard management for status epilepticus and seizure applies (as discussed in Chap. 2), followed by treatment of the underlying tumor which can include surgical resection, chemotherapy, radiation or a combination of all of them.

When a tumor is identified, based on the appearance, primary versus metastatic disease should be considered. CT scans chest, abdomen, and pelvis; mammogram and testicular ultrasound should be considered in cases of suspected metastasis in which the primary tumor is unknown. PET scanning is another valid option.

Pituitary Apoplexy

New-onset sudden severe thunderclap headache triggers concern for sudden hemorrhage or infarction into the pituitary gland, also known as pituitary apoplexy. The reason for apoplexy remains controversial though the size of the adenoma in addition to pregnancy and head trauma are considered to be risk factors. Imaging often reveals hyperintensity within the sella on CT scan without contrast indicating hemorrhage. MRI may reveal heterogeneity within the sella. In addition to headache, patients may also develop cranial neuropathies, specifically ophthalmoparesis. All patients with suspected apoplexy should have the following serum studies evaluated: complete blood count, electrolyte panel, and pituitary panel. Formal visual fields may be tested once the patient is stable. Management requires a multidisciplinary approach, including neurosurgery and endocrinology, due to the life-threatening hypotension that can result from sudden cortisol deficiency. In cases of prolactinoma, a dopamine agonist agent may be implemented in order to shrink the tumor. Treatment typically includes hydrocortisone in order to avoid adrenal crisis. Surgical intervention is typically aimed at the reduction of mass effect in the region to improve cranial nerve function. If the patient's symptoms are mild, close observation and medical management are recommended (Fig. 6.3).

Treatment-Related Neurologic Emergencies

Neurologic Emergencies Related to Radiation Therapy

Radiation therapy is unequivocally beneficial in regard to overall survival of patients with glioma and CNS metastases. Despite its benefit, radiation may cause devastating untoward effects, including radiation necrosis as well as panhypopituitarism,

Fig. 6.3 MRI of the brain (FLAIR sequence, axial view) demonstrates changes typical of pituitary apoplexy

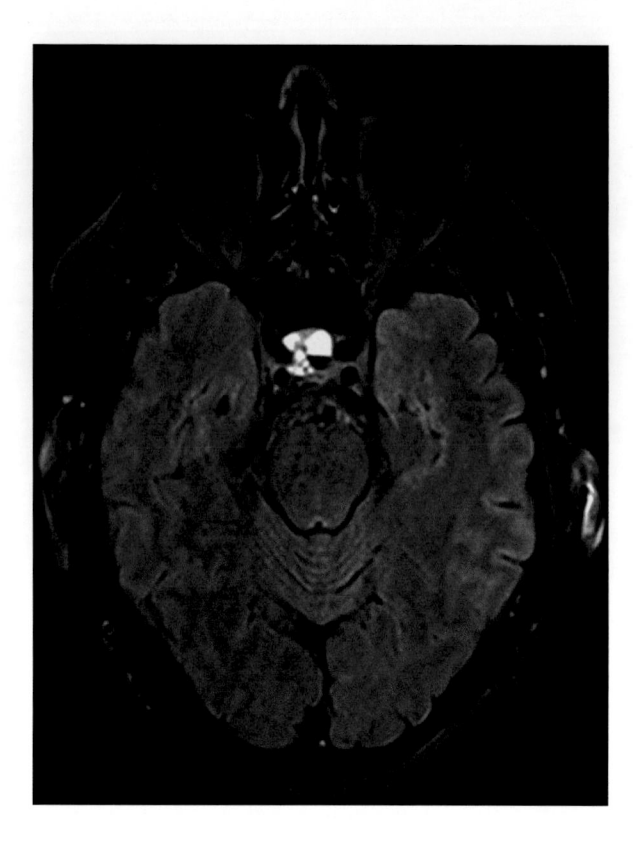

cerebral atrophy, leukoencephalopathy, gliosis, vascular anomalies, and secondary neoplasms months to years following treatment. Given their prevalence, the clinician should anticipate these adverse effects when evaluating patients with prior cranial or spinal irradiation.

Following (or in some cases, during) fractionated radiotherapy treatment, radiation-induced inflammation and necrosis may result in parenchymal swelling with subacute progression of new neurologic deficits. Within 10 days of the start of radiation, patients may develop symptomatic cerebral edema, initially manifesting as fatigue, appetite changes, and sleep disturbance. In extreme cases, if unchecked, radiation-induced cerebral edema can result in mass effect with increased intracranial pressure, brain compression and herniation, coma, and death. The onset of radiation necrosis varies by radiation modality, and may appear more rapidly in the setting of stereotactic radiosurgery (e.g., within 2–4 months). Contrast-enhancing mass lesions may appear within 6–18 months or treatment with conventional forms of radiation therapy, reflecting the development of radiation-induced white matter necrosis.

The incidence of radiation-induced necrosis in the treatment of primary brain tumors is between 3–24%, and it can be as high as 68% in patients treated with stereotactic radiosurgery for brain metastases [4]. Risk of cerebral from radiation necrosis is contingent upon the dose of radiation, the fraction size, and the subsequent administration of chemotherapy. With concurrent chemotherapy for malignant gliomas, the incidence increases by threefold. Re-irradiation or additional boost radiation treatment by stereotactic radiotherapy further increases the risk of cerebral radiation necrosis.

Pathologically, radiation necrosis is characterized by coagulation and liquefaction in the white matter, with capillary collapse and vessel hyalinization. The leading hypothesis for the cause of radiation necrosis is direct primary injury to the blood vessels causing subsequent parenchymal injury. Angiogenesis and inflammation may contribute to a synergistic and malignant cycle, leading to the progression of radiation necrosis.

Corticosteroids, antiplatelet agents, anticoagulants, hyperbaric oxygen, high-dose vitamins, and surgery have been used to combat radiation necrosis. The development of effective therapies for symptomatic radiation necrosis has been hampered by an incomplete understanding of the pathophysiology of this disorder. Several studies have demonstrated that bevacizumab, a monoclonal antibody against vascular endothelial growth factor (VEGF), is an effective treatment for radiation necrosis in brain regardless of the original tumor type. Clinical trials are ongoing [5].

Post-radiation Vasculopathy

Radiation may induce a delayed vasculopathy, hypothesized to be secondary to endothelial or vasa vasorum injury, that may result in delayed cerebral infarction and vascular proliferative lesions such as capillary telangiectasias and cavernoma. Radiation-induced vasculopathy affects medium and large vessels, resulting in symptomatic cerebrovascular disease years (0.4–10) after exposure [6]. Animal models suggest that radiation induces acute endothelial injury followed by chronic inflammation, and injury to the vasa vasorum. These changes, in turn, may result in accelerated atherosclerosis, leading to focal narrowing of the vessel lumen. Most ischemic strokes after brain radiation are related to this process. Cerebral infarction secondary to direct vascular compression from an intracranial tumor is exceedingly rare and often associated with rapid tumor expansion or hemorrhage. So far, no trials have adequately assessed medical treatment options for primary or secondary stroke prevention in patients who have received head/neck radiation.

In the setting of acute stroke with a known or suspected intracranial neoplasm, intravenous thrombolysis is deemed contraindicated due to the increase of symptomatic intracranial hemorrhage (sICH), according to current guidelines [7]. The actual risk of administering thrombolysis to patients with acute ischemic stroke and brain tumor is not well known. In practice, patients with known brain malignancy are often not treated with intravenous thrombolysis due to the perceived higher risk for intracranial hemorrhage, lower life expectancy, and often the uncertainty of diagnosis within the acute time window. Yet, published experience on patients with intracranial malignancy undergoing thrombolysis is limited to case reports of favorable outcomes without symptomatic intracranial hemorrhage except for one case (a patient with an undiagnosed temporal lobe glioblastoma multiforme). Based on this data, it appears that thrombolysis can be safe in some patients with intracranial neoplasms, particularly if small and extra-axial. Mechanical embolectomy represents a valid option in patients with intracranial tumors who have preserved daily function and life expectancy of at least 1–2 years [8, 9]. The clinical trials that demonstrated the efficacy of embolectomy for patients with large vessel occlusion did not specifically exclude patients with intracranial malignancy. The decision to utilize acute stroke treatments should be made on a case by case basis, estimating the balance of the risk of hemorrhage in relation to the chances of functional recovery.

SMART Syndrome

A spectrum of acute late-onset complications of brain irradiation consisting of typically reversible focal neurologic deficits, seizures, and imaging abnormalities have been reported and classified as Stroke Like Migraine Attacks after Radiation Therapy (SMART), peri-ictal pseudoprogression, (PIPG) and Acute Late-onset Encephalopathy after Radiotherapy (ALERT) [10, 11].

Stroke-Like migraine attacks after radiation therapy (SMART) is a clinical entity caused by transient hemispheric dysfunction and often manifesting with visuospatial deficits, confusion, aphasia, lateralized sensory, or motor deficits, often (but not always) followed by severe headache and occasionally seizures in patients with a history (usually 2–10 years prior) of external beam radiation therapy to the brain parenchyma. Symptoms are paroxysmal and generally reversible, but headache can be prolonged. MRI characteristically demonstrates cortical swelling and diffuse or patchy unilateral contrast enhancement usually corresponding to the previous radiation field.

The etiology is poorly understood, but it is felt to be a form of vascular dysfunction akin to that implicated in radiation necrosis. Postulated mechanisms abound regarding the underlying pathophysiology. A small series of patients with SMART who underwent perfusion scans peri-ictally demonstrated regional hyperperfusion preceding the appearance of cortical abnormalities on MRI, which suggests transient impaired cerebral autoregulation. Yet, another case series reported hemispheric hypoperfusion in two patients with recurrent episodes of SMART, followed by abrupt resolution with L-arginine [12, 13]. The rarity of SMART suggests a genetic predisposition. It has also been postulated that radiation could induce cortical hyperexcitability analogous to hemiplegic migraine. The minimum dose of radiation required to elicit SMART is uncertain.

Work-up for suspected SMART syndrome should include an MRI brain. CSF analysis, EEG, MRA, serum lactic acid level, and blood pressure monitoring are all worth consideration. Of note, conventional angiography has previously been described as a trigger for SMART, and consequently MRA is the vessel imaging modality of choice.

To date, there is no evidence to guide treatment. Corticosteroids, antiplatelet agents, propranolol, and verapamil have all been used with uncertain benefit. Seizures should be treated as per usual standards. Seizure control and prevention may be particularly important in patients with SMART because their underlying endothelial dysfunction may put them at increased risk of cortical infarction and laminar necrosis with increased metabolic demand.

Emergencies Related to Systemic Therapies

Chemotherapeutic agents are the backbone of modern oncology. The use of chemotherapy is associated with a number of well-described and predictable neurologic sequelae including direct neuronal toxicity manifesting as acute encephalopathy, cerebellar dysfunction, aseptic meningitis, and myelopathy. Chemotherapy-associated encephalopathy as a result of direct neuronal toxicity, ischemic infarction, or cerebral hemorrhage may be encountered in emergency neurologic consultations of patients undergoing treatment for malignancy. In addition to direct neurotoxic effects, cytotoxic chemotherapies may result in severe bone marrow suppression that increases the risk of opportunistic infection and they may also produce endothelial injury and dysfunction resulting in posterior reversible encephalopathy syndrome, cerebral ischemia, or hemorrhage.

Acute encephalopathy may manifest as a decline in mental status with or without focal neurologic signs (e.g., aphasia), which are usually reversible. Brain imaging, including MRI, is usually normal, and EEG usually only shows slowing of the background [14]. Several chemotherapeutic agents are associated with encephalopathy, including methotrexate, cyclophosphamide, vincristine, cyclosporine, fludarabine, cytarabine, 5-fluorouracil, cisplatin, and the interferons; but the incidence of acute encephalopathy is most frequent with ifosfamide. Ifosfamide is an alkylating drug used to treat several systemic malignancies, including germ cell testicular cancer and sarcomas. Ifosfamide can penetrate the blood-brain barrier and causes encephalopathy in 10–40% of patients receiving high-dose intravenous regimens. Treatment is conservative, though there are reports of rapid improvement after the administration of methylene blue. Cyclophosphamide is an analog of ifosfamide and there are similar but less frequent reports of encephalopathy with its use.

High-dose methotrexate, defined as a dose higher than 500 mg/m^2, can cause acute (also subacute or chronic) neurotoxicity and leukoencephalopathy. The most likely mechanisms are disruption of folate metabolism or direct neuronal damage. Acute or subacute onset neurotoxicity may manifest with focal neurologic deficits, encephalopathy or seizures. The incidence of acute methotrexate neurotoxicity ranges from 3–10% and varies with route of administration and dose. Neurotoxicity is frequently seen 10–12 days after intrathecal methotrexate administration. Treatment consists of drug withdrawal and supportive care. Intrathecal or intraventricular chemotherapy administration (e.g., methotrexate or cytarabine) may also be associated with aseptic meningitis. These symptoms are typically self-limited and can be prevented or abated with supportive therapy (e.g., dexamethasone).

The alternative diagnosis of Wernicke encephalopathy should be considered during the evaluation of patients who develop encephalopathy in the setting of chemotherapy, because the hypermetabolic state of patients with cancer coupled with the emetogenic potential of chemotherapeutics substantially increases the risk of malnutrition and critical thiamine deficiency. Additionally, cytotoxic drugs to treat malignancies (as well as organ rejection) are well-known triggers of posterior reversible encephalopathy syndrome (PRES) characterized by encephalopathy, seizures with potential for status epilepticus, headache, visual disturbance, and focal neurologic deficits. Antineoplastic agents most often implicated in the pathogenesis of PRES include antiangiogenic drugs that antagonize the action of VEGF, such as bevacizumab, sunitinib, and sorafenib (Tables 6.1 and 6.2) [15].

Table 6.1 Symptoms associated with posterior reversible encephalopathy syndrome (PRES)

Encephalopathy	50–80%
Seizure	60–75%
Headache	50%
Visual disturbances	33%
Focal neurological deficit	10–15%
Status epilepticus	5–15%

Table 6.2 Potential acute neurologic complications associated with chemotherapy agents

Agent	Indication	Relevant toxicity
Ifosfamide	Germ cell testicular cancer, sarcomas	Encephalopathy (10–40% of pts)
Cyclophosphamide	Lymphomas	Encephalopathy
Methotrexate	Lymphoma, intrathecal therapy for leptomeningeal metastases	Acute encephalitis, aseptic meningitis, leukoencephalopathy, myelopathy
5-Fluorouracil	Breast and gastrointestinal tract cancers	Acute cerebellar syndrome, leukoencephalopathy
Cytarabine	Leukemia, lymphoma, intrathecal therapy for leptomeningeal metastases	Acute encephalopathy, acute cerebellar syndrome, aseptic meningitis, myelopathy
Temozolomide	Glioma, melanoma	Thrombocytopenia, lymphopenia
Lomustine	Glioma	Thrombocytopenia, lymphopenia, neutropenia
Procarbazine	Glioma	Serotonin syndrome
VEGF antagonists (bevacizumab, sunitinib, sorafenib)	Glioma, RCC, GIST, pNET, HCC, thyroid carcinoma	PRES

Abbreviations: *VEGF* vascular endothelial growth factor, *RCC* renal cell carcinoma, *GIST* gastrointestinal stromal tumor, *pNET* primitive neuroectodermal tumor, *HCC* hepatocellular carcinoma, *PRES* posterior reversible encephalopathy syndrome

Targeted Therapies

Bevacizumab, a medication frequently used for the treatment of recurrent glioma and symptomatic radiation necrosis, increases the risk of arterial thrombotic events including stroke, as well as hemorrhage. Bevacizumab has also been associated with higher risk of spontaneous bowel perforation and delayed wound healing. Clinically significant intracranial hemorrhage occurs in 1–2% of patients with glioblastoma being treated with bevacizumab. As a result, bevacizumab is relatively contraindicated in patients with the history of intracranial hemorrhage. That said, the strength of the association of bevacizumab with intracranial hemorrhage was questioned by trials in which bevacizumab was used as an early strategy to treat glioblastoma; in these studies, bevacizumab administration did not appear to increase the risk of hemorrhage.

Patients with an acute presentation of symptomatic intracranial hemorrhage require ICU admission, blood pressure control (no data on goal), serial imaging to monitor hematoma stability, and reversal of anticoagulation if pertinent. Plasma exchange to remove the monoclonal antibody is theoretically possible, but of uncertain value.

Off target immune-related adverse effects are an increasingly recognized complication of immune checkpoint inhibitors used for the treatment of solid tumors. The incidence of neurological immune-related adverse events is low, ranging from 0.4 to 4.2% [16]. The clinical spectrum of these disorders is remarkably heterogeneous. Headache, encephalopathy, meningitis, meningoradiculoneuritis, polyradiculoneuropathies, transverse myelitis, inflammatory myopathy, necrotizing myopathy, myasthenia gravis, PRES, and cranial or peripheral neuropathies (e.g., inflammatory enteric neuropathy, bilateral phrenic neuropathies) have all been described in association with various checkpoint inhibitors. In clinical studies, the median time to neurologic symptom onset was approximately 6 weeks, with the majority of neurological complications occurring during the induction phase. Yet, neurological adverse events have also been reported several weeks or months after the last dose. In the majority of cases, drug interruption and initiation of corticosteroids affords at least some degree of neurological recovery.

CAR-T

Chimeric Antigen Receptor T-cell (CAR-T) therapy combines recognition of an antibody with the effector function of a T cell. CAR-T therapy has emerged as a potent and potentially curative therapy in hematological malignancies with two products being FDA approved in 2017. Numerous ongoing pre-clinical and clinical trials are testing CAR-T for other malignancies, including glioblastoma [17]. Many patients experience a transient neurotoxicity syndrome after the infusion of CAR-T, often in synchrony with symptoms of cytokine response syndrome (CRS). The pathophysiology is poorly understood. Rare cases of fulminant brain edema have also been reported.

The two CD-19 targeted CAR-Ts currently approved for clinical use are tisagenlecleucel and axicabtagene ciloleucel. In clinical trials, neurotoxicity was seen in 15% of patients who received tisagenlecleucel, and 28% of patients who received axicabtagene ciloleucel. Thus far, the only identified predisposing risk factor is a history of neurologic disorder (e.g., seizures). Treatment strategies currently include tocilizumab and dexamethasone. When present, brain edema and seizures should be treated as per usual standards.

Cardinal Messages
- Tumor-related vasogenic edema can be very responsive to steroid therapy and therefore steroids should be started in patients with symptomatic peritumoral swelling.
- New-onset seizure or status epilepticus in a patient with known cancer should be worked up for new brain metastasis, CNS infection, or inflammation, as well as metabolic derangements related to cancer therapy.
- Acute back pain in a cancer patient, particularly when associated with neurological deficits, can be related to epidural spinal cord compression and requires emergent imaging and intervention by neurosurgery and radiation oncology to limit neurologic morbidity.
- Severe sudden-onset headache followed by cranial neuropathies (specifically ophthalmoparesis) raises suspicion for pituitary apoplexy.
- Radiation necrosis may result in delayed neurological complications, including brain ischemia. Treatment with steroids should be attempted in these cases.
- Encephalopathy can be associated with many systemic regimens for cancer treatment. In all cases, holding the therapy and providing supportive care is recommended.
- CAR-T can be associated with severe acute neurotoxicity in the setting of cytokine release syndrome. If suspected, initiate dexamethasone, consider tocilizumab, and exclude seizures and brain edema.

References

1. Jo JT, Schiff D. Management of neuro-oncologic emergencies. Handb Clin Neurol. 2017;141:715–41.
2. Scott BJ. Neuro-oncologic emergencies. Semin Neurol. 2015;35(6):675–82. Epub 2015 Nov 23
3. Baldwin KJ, Zivković SA, Lieberman FS. Neurologic emergencies in patients who have cancer: diagnosis and management. Neurol Clin. 2012;30(1):101–28, viii. Epub 2011 Oct 14.
4. Giglio P, Gilbert MR. Cerebral radiation necrosis. Neurologist. 2003;9:180–8. [PubMed].
5. Levin VA, Bidaut L, Hou P, et al. Randomized double-blind placebo-controlled trial of bevacizumab therapy for radiation necrosis of the central nervous system. Int J Radiat Oncol Biol Phys. 2011;79(5):1487–95.

6. Glantz MJ, Burger PC, Friedman AH, et al. Treatment of radiation-induced nervous system injury with heparin and warfarin. Neurology. 1994;44:2020–7. [PubMed].
7. Ferriero DM, Fullerton HJ, Bernard TJ, Billinghurst L, Daniels SR, DeBaun MR, deVeber G, Ichord RN, Jordan LC, Massicotte P, Meldau J, Roach ES, Smith ER, American Heart Association Stroke Council and Council on Cardiovascular and Stroke Nursing. Management of stroke in neonates and children: a scientific statement from the American Heart Association/American Stroke Association. Stroke. 2019;50(3):e51–96.
8. Kreisl TN, Toothaker T, Karimi S, DeAngelis LM. Ischemic stroke in patients with primary brain tumors. Neurology. 2008;70(24):2314–20.
9. Fugate JE, Rabinstein AA. Absolute and relative contraindications to IV rt-PA for acute ischemic stroke. Neurohospitalist. 2015;5(3):110–21.
10. Black DF, Bartleson JD, Bell ML, Lachance DH. SMART: stroke-like migraine attacks after radiation therapy. Cephalalgia. 2006;26(9):1137–42.
11. Black DF, Morris JM, Lindell EP, et al. Stroke-like migraine attacks after radiation therapy (SMART) syndrome is not always completely reversible: a case series. AJNR Am J Neuroradiol. 2013;34(12):2298–303.
12. Olsen AL, Miller JJ, Bhattacharyya S, Voinescu PE, Klein JP. Cerebral perfusion in stroke-like migraine attacks after radiation therapy syndrome. Neurology. 2016;86(8):787–9.
13. Wai K, Balabanski A, Chia N, Kleinig T. Reversible hemispheric hypoperfusion in two cases of SMART syndrome. J Clin Neurosci. 2017;43:146–8. Epub 2017 Jun 20.
14. Di Stefano AL, Berzero G, Vitali P, et al. Acute late-onset encephalopathy after radiotherapy: an unusual life-threatening complication. Neurology. 2013;81(11):1014–7.
15. Fugate JE, Rabinstein AA. Posterior reversible encephalopathy syndrome: clinical and radiological manifestations, pathophysiology, and outstanding questions. Lancet Neurol. 2015;14(9):914–25.
16. Cuzzubbo S, Javeri F, Tissier M, Roumi A, Barlog C, Doridam J, Lebbe C, Belin C, Ursu R, Carpentier AF. Neurological adverse events associated with immune checkpoint inhibitors: review of the literature. Eur J Cancer. 2017;73:1–8. Epub 2017 Jan 5. Review.
17. Petersen CT, Krenciute G. Next generation CAR T cells for the immunotherapy of high-grade glioma. Front Oncol. 2019;9:69. eCollection 2019.

Chapter 7
Severe Infections of the Central Nervous System

Micah D. Yost and Michel Toledano

> **Diagnostic Keys**
> - The complete triad of fever, nuchal rigidity, and headache is only present in about half of patients presenting with meningitis.
> - Initiation of antibiotics reduces the yield of CSF Gram stain and culture.
> - CSF pneumococcus antigen can help diagnose pneumococcal meningitis when Gram stain and cultures are negative.
> - CSF HSV PCR can be negative if obtained early in the course of the disease.
> - MRI is highly sensitive for the diagnosis of HSV-1 encephalitis.
> - Headache and focal neurologic signs are the most common presentation of a cerebral abscess. Fever occurs in about half of the patients.
> - PML-IRIS in HIV patients usually occurs weeks after the initiation of anti-retroviral therapy. MRI imaging can demonstrate vasogenic edema and speckled gadolinium enhancement.

M. D. Yost · M. Toledano (✉)
Department of Neurology, Mayo Clinic, Rochester, MN, USA
e-mail: toledano.michel@mayo.edu

Treatment Priorities
- Blood and CSF cultures should be obtained before initiating antibiotics, but antibiotics should be started without delay if unable to obtain lumbar puncture in a timely manner.
- Intravenous dexamethasone should be initiated prior to or concurrently with antibiotics in patients suspected of having pneumococcal meningitis.
- Repeated lumbar punctures may be required to manage increased intracranial pressure in patients with cryptococcal meningitis.
- Acyclovir should be started empirically if HSV encephalitis is suspected as delays in treatment result in worse prognosis.
- If clinical suspicion for HSV encephalitis is high, Acyclovir should be continued even if first HSV PCR is negative.
- The management of cerebral abscesses is guided by the number and location of the lesions.
- Corticosteroids is used to treat PML-IRIS, although data supporting efficacy are lacking.

Prognosis at a Glance
- The prognosis of acute bacterial meningitis is favorable with the prompt initiation of appropriate antibiotic therapy. Yet, any treatment delays can have life-threatening consequences.
- Coma, late initiation of acyclovir, and the presence of restricted diffusion on brain MRI are associated with worse prognosis in patients with HSV-1 encephalitis.
- Aggressive antiretroviral treatment has improved the prognosis of HIV patients presenting with opportunistic CNS infections, but IRIS can be a major complication in these cases.

Introduction

In spite of advances in diagnosis and treatment, infections of the central nervous system (CNS) still result in significant morbidity and mortality. Early recognition of an infectious syndrome and initiation of treatment improves outcome. Choosing appropriate diagnostic studies can expedite diagnosis, avoid exposure to unnecessary invasive testing, and reduce costs of care. Awareness and early detection of known complications of CNS infections can decrease morbidity. In this chapter, we review common and rare infections that can result in severe neurologic compromise. We use a syndromic approach, emphasizing the practical aspects of diagnosis and management.

Meningitis

Bacteria

Inflammation of the meninges is known as meningitis. Bacterial meningitis typically presents more acutely than other forms of meningitis. The triad of neck stiffness, fever, and headache occurs in less than half of the patients, but most patients will have at least two out of four symptoms including fever, headache, neck stiffness, and altered level of awareness [1]. Photophobia is common. Confusion, agitation, focal neurological signs, and seizures can occur, but they are more suggestive of encephalitis. While almost any bacteria can cause meningitis, the most common culprits in adults living in developed countries are *Streptococcus pneumoniae* and *Neisseria meningitides*. *Listeria* should be considered in patients who are immunocompromised or over the age of 50 years. *Pseudomonas* and *Staphylococcus* can cause meningitis in patients with recent neurosurgical procedure or cerebrospinal fluid shunt placement.

Lumbar puncture is the most important diagnostic test in acute meningitis, but blood cultures should always be obtained as they can be positive in a substantial proportion of cases (Fig. 7.1). Patients with seizures, focal neurologic findings, papilledema, or encephalopathy should undergo brain imaging prior to lumbar puncture, as should immunocompromised patients. Opening pressure is usually elevated in bacterial meningitis. Cerebral spinal fluid (CSF) studies should include protein, glucose, cell count with differential, Gram stain, bacterial culture, and lactate. Most patients with bacterial meningitis have one of the following CSF markers; protein >200 mg/dL, glucose <40 mg/dL or CSF: serum glucose ratio ≤ 0.4, and a white blood cell count (WBC) count >2000 (range 100–10,000) cells/mm^3 with a percentage of neutrophils usually greater than 80%. A CSF lactate >3.5 mmol/L favors a diagnosis of bacterial over viral meningitis [2, 3]. Prior administration of antimicrobials tends to have minimal immediate effects on CSF parameters but significantly reduce the yield of Gram stain and culture. Whenever possible, CSF should be obtained prior to or concurrently with the initiation of empiric antimicrobials. However, antimicrobials should not be held while awaiting the completion of diagnostic studies if delays are expected.

Empiric treatment for bacterial meningitis consists of a third-generation cephalosporin such as ceftriaxone and vancomycin (Table 7.1). Ampicillin is used in immunocompromised patients and those over the age of 50 years to cover for *Listeria monocytogenes*. In developed countries, intravenous dexamethasone is given before or concurrently with the initial dose of antibiotics because it has been associated with reduced morbidity in a trial of patients who predominantly had pneumococcal meningitis [4]. Dexamethasone need only be continued if microbiological studies are suggestive of *Pneumococcus*. Patients with meningitis in the setting of head trauma, recent neurosurgery, or those with impaired cellular immunity

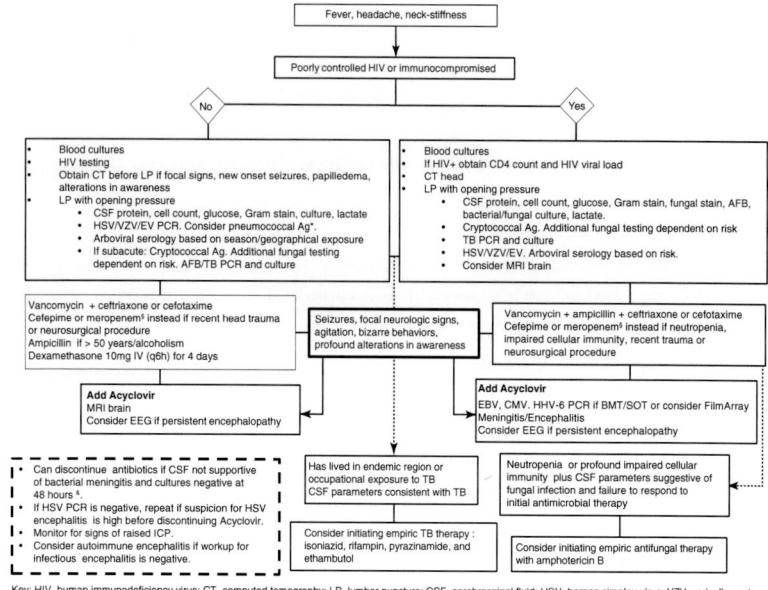

Fig. 7.1 Initial management in patients presenting with meningitis or meningoencephalitis

require coverage for Gram-negative organisms [5]. In these cases, ceftriaxone should be replaced by cefepime or meropenem, although the latter should be used with caution, as it lowers seizure threshold. When possible, antibiotic coverage should be narrowed based on culture and susceptibilities.

Neurologic complications of bacterial meningitis include cerebral venous sinus thrombosis, hydrocephalus, hearing loss, aneurysm formation, ventriculitis, abscess formation, and seizures. These may present anytime during the course of infection, up to and including the immediate period following the completion of therapy. Independent factors that have been shown to be associated with worse outcome include hypotension, delay in diagnosis and initiation of treatment, seizures, hydrocephalus, poor cellular response in the CSF (<500 cells/mm^3), and altered mental status [1, 6]. Bacterial meningitis can also cause a secondary vasculitis, leading to ischemic stroke. Patients with pneumococcal meningitis can suffer catastrophic delayed ischemic events involving the brainstem and deep gray matter days to weeks after initial recovery (Fig. 7.2). The mechanism of this is unclear, but pathology has suggested an inflammatory vasculitis [7]. Steroids have been used to treat

Table 7.1 Bacterial meningitis

Patient age and other factors	Most likely organisms	Empiric treatment
<30 days	S. agalactiae, E. coli, L. monocytogenes	Ampicillin plus aminoglycoside plus cefotaxime or ceftazidime
1 month—2 years	S. pneumoniae, N. meningitidis, H. influenzae, S. agalactiae, E. coli	Vancomycin 60 mg/kg q6h (max 4 g/day) plus ceftriaxone 100 mg/kg q12h (max 4 g/day) or cefotaxime 300 mg/kg q8h (max 12 g/day)
2—50 years	S. pneumoniae, N. meningitidis	Vancomycin 15–20 mg/kg IV q12h plus ceftriaxone[a] 2 g IV q12h or cefotaxime 2 g IV q6h
>50 years	S. pneumoniae, N. meningitidis, aerobic gram-negative bacilli, L. monocytogenes	Vancomycin 15–20 mg/kg IV q12h plus ceftriaxone 2 g IV q12h or cefotaxime 2 g IV q6h plus ampicillin[b] 2 g IV q4h
Immunocompromised patient	S. pneumoniae, P. aeruginosa, N. meningitidis, L. monocytogenes, aerobic gram-negative bacilli	Vancomycin 15–20 mg/kg IV q12h plus ampicillin 2 g IV q4h plus either cefepime[c] 2 g IV q12h or meropenem[d] 2 g IV q8h
Neurosurgery patient or patient with a shunt	S. aureus, aerobic gram-negative bacilli, coagulase-negative staph, P. acnes	Vancomycin 15–20 mg/kg q12h plus either cefepime 2 g IV q12h ceftazidime 2 g IV q8h or meropenem 2 g IV q8h

Key: *IV* intravenous

[a]In immunocompetent patients with severe beta-lactam allergy, moxifloxacin 400 mg IV daily can be substituted

[b]Trimethoprim-sulfamethoxazole 5 mg/kg IV (based on trimethoprim component) every 6–12 hours can be used as a substitute for ampicillin

[c]In immunocompromised patients with severe beta-lactam allergy and in whom meropenem is contraindicated, aztreonam 2 g IV q8h or ciprofloxacin 400 mg IV q12h can be use as substitutes

[d]Meropenem lowers seizure threshold. Avoid if possible in patients presenting with seizures or in patients with increased seizure risk such as those presenting with mass lesions or meningoencephalitis

this form of vasculitis, but evidence demonstrating efficacy is lacking. New focal findings, alterations in the level of awareness, or worsening headache after a few days of therapy should prompt appropriate imaging studies. Computed tomography (CT) head is sufficient to assess for evolving hydrocephalus or hemorrhage, but magnetic resonance imaging (MRI) should be obtained to rule out ischemia or abscess. CT or MR venography is necessary to rule out venous thrombosis.

As with other bacterial meningitides, syphilitic meningitis can cause an infectious vasculitis that can result in ischemia of the brain or spinal cord (meningovascular syphilis). Syphilitic meningitis, which is caused by *Treponema pallidum*, most commonly occurs within the first year of infection, but can also occur later

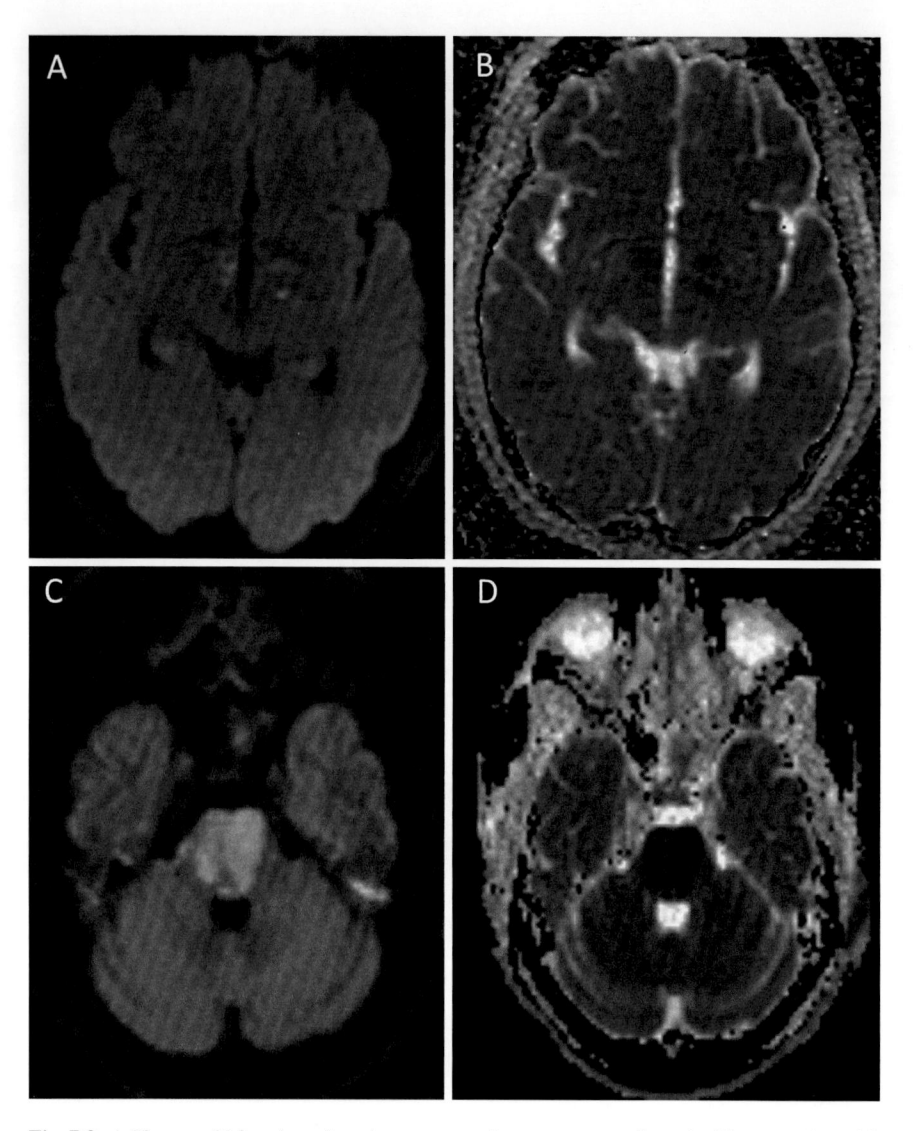

Fig. 7.2 A 58-year-old female undergoing treatment for pneumococcal meningitis presenting with new-onset encephalopathy. MRI brain showed restricted diffusion in deep gray matter structures (**a, b**) consistent with ischemic infarct. CT venogram (not shown) was negative for venous thrombosis. Three days later, she developed further deterioration in her mental status and repeat MRI showed a large area of restricted diffusion in the pons (**c, d**)

(Table 7.2). CSF protein is typically between 100 and 400 mg/dL and CSF lymphocyte counts are generally between 200 and 400 cells/mm3. CSF VDRL is almost always reactive, but serum treponemal and non-treponemal studies should always be obtained concurrently [8].

Table 7.2 Neurosyphilis

Neurosyphilis	Clinical manifestations	Diagnosis	Treatment	Post-treatment monitoring
Early neurosyphilis	Meningitis (asymptomatic or symptomatic), meningovascular disease (stroke), otologic or ocular disease (uveitis, keratitis, retinitis, and optic neuritis)	Serum treponemal and non-treponemal tests. CSF VDRL	Preferred: Penicillin G 2.4 million units intramuscular once daily plus probenecid 500 mg orally four times a day; all above regimens for 10–14 days Alternative: Desensitize to penicillin if allergic, or use ceftriaxone 2 g IV daily for 10–14 days	Neurologic exam and LP 3–6 months after completion of Tx and every 6 months thereafter until pleocytosis resolves and VDRL is non-reactive
Late neurosyphilis	Tabes dorsalis (dorsal column predominant myelitis), general paresis (dementia)			

Key: *VDRL* venereal disease research laboratory, *LP* lumbar puncture, *Tx* treatment

Tuberculosis

Tuberculous meningitis should be considered in individuals from high-prevalence countries, as well as in immunocompromised patients. In addition to the common symptoms of meningitis such as fever, headache, and photophobia, these patients can present with hydrocephalus, strokes, and cranial neuropathies as tuberculosis typically causes a basilar meningitis. Onset is usually slower than bacterial meningitis, with patients presenting with weeks of malaise, low-grade fevers, fatigue, and headache, followed by the development of frank meningeal signs. At this stage, patients can rapidly deteriorate and evolve to stupor and coma within days.

A positive tuberculin skin test or an interferon-gamma release assay (IGRA) suggests past exposure to mycobacterium but is not diagnostic of tuberculous meningitis; conversely, a negative result does not exclude the diagnosis. CSF generally shows high protein (100–500 mg/dL) and lymphocytic pleocytosis (50–1000 cells/mm^3) although neutrophils can predominate early in the course of disease. Hypoglycorrhachia is typically present. Acid-fast bacilli staining and cultures have low sensitivity, but serial lumbar punctures (up to 3) greatly improve diagnostic yield. Nucleic amplification assays have a rapid turnaround time and high specificity, but only moderate sensitivity.

For patients not known to be infected with a resistant strain, treatment involves quadruple therapy (isoniazid, rifampin, pyrazinamide, and ethambutol) for 2 months, followed by rifampin and isoniazid therapy for at least 7 months. All patients who do not have HIV-coinfection should receive adjunctive corticosteroid therapy.

Empiric treatment should be initiated while awaiting confirmatory studies in patients from endemic regions in whom tuberculous meningitis is suspected on clinical grounds.

Fungal

Fungal meningitis also tends to present subacutely with predominant basilar features. CSF will typically show an elevated protein with very low glucose. Lymphocytic pleocytosis is most common, but neutrophilic and even eosinophilic pleocytosis can occur. Regional exposure and immune status should be considered when analyzing the likelihood of specific fungi (Table 7.3).

Cryptococcus is the most common cause of fungal meningitis, especially in patients who are immunocompromised. Diagnosis is made with a positive CSF cryptococcal antigen. Patients with elevated opening pressures should undergo serial lumbar punctures, and may ultimately require drain or shunt placement for management. Standard treatment for *Cryptococcus* includes induction with amphotericin B and flucytosine for 2 weeks, and longer if CSF cultures remain positive or there is no significant clinical improvement. This is followed by consolidation therapy with high-dose fluconazole for a minimum of 8 weeks, and then a lower dose of fluconazole maintenance for a minimum of 1 year [9].

Viral

Viral meningitis, while more common than bacterial meningitis, is typically less severe and self-limited. The most common viral agents causing meningitis are enteroviruses, varicella zoster virus (VZV), herpes simplex virus (HSV)-2, and arboviruses (Table 7.4). Lumbar puncture is necessary in these patients, as history and physical exam cannot reliably distinguish between viral and bacterial meningitis. CSF typically shows mildly to moderately elevated protein, as well as mild to moderate lymphocytic pleocytosis, although neutrophils can predominate early on. Glucose is most commonly normal, though it can be low in some cases. Treatment is usually supportive, but intravenous acyclovir is used in the treatment of VZV meningitis. The efficacy of acyclovir in HSV-2 meningitis is uncertain but it is usually given in this setting.

Table 7.3 Fungal infections

Fungal infections of the CNS	Neurological presentation	Risk factors	Imaging	Diagnosis	Treatment
Cryptococcus spp. (*neoformans, gatti*)	Meningoencephalitis, space-occupying lesion (cryptococcoma)	HIV, biologicals, immunomodulatory agents	Meningeal enhancement, cryptococcomas Absence of radiographic hydrocephalus in spite of very elevated ICP	CSF Ag, cx, India ink stain	Induction: AmB + flucytosine; Consolidation and maintenance: fluconazole
Aspergillus	Abscess, vasculopathy	Hematologic malignancies, neutropenia, BMT, SOT, neurosurgical intervention, spinal injections	Focal mass lesion, hemorrhagic and/or ischemic stroke	Galactomannan (*Aspergillus* Ag) and PCR, CSF cultures are not sensitive	Voriconazole, corticosteroids may be effective; surgery may be necessary
Non-aspergillus molds (e.g., *Mucorales*, *Fusarium*)	Abscess, meningitis, rhino-orbital-cerebral disease (mucorales), latter can be complicated by cavernous sinus syndrome, internal carotid artery thrombosis	HIV, IVDU, diabetes, corticosteroids, deferoxamine, iron overload, hematologic malignancy, BMT, SOT, malnutrition	Focal lesions, hemorrhage, orbital edema, CST	For Mucor: histopathology, PCR on tissue, Cx. BDG[a] not sensitive. Other molds: Cx, PCR, BDG[a]	Mucorales: AmB followed by an azole
Candida spp.	Meningoencephalitis	IVDU, neurosurgical intervention, spinal injection, SOT, premature birth, intravascular devices	Meningeal enhancement or microabscesses on MRI	CSF Cx, BDG[a]	AmB sometimes with flucytosine, deescalate to fluconazole

(continued)

Table 7.3 (continued)

Fungal infections of the CNS	Neurological presentation	Risk factors	Imaging	Diagnosis	Treatment
Dimorphic fungi (blastomycosis, histoplasmosis, coccidiomycosis, paracoccidoimycosis)	Meningitis, meningoencephalitis, myelitis, abscess	*Blasto/Histo*: States bordering the Mississippi and Ohio River basins *Cocci*: Deserts of southwestern USA *Paracocci*: Central and South America HIV, biologicals, steroids, transplant patients, extremes of age	Meningeal enhancement, abscess, hydrocephalus	CSF, serum, and urine Ag test for blasto and histo; CSF serology; CSF PCR; Cx	*Blasto/Histo*: AmB, followed by an azole *Cocci*: Fluconazole or itraconazole and consider steroids *Paracocci*: AmB followed by TMP-SMX

Key: *HIV* human immunodeficiency virus, *ICP* intracranial pressure, *CSF* cerebrospinal fluid, *Cx* culture, *Ag* antigen, *AmB* amphoteric B, *BMT* bone marrow transplant, *SOT* solid organ transplant, *PCR* polymerase chain reaction, *IVDU* intravenous drug use, *CST* cavernous sinus thrombosis, *BDG* (1–3)-β[beta]-D-Glucan, *TMP-SMX* Trimethoprim-Sulfamethoxazole

[a](1–3)-β[beta]-D-Glucan is insensitive for *Cryptococcus*, *Mucorales*, and *Blastomyces dermatitidis*. Exposure to antibiotics such as piperacillin-tazobactam and ampicillin can result in false positive results

Table 7.4 Viral meningitis

Viral meningitis	Diagnosis	Characteristic features
Enteroviruses	CSF PCR	Most common cause of viral meningitis
Human immunodeficiency virus (HIV)	Serology, serum/CSF viral load	Typically occurs during primary HIV infection
Herpes simplex virus (HSV)	CSF PCR	HSV-2 can cause monophasic or recurrent "Mollaret's" meningitis Most patients with HSV-2 meningitis do not have a known history of genital herpes Can consider treating with acyclovir, particularly in the immunosuppressed, although can be self-limiting No evidence to support prophylactic valacyclovir in cases of recurrent meningitis
Lymphocytic choriomeningitis virus (LCMV)	Serology, CSF cell culture	Excreted in the urine and feces of rodents, contracted through direct contact or aerosol, hypoglychorachia in 20–30%, WBC count may be >1000/uL
Varicella zoster virus (VZV)	CSF PCR, IgG serum/CSF index	Responds to acyclovir

Key: *CSF* cerebral spinal fluid, *PCR* polymerase chain reaction, *IV* intravenous, *WBC* white blood cell

Encephalitis

Inflammation of the brain parenchyma is known as encephalitis. Individuals can present with fever, headache, focal neurologic findings, seizures, and encephalopathy. Many pathogens are known to cause encephalitis, with a majority of infectious cases being due to viruses. Historically, encephalitis was synonymous with infection, but autoimmune causes are increasingly being recognized. In this section, we review common infectious causes.

Herpes Simplex Virus

The most common cause of sporadic infectious encephalitis is herpes simplex virus [10] (Table 7.5). A majority of cases are caused by HSV-1 but around 10% are caused by HSV-2 [11]. Fever, encephalopathy, aphasia, and other focal neurologic signs are the most distinctive presenting features. Up to two-thirds of patients may have seizures at the time of presentation. Non-convulsive status epilepticus can occur with HSV and other encephalitides. Clinicians should have a low threshold for obtaining an electroencephalogram (EEG) in patients with encephalitis and persistent alterations in alertness or awareness.

Table 7.5 Herpes virus–associated encephalitis

Herpes Viruses	Clinical presentation	Predisposing factors	Diagnosis	Treatment
HSV-1	Meningoencephalitis		PCR, MRI (asymmetric, bitemporal, insular, inferior frontal T2 hyperintensity with variable enhancement)	Acylovir
HSV-2	Meningoencephalitis. Can also cause isolated meningitis (see Table 7.3)	Immunocompromised	PCR	Acylovir
VZV	Meningoencephalitis, vasculopathy resulting in ischemic and hemorrhagic infarctions	Immunocompromised	PCR, IgG serum/CSF index	Acyclovir
CMV	Encephalitis, radiculomyelitis, retinitis	Immunocompromised	PCR, quantitative serum PCR to follow treatment effect and help determine severity	Ganciclovir, foscarnet followed by valganciclovir
HHV-6	Limbic encephalitis	Immunocompromised, especially bone marrow and solid organ transplant patients	PCR	Ganciclovir, foscarnet
EBV	Encephalitis	Immunocompromised	PCR	Supportive

Key: *HSV* herpes simplex virus, *VZV* varicella zoster virus, *CMV* cytomegalovirus, *HHV6* human herpes virus 6, *EBV* Epstein-Barr virus, *PCR* polymerase chain reaction, *MRI* magnetic resonance imaging, *IVIG* intravenous immunoglobulin, PLEX plasma exchange

CSF HSV polymerase chain reaction (PCR) is both highly sensitive and specific and usually establishes the diagnosis, although it can be negative if obtained very acutely [11]. If suspicion is high, repeated CSF examination after 24–72 hours should be diagnostic. CSF PCR remains positive for up to 2 weeks, but sensitivity decreases after 7 days of treatment.

MRI shows markedly asymmetric but usually bilateral T2 weighted signal abnormalities with or without gadolinium enhancement in mesiotemporal structures, insular cortices, and inferolateral frontal lobes (Fig. 7.3). Though MRI findings are not pathognomonic, more than 90% of patients have MRI abnormalities 48 hours after symptom onset, with closer to 100% between the 3rd and 10th day [12]. In addition to its very high sensitivity, brain MRI offers important prognostic information in patients with HSV-1 encephalitis; the presence of diffusion restriction is associated with worse recovery [13]. EEG will often show lateralized periodic discharges. Treatment is acyclovir at a dose of 10 mg/kg for 14–21 days. Prognosis is

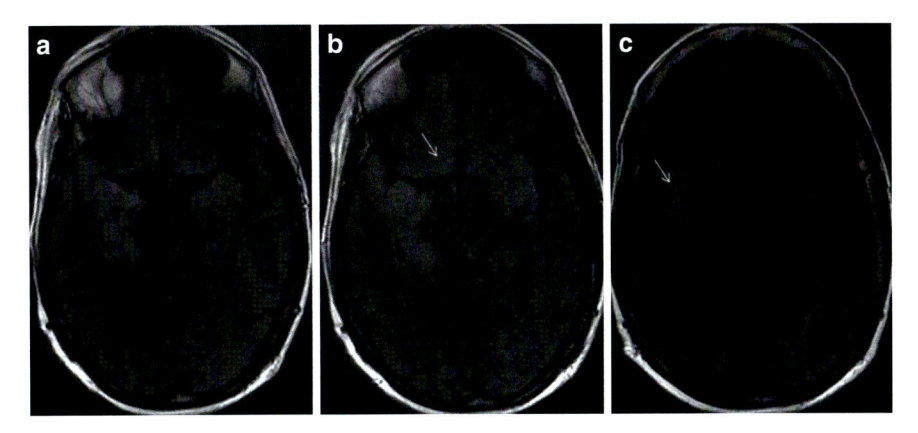

Fig. 7.3 (a–c) A 63-year-old female with HSV encephalitis. MRI brain performed 48 hours after symptom onset shows T2 FLAIR signal abnormality in the right greater than left mesiotemporal structures (**a, b**), left orbitofrontal region (arrow) (**b**), and right insular cortex (arrow) (**c**)

worsened by any delays in the initiation of antiviral treatment. Following treatment, a minority of patients can develop post-infectious encephalitis with antibodies against the N-methyl-D-aspartate (NMDA) receptor [14].

Other Herpes Viruses

VZV is another cause of encephalitis, especially in immunocompromised patients. VZV is also known to cause meningitis, vasculopathy, and myelitis. CNS complications are often associated with cutaneous manifestations, though CNS disease can occur in isolation. Imaging may show leptomeningeal enhancement, as well as hemorrhagic or ischemic lesions. VZV menigoencephalitis can be associated with small-vessel vasculitis, but a post-viral delayed (by days to months) vasculopathy resulting in ischemic stroke and affecting larger caliber vessels may also occur. CSF VZV PCR is the test of choice in early disease, but VZV IgG serum:CSF index can be helpful in chronic infections, particularly those with delayed vasculopathy. Intravenous acyclovir is used in VZV meningoencephalitis and delayed vasculopathy, although studies demonstrating efficacy are lacking.

Cytomegalovirus (CMV) can cause encephalitis in immunocompromised hosts, though it more commonly causes polyradiculitis or retinitis.

Epstein-Barr virus (EBV) may cause encephalitis in both immunocompromised and immunocompetent patients. However, caution is needed when interpreting tests results as CSF EBV PCR positivity can be seen in the setting of CNS inflammation or infection by a different pathogen, presumably due to trafficking of latently infected leucocytes into the intrathecal space [15]. CSF EBV PCR positivity can also be seen with CNS lymphoproliferative disorders. A diagnosis of EBV encephalitis should be made only after other potential causes have been excluded.

Human herpes virus (HHV)-6 can cause limbic encephalitis, primarily among solid organ and hematopoietic cell transplant recipients [16]. Yet, as in the case with EBV, HHV-6 causes latent infection of peripheral mononuclear cells, and a positive PCR does not necessarily reflect active infection. Also, inherited chromosomally integrated HHV-6 is found in about 1% of the population, and these patients can have high levels of viral DNA in blood and CSF in the absence of active infection. In general, the diagnosis of HHV-6 encephalitis should be made with particular caution, only in the correct clinical setting and once other possible etiologies have been ruled out.

Enteroviruses

The most common manifestation of enterovirus is meningitis, but some patients present with encephalitis [17]. Brainstem encephalitis with associated autonomic dysfunction and myoclonus can occur with EV71 and has high morbidity, especially in the pediatric population. Enteroviral meningoencephalitis tends to be less severe in adults, although fatal cases have been reported in association with chimeric anti-CD20 monoclonal therapies such as rituximab or patients with primary humoral immunodeficiency. Intravenous immunoglobulin (IVIG) may be considered in these cases.

Arboviruses

Arboviruses (Bunyaviridae, Togaviridae, Reoviridae, and Flaviviridae) are spread by arthropod vectors, typically mosquitos and ticks, and the incidence of various infections varies greatly with geographic region and seasonal exposure (Table 7.6).

West Nile virus is endemic to the whole continental United States, where it is the most common arboviral infection. Patients who are immunosuppressed or over the age of 65 are at the highest risk for developing neuroinvasive disease, which occurs in less than 1% of individuals infected by the virus [18]. In addition to encephalitis, the virus can cause meningitis or myelitis with acute flaccid paralysis and presentations often overlap. Encephalitis is more common in older patients, with meningitis being more common in younger patients. MRI can show abnormalities in the diencephalon, basal ganglia, brainstem, leptomeninges, and anterior horns of the spinal cord. Testing for arthropod-borne viral encephalitides should include IgM and IgG in the CSF, as CSF PCR is specific but not sensitive. Serology can be negative early in the infection, and should be repeated if there is a high index of suspicion and no other cause for encephalitis is found. Early prognosis of severe cases of neuroinvasive West Nile virus infection is poor, but slow recovery over time is possible [19].

Table 7.6 Arthropod-borne CNS infections

Virus	Clinical presentation	Diagnosis	Vector	Geographic distribution
Flaviviruses				
West Nile virus	Meningoencephalitis, brainstem encephalitis, meningitis, myelitis	CSF serology	Mosquitos	North America, Asia, Africa
Dengue virus	Meningoencephalitis, hemorrhagic fever, shock, thrombocytopenia, leukopenia	PCR and serology	Mosquitos	Asia, Africa, South and Central America
Powassan virus	Meningoencephalitis	CSF serology	Ticks	Northern USA, Canada, Europe
Tick-borne encephalitis	Meningoencephalitis	CSF serology	Ticks	Europe, Asia
Murray Valley virus	Meningoencephalitis	CSF serology	Mosquitos	Australia
St. Louis virus	Meningoencephalitis, brainstem encephalitis,	CSF serology	Mosquitos	North America
Japanese virus	Meningoencephalitis	CSF serology	Mosquitos	Asia
Togaviruses				
Chikungunya virus	Meningoencephalitis	PCR, serology	Mosquitos	Africa, Asia, Europe
Venezuelan, Eastern, and Western equine encephalitis	Meningoencephalitis, hyponatremia	CSF serology	Mosquitos	Americas
Reoviruses				
Colorado Tick fever	Meningoencephalitis, leukopenia	CSF serology	Ticks	Western USA
Bunyaviruses				
La Crosse encephalitis	Meningoencephalitis, hyponatremia	CSF serology	Mosquitos	Central and Eastern USA
Toscana virus	Meningoencephalitis	CSF serology	Sandflies	Europe
Rhabdoviruses				
Chandipura virus	Meningoencephalitis	CSF serology	Sandflies, mosquitos	India, Africa

Key: *CSF* cerebral spinal fluid, *PCR* polymerase chain reaction

Other arboviruses of note in North America include Saint Louis, LaCrosse, and Powassan viruses which may present in similar fashion (Fig. 7.4). The likelihood of infection is highly dependent on risk of exposure, and this should be taken into account before testing as false positive results can occur.

Fig. 7.4 (a–c) A 56-year-old female with Powassan virus encephalitis presented with fever, hemiparesis, and parkinsonism. MRI brain showed T2 FLAIR signal abnormality involving the left deep gray nuclei (**a**) and restricted diffusion of the left thalamus (arrow) (**b, c**)

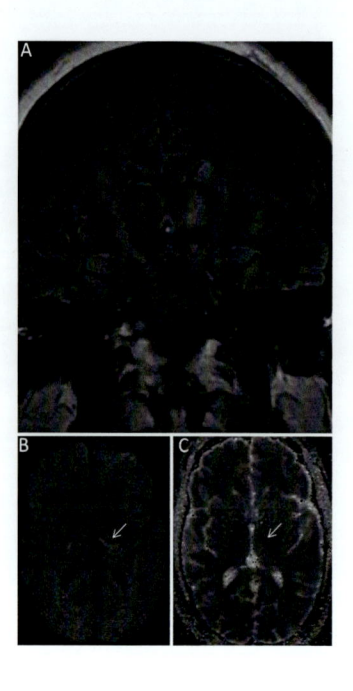

Rabies

Rabies is caused by a number of different species of neurotropic viruses in the Rhabdoviridae family, genus Lyssavirus. The virus is transmitted to humans by bites from animal vectors. There are two clinical forms of the disease: ENCEPHALITIC rabies (80% of cases) and paralytic rabies. The onset of symptoms is between 20 and 90 days from exposure, but incubation periods longer than a year have been documented. The earliest neurologic manifestations are usually paraesthesia, pain, and pruritus near the site of exposure. In encephalitic rabies, this is followed by episodes of hyperexcitability, hallucinations, confusion, and dysautonomia. Hydrophophia, characterized initially by dysphagia, followed by an overwhelming fear of water based on involuntary pharyngeal muscle spasms when attempting to drink, is virtually pathognomonic. In paralytic rabies, there is early prominent weakness which initially may only affect the bitten limb but invariably progresses to involve other limbs and bulbar muscles and can resemble Guillain-Barre syndrome. In both forms, progressive neurologic deterioration leads to paralysis, coma, and death.

MR imaging shows areas of increased T2 signal in the hippocampus, hypothalamus, and brainstem. Diagnosis is based on a combination of several tests. Serology can be tested in serum and CSF. Reverse transcription (RT)-PCR can be done on saliva. Skin biopsy from the nape of the neck is examined for rabies antigen in the cutaneous nerves at the base of hair follicles. There is no proven treatment for rabies, although development of the disease can be prevented with post-exposure rabies prophylaxis.

Bacteria and Parasites

Though bacterial encephalitis can occur in isolation, it most often accompanies advanced meningitis (Table 7.7). *Mycoplasma pneumoniae* has been associated with encephalitis in young adults and children. A post-infectious immune-mediated inflammatory response may be responsible, although the mechanism remains unclear. IgM and PCR for *M. pneumoniae* in the CSF supports this diagnosis. *Listeria* is known to cause a rhomboencephalitis. These patients may present with brainstem or cerebellar signs such as vertigo, cranial neuropathies, ataxia, or bulbar weakness.

Rocky Mountain spotted fever is a potentially lethal tick-borne disease associated with encephalitis that occurs primarily in children. MRI can show multiple small infarcts in the periventricular and subcortical white matter known as a "starry sky" appearance [20]. This is an important diagnosis to consider as it is one of the few causes of infectious encephalitis with a specific treatment. PCR testing is limited due to low sensitivity, and serology is the test of choice. Doxycycline is the first-line treatment.

Although not strictly a cause of encephalitis, malaria is another important pathogen to consider in patients presenting with fever and encephalopathy. In adults, cerebral malaria is more common in non-immune individuals than those living in endemic areas and it should be suspected in travelers returning from endemic regions. It is almost always associated with *Plasmodium falciparum* infection. Risk factors for cerebral malaria include extremes of age, immunosuppression, pregnancy, and splenectomy. A prodrome of irregular fevers, malaise, abdominal pain, headache, anorexia, and vomiting is followed in approximately 7 days by encephalopathy, seizures, and eventually coma. Retinal hemorrhages are common. CSF is bland but opening pressure is often elevated at the time of diagnosis, and cerebral edema is a significant contributor to the morbidity and mortality associated with this condition. Diagnosis is based on blood smear in combination with appropriate history. Treatment can be complicated and involves antimalarial therapy, as well as seizure control and management of intracranial pressure.

Myelitis

The presentation of infectious myelitis varies depending on the spinal cord level and location. Most cases are caused by viruses, either by the reactivation of latent infection or in the setting of primary infection. Latent viruses cause myelitis by retrograde spread along sensory nerves from dorsal root ganglia to the spinal cord. Signs and symptoms include pain, weakness, sensory changes, and urinary retention among others. VZV typically causes a rash at the time of myelitis. HSV-2 can cause a sacral myeloradiculitis presenting days to weeks after anogenital infection which is associated with severe pain, as well as urinary retention, decreased rectal tone,

Table 7.7 Bacterial and parasitic causes of meningoencephalitis

Bacterial and parasitic causes of encephalitis	Exposure	Clinical course	Diagnosis	Treatment
Rocky mountain spotted fever	Tick exposure, most common in children	Encephalitis	Serology, MRI may show a "starry sky" appearance due to multiple small white matter infarcts	Doxycycline
Naegleria fowleri	Inhalation or direct olfactory contact with water usually while swimming, most common in children	Primary amebic meningitis, rapidly progressive meningoencephalitis with a course similar to acute bacterial meningitis	CSF may show a hemorrhagic pleocytosis with elevated opening pressure and protein with low glucose; wet mount preparation may show free-swimming organisms, CSF PCR	Most commonly amphotericin plus rifampin, may also add azoles or macrolides, prognosis is usually very poor, optimal treatment remains unclear
Acanthamoeba	Commonly found in the environment, transmitted through inhalation or direct skin contact, most commonly occurs in immunosuppressed patients, has been associated with contact lens use	Subacute-chronic meningoencephalitis with space-occupying lesions	CSF pleocytosis with elevated protein and low or normal glucose, CSF PCR, histopathology	Amphotericin B or clotrimazole, CSF diversion or surgery may be necessary, optimal regimen remains unclear, prognosis is usually poor
Balamuthia mandrillaris	Disease is often associated with various outdoor activities causing dust and soil exposure, most common in immunosuppressed patients, though disease can occur in immunocompetent patients as well	Subacute-chronic granulomatous meningoencephalitis, may have single or multifocal space-occupying mass lesions which commonly involve the diencephalon and brainstem, may have chronic granulomatous skin lesions	Histopathology, PCR	Pentamidine, clarithromycin, sulfadiazine, and fluconazole, CSF diversion or surgery may be necessary, optimal regimen remains unclear, prognosis is usually poor

Coxiella burnetii (Q fever)	Exposure to placental tissue, parturient fluids, or newborn animals of cats, sheep, and goats, more common in adults than children	Encephalitis	Serology and PCR	Doxycycline Fluoroquinolones, TMP-SMX are also options
Toxoplasmosma	Environmental exposure in the setting of immunosuppression	Encephalitis, focal neurologic deficits, seizures	Serology, MRI (usually multiple, ring enhancing, edema), biopsy	Multiple options including regimen of sulfadiazine, pyrimethamine, and leucovorin
Bartonella	Lice	Encephalitis	PCR and serology, serology should not be used alone to make the diagnosis, culture is definitive but not sensitive	Doxycycline plus gentamycin
Leptospira	Animal exposure, infected soil	Encephalitis, meningitis	Serology, PCR, microscopic agglutination test	IV Penicillin, IV doxycycline, ceftriaxone, or cefotaxime
Mycoplasma	Respiratory, possible post-infectious autoimmune phenomenon	Encephalitis, meningitis, myelitis, most common in children and adolescents	Serum and CSF serology and PCR	Macrolides, fluoroquinolones or doxycycline, as well as steroids, and plasma exchange have been used

Key: *CSF* cerebral spinal fluid, *PCR* polymerase chain reaction, *MRI* magnetic resonance imaging, *IV* intravenous, *TMP-SMX* Trimethoprim-Sulfamethoxazole

and possibly weakness. Treatment frequently includes acyclovir and corticosteroids, though data are largely anecdotal [21].

Unbiased Testing

The selection of diagnostic tests in patients with meningoencephalomyelitis should be based on immune status and exposure history. However, the differential diagnosis is broad and a specific cause is not identified in close to 50% of cases. A variety of tests not targeting a specific pathogen are increasingly becoming available to clinicians (Table 7.8). Some, like the FilmArray Meningitis/Encephalitis panel, utilize nucleic acid amplification to simultaneously test for 14 pathogens. Others, like 16s rRNA, are used to detect the presence of *any* bacteria in a sample. Metagenomic next-generation sequencing of CSF and brain tissue samples can potentially detect the presence of DNA or RNA sequences of all previously catalogued and sequenced pathogens. Utility, cost, and availability vary for these tests, but they are likely to become part of diagnostic algorithms in the near future.

Space-Occupying Lesions

Bacteria

Bacterial abscesses can present as mass lesion(s) without fever or other systemic signs. Common etiologies include spread from contiguous infections (meningitis, dental, otogenic), trauma, surgical procedures, and hematogenous spread (Table 7.9). Patients present with daily persistent headache, focal neurological findings, and seizures. Fever occurs in only 50% of patients at presentation. MRI shows one or multiple ring-enhancing lesions, usually at the gray-white junction, with or without associated edema. Central diffusion restriction is common and can help distinguish an abscess from other ring-enhancing brain lesions (Table 7.10). They are commonly caused by anaerobic, *Streptococcal,* and *Staphylococcal* species [22]. *Nocardia species* can cause cerebral abscesses in the immunocompromised (Fig. 7.5). Management is guided by number of lesions and location of the abscess, but includes antibiotics as well as neurosurgical intervention (stereotactic or open aspiration) for source control when possible (Fig. 7.6). Extra-axial fluid collections, such as subdural empyema and epidural abscess, can form as a result of bacterial infection, and require surgical drainage in addition to antibiotic therapy. Although subdural and epidural collections can be seen on CT, MRI is more sensitive (Fig. 7.7).

Table 7.8 Tests not targeting specific pathogens

Assay	Function	Utility
FilmArray Meningitis/Encephalitis (ME) Panel	Real-time multiplex PCR that can simultaneously detect 14 pathogens: *E. coli* K1, *H. influenzae, Listeria monocytogenes, Neisseria meningitidis, S. pneumoniae, S. agalactiae*, CMV, VZV, HSV 1 & 2, HHV-6, enterovirus, human parechovirus, and *Cryptococcus neoformans/Cryptococcus gattii*	Fast turnaround time with potential to decrease unnecessary antimicrobial exposure Sensitivities and specificities vary for individual pathogens but most >90%, although lower for *Cryptococcus* Both false positive and false negative results occur No antibiotic susceptibilities Testing may be unnecessarily broad for immunocompetent adults but could prove useful in immunocompromised hosts, as well as those who have been previously treated with antibiotics
16S rRNA PCR with reflex sequencing	Detection of 16S rRNA gene polymerase which is highly preserved in bacteria (including mycobacteria) is followed by sequencing of the amplified product, enabling a diagnosis	Sensitivity and specificity ~90% Useful for identifying bacteria in partially treated meningitis or culture negative meningoencephalitis No antibiotic susceptibilities
(1–3)-β[beta]-D-Glucan (Fungitell)	(1–3)-β[beta]-D-Glucan is a cell wall polysaccharide present in most fungi (excepting cryptococci, the zygomycetes, and *Blastomyces dermatitidis*)	Sensitivity and specificity in serum varies depending on population (highest among immunocompromised). Few studies assessing utility in CSF May be used as an adjunct in early detection of fungal infection Not sufficient to rule out CNS fungal infection if negative Exposure to antibiotics like piperacillin-tazobactam and ampicillin can cause false positive results
Metagenomic next-generation sequencing	All DNA and RNA in CSF or brain tissue sample are sequenced without need for prior culturing. Results can be compared to databases of all known microorganisms	Can potentially detect any pathogen (bacteria, virus, fungus, and parasite) in a clinical sample Useful in cryptogenic meningoencephalitis Not widely available Remains costly May be overly sensitive

Key: *CMV* cytomegalovirus, *VZV* varicella zoster virus, *HSV* herpes zoster virus, *HHV* human herpes virus, *CSF* cerebral spinal fluid, *CNS* central nervous system, *PCR* polymerase chain reaction, *RNA* ribonucleic acid, *DNA* deoxyribonucleic acid

Table 7.9 Bacteria causing abscesses

Bacterial source/immune status	Specific microorganisms
Odontogenic source	Streptococci, Haemophilus, Bacteroides, Prevotella, Fusobacterium
Otogenic sources	Streptococci, Pseudomonas aeruginosa, Bacteroides, Enterobacteriaceae
Paranasal sinuses	Streptococcus, Haemophilus, Bacteroides, Fusobacterium
Lungs	Streptococcocus, Fusobacterium, Actinomyces
Urinary tract	Pseudomonas aeruginosa, Enterobacter
Congenital cardiac malformations	Streptococcus species
Endocarditis	Viridans streptococci, Staphylococcus aureus
Penetrating head trauma	Staphylococcus aureus, Clostridium, Enterobacter
Neurosurgical procedures	Staphylococcus, Streptococcus, Pseudomonas aeruginosa, Enterobacter
Immunocompromised	Toxoplasma gondii, Listeria monocytogens (brainstem abscesses), Nocardia asteroids, Aspergillus, Cryptococcus neoformans, Candida

Table 7.10 Imaging characteristics and differential of solitary mass suspicious for bacterial abscess

	Abscess	Tumefactive MS	Glioma	Metastases	Lymphoma
Edema	+/+++	+/++	High grade: +++ Low grade: +	+/++	+/+++
T1W	Isointense	Hypointense	Heterogeneous	Heterogeneous	Hypointense
T2W	Hyperintense	Hyperintense	High grade: Heterogeneous Low grade: Hyperintense	Heterogeneous	Hyperintense
Ring enhancement	Ring	Ring or C-shaped arc open to gray matter	High grade: Ring Low grade: Rare	Ring/incomplete arc	Ring/incomplete arc
DWI	Central	Peripheral (rim)	Heterogeneous	Heterogeneous	Central/peripheral

Key: *MS* multiple sclerosis, *GM* gray matter, *DWI* diffusion-weighted imaging

CSF studies are usually not helpful unless there is associated meningitis, and lumbar puncture may be contraindicated due to mass effect. Blood cultures should be obtained but definitive diagnosis is based on microbiology from neurosurgical samples. Empiric antibiotics should include anaerobic coverage with the addition of metronidazole to vancomycin and a third-generation cephalosporin.

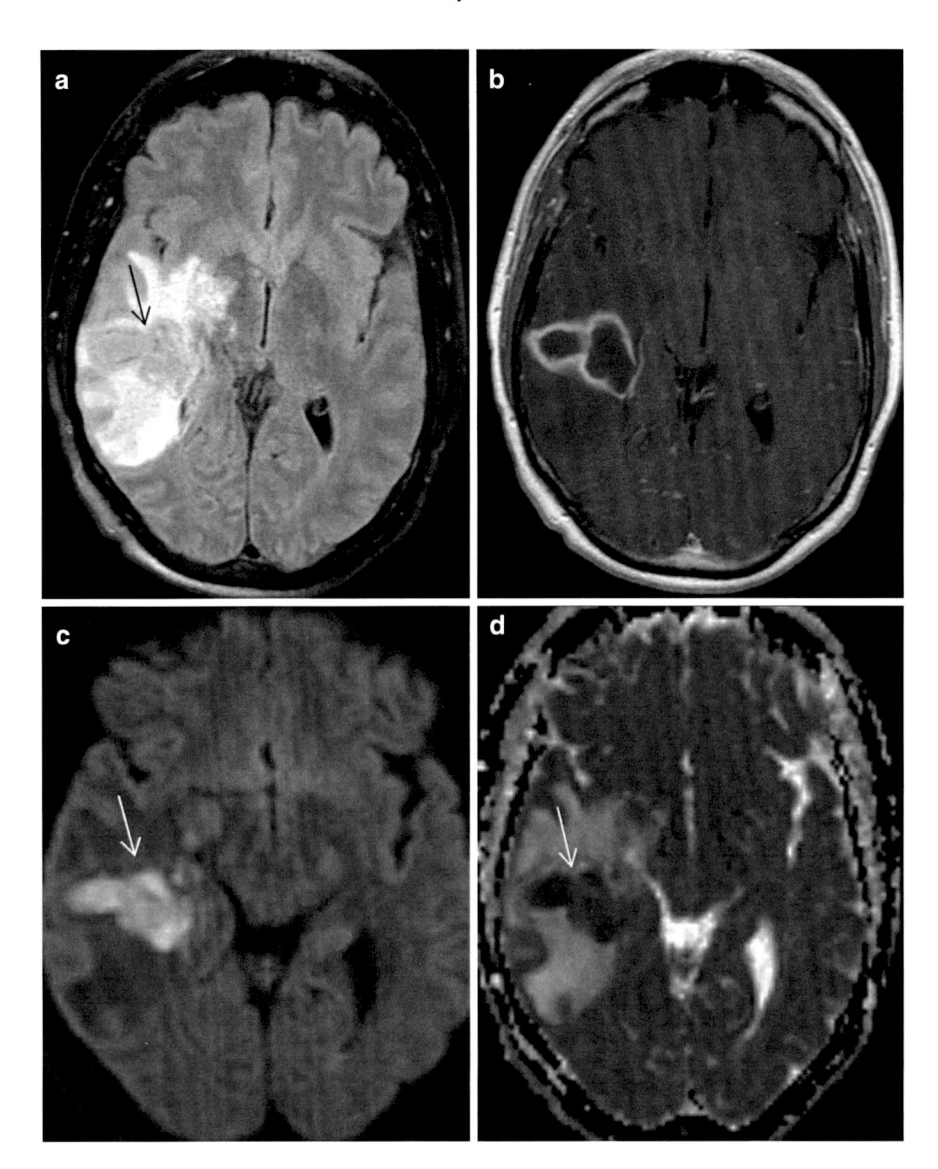

Fig. 7.5 (**a–d**) A 50-year-old male with a history of autologous stem cell transplant and graft-versus-host disease on chronic immunosuppression presented with 5 days of severe headache and confusion. MRI brain showed a loculated T2 isointense mass lesion in the right temporal lobe with extensive vasogenic edema (arrow) (**a**), ring enhancement (**b**), and central restricted diffusion (**c**, **d**) (arrows). Cultures from biopsy grew *Nocardia* spp.

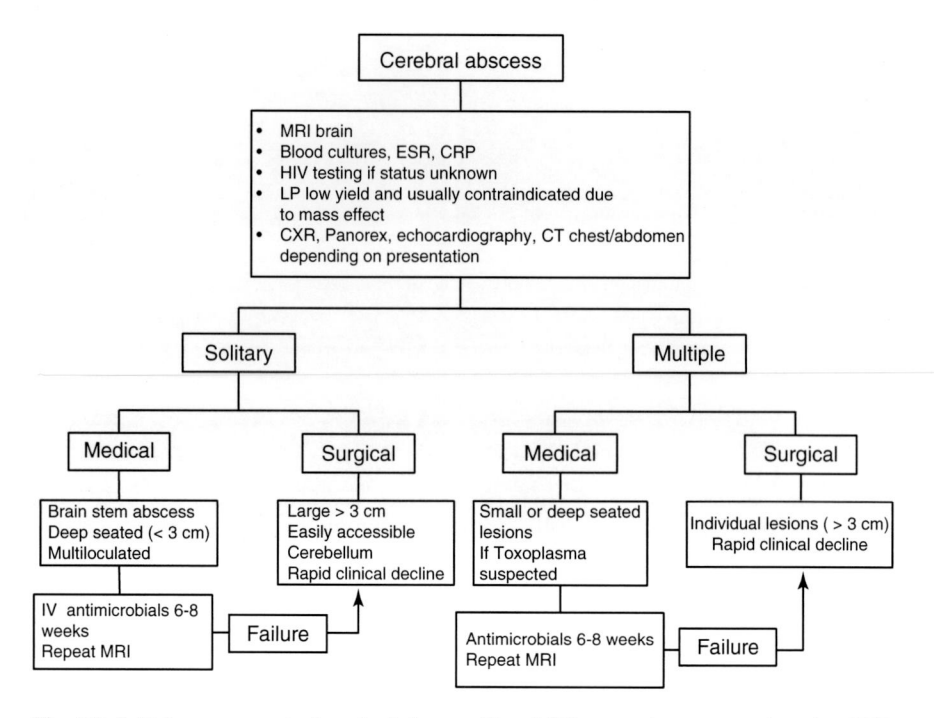

Fig. 7.6 Initial management of cerebral abscess. Key: MRI magnetic resonance imaging, ESR sedimentation rate, CRP C-reactive protein, HIV human immunodeficiency virus, LP lumbar puncture, CT computed tomography, CXR chest X-ray. (Modified with permission from Figure 32.2 in "Chapter 32 Brain Abscess." *The Practice of Emergency and Critical Care Neurology*. Wijdicks, E FM. Oxford University Press, 2010, pg. 465)

Fungal

Fungi can cause abscesses in the CNS, and usually present in the setting of immunosuppression (Table 7.3). Aspergillus species can cause CNS infection through hematologic spread, spread from nearby structures such as the paranasal sinuses, surgical interventions, or fungal endocarditis. The most common presentation for CNS aspergillosis is mass lesions (aspergillomas). It can also cause cerebral infarction, spinal cord invasion, and rarely isolated meningitis. CSF aspergillus antigen (galactomannan) can be diagnostic if positive, but brain biopsy may be required.

Suggestive CSF parameters, evidence of fungal infection elsewhere in the body, or failure to respond to antibiotics in the setting of immunosuppression should raise suspicion that the abscess is fungal and prompt consideration of initiating empiric antifungal therapy.

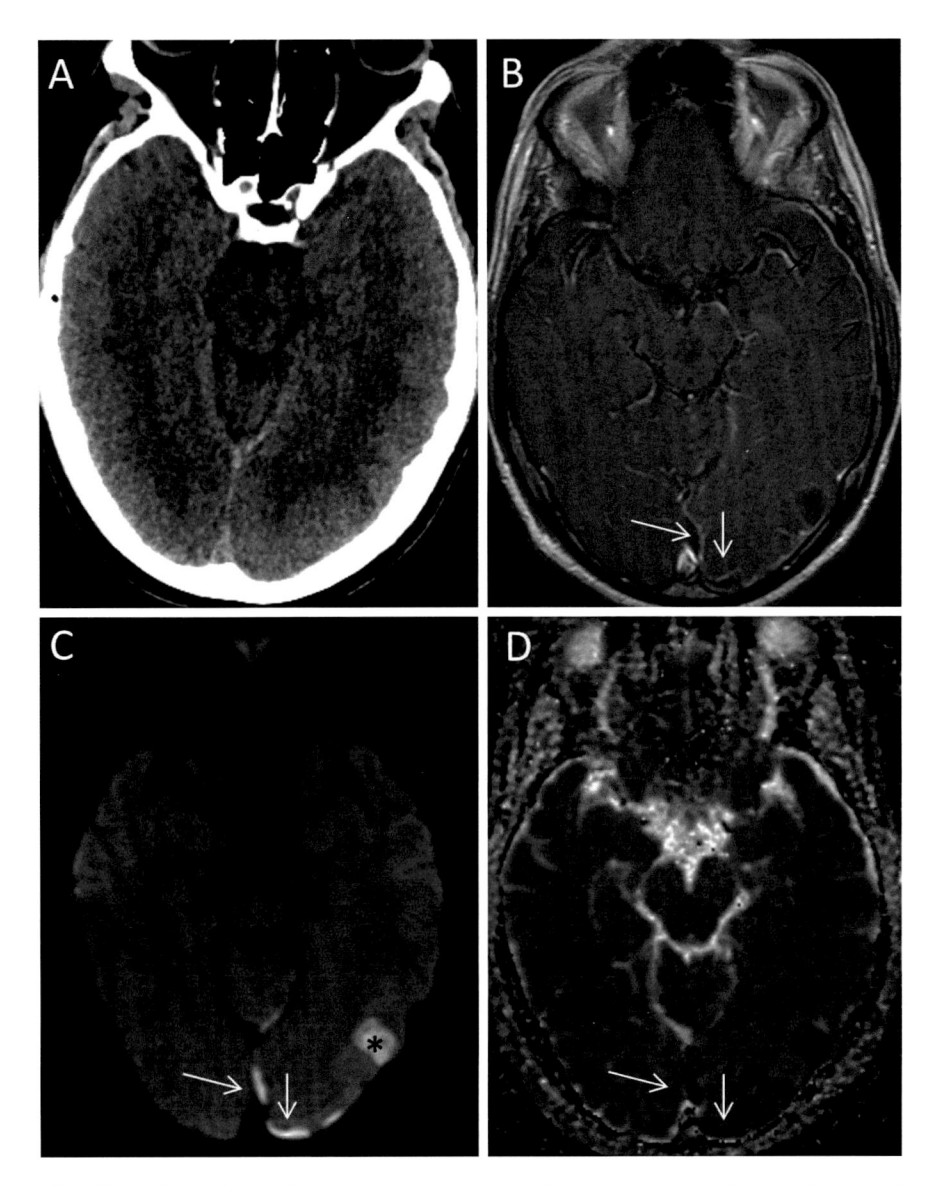

Fig. 7.7 (**a–d**) A 55-year-old male presenting with headache, nausea, vomiting, confusion, and focal findings on exam. CT done at admission was unremarkable (**a**). T1 gadolinium images (**b**) revealed left hemispheric leptomeningeal enhancement (black arrows), a ring-enhancing lesion (asterisk), and associated subdural fluid collections (white arrows). The subdural collections demonstrated restricted diffusion (white arrows, **c** and **d**), as did the ring-enhancing lesion (asterisk), consistent with a diagnosis of subdural empyema and associated abscess. The patient underwent craniotomy for empyema evacuation and abscess debridement. Blood and CSF cultures were negative but operative cultures grew *Streptococcus anginosus* (not shown)

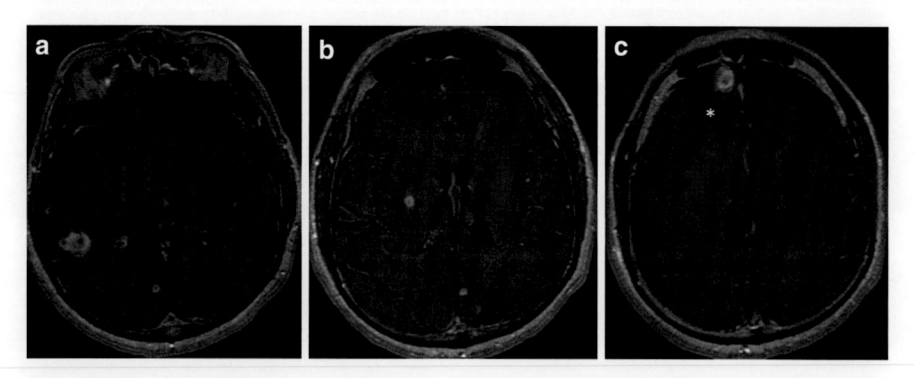

Fig. 7.8 (**a–c**) A 48-year-old recently HIV-positive male with CNS toxoplasmosis. MRI brain shows multiple ring-enhancing lesions located in the cortex, juxtacortical white matter, and deep gray matter (**a–c**). A right frontal lesion is associated with significant vasogenic edema (asterisk)

Parasites

Parasitic causes of CNS mass lesions include toxoplasmosis, cysticercosis, and *Balamuthia mandrillaris*. *Toxoplasma gondii* is an intracellular parasite, which humans acquire through ingesting oocytes. The infection can remain dormant, and typically presents in immunosuppressed individuals with multiple ring-enhancing lesions in the deep gray matter or at the gray-white junction with significant edema (Fig. 7.8). Seizures are common, as are headaches, encephalopathy, focal neurologic deficits, and hyperkinetic movement disorders. Diagnosis can frequently be made with neuroimaging and serology in patients with an appropriate history, though biopsy is sometimes required. Treatment involves correcting the underlying immunosuppression, as well as antiparasitic therapy. Initial treatment is typically a 6-week course of sulfadiazine, pyrimethamine, and leucovorin [23].

Human Immunodeficiency Virus (HIV)

HIV can manifest as a self-limiting meningoencephalitis during acute infection. Patients can also develop myelitis during this stage, though this is less common. A variety of immune-mediated nervous system complications can also accompany HIV infection, including cranial neuropathies, as well as demyelinating or axonal polyradiculoneuropathies.

As CD4 T-cell counts decline, patients are at risk of developing opportunistic infections, as well as malignancies, such as CNS lymphoma. Progressive multifocal leukoencephalopathy (PML) is a severe demyelinating disease of the CNS caused by the reactivation of the John Cunningham (JC) virus mostly in immunocompromised patients. In HIV patients it is usually seen in those with CD4 counts <200 mm^3.

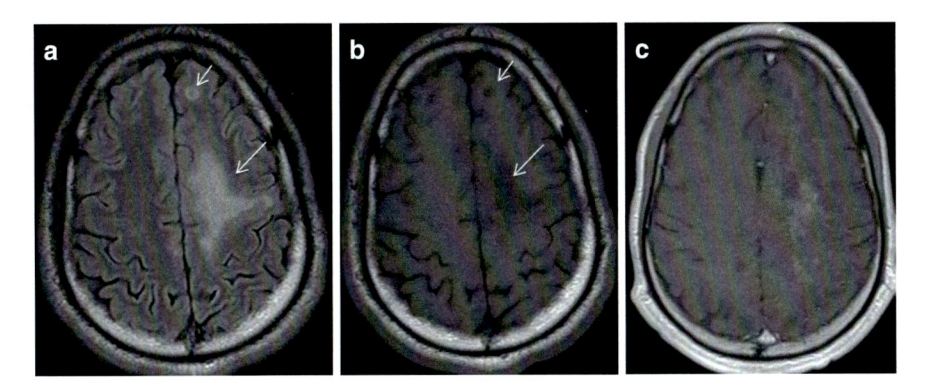

Fig. 7.9 A 25-year-old male presented with progressive right hemiparesis and aphasia. MRI brain revealed two discrete T2 hyperintense lesions in the left frontal subcortical white matter (**a**) with associated T1 hypointensity (**b**) (arrows). CSF studies confirmed a diagnosis of progressive multifocal leukoencephalopathy and he was found to be HIV positive. Four weeks after initiation of antiretroviral therapy he developed worsening aphasia and hemiparesis. Repeat MRI brain revealed speckled gadolinium enhancement involving the previously identified left frontal lesions (**c**) consistent with IRIS

Presentation is characterized by the insidious onset of progressive focal neurological deficits, cognitive changes, hemianopia, and ataxia. MRI usually shows asymmetric multifocal areas of white matter T2 signal change with associated T1 hypointensity and without mass effect (Fig. 7.9). Solitary lesions can occur. Gadolinium enhancement and edema can be present in patients who are not profoundly immunocompromised and in those with immune reconstitution inflammatory syndrome (IRIS). CSF JC PCR has high sensitivity and specificity; but, after two negative results, brain biopsy should be pursued if suspicion remains high. The main treatment is to restore immune function. In HIV patients, the initiation of antiretroviral therapy can lead to recovery in about 50% but the course is usually complicated by IRIS and neurologic sequelae are common.

CNS IRIS is defined by a pathologic inflammatory response to either a recently treated (paradoxical) or a previously undiagnosed (unmasked) opportunistic infections. IRIS results from the restoration of a dysregulated immune response against pathogen-specific antigens. In HIV, IRIS is characterized by paradoxical clinical deterioration following the initiation of antiretroviral therapy. IRIS commonly occurs in response to opportunistic organisms, such as *Mycobacterium tuberculosis*, *Cryptococcus neoformans*, or JC virus [24]. Paradoxical worsening, manifesting as alterations in consciousness, focal deficits, cranial neuropathies, and seizures, occurs 3–5 weeks after the initiation of antiretroviral therapy but can develop months after treatment. Brain imaging varies depending on the underlying infection but associated gadolinium enhancement and edema are common. Corticosteroids are used as treatment but data demonstrating efficacy is lacking. Initiating treatment of the opportunistic infection weeks before antiretroviral therapy is recommended and reduces, but does not eliminate, the chances of developing IRIS.

Cardinal Messages
- CNS infections carry significant morbidity and mortality. Prompt recognition and initiation of therapy improves outcome.
- The full triad of headache, neck stiffness, and fever occurs in less than half of patients with meningitis.
- Initiation of antibiotics reduces the yield of CSF Gram stain and culture. However, antibiotics should not be held when delays in diagnostic testing are expected.
- Although confusion, agitation, focal neurologic signs, and seizures can occur in meningitis, they are suggestive of parenchymal involvement and should prompt initiation of empiric coverage for HSV encephalitis.
- The differential of encephalitis is broad and includes both infectious and autoimmune etiologies.
- Headache and focal neurologic signs are the most common presentation of a cerebral abscess. Fever occurs in about half of the patients.
- Initiation of antiretroviral therapy has improved mortality in HIV-associated PML, but IRIS and neurologic sequelae are common.

References

1. van de Beek D, de Gans J, Spanjaard L, Weisfelt M, Reitsma JB, Vermeulen M. Clinical features and prognostic factors in adults with bacterial meningitis. N Engl J Med. 2004;351(18):1849–59.
2. Huy NT, Thao NT, Diep DT, Kikuchi M, Zamora J, Hirayama K. Cerebrospinal fluid lactate concentration to distinguish bacterial from aseptic meningitis: a systemic review and meta-analysis. Crit Care. 2010;14(6):R240.
3. Sakushima K, Hayashino Y, Kawaguchi T, Jackson JL, Fukuhara S. Diagnostic accuracy of cerebrospinal fluid lactate for differentiating bacterial meningitis from aseptic meningitis: a meta-analysis. J Infect. 2011;62(4):255–62.
4. de Gans J, van de Beek D, European Dexamethasone in Adulthood Bacterial Meningitis Study Investigators. Dexamethasone in adults with bacterial meningitis. N Engl J Med. 2002;347(20):1549–56.
5. Tunkel AR, Hartman BJ, Kaplan SL, Kaufman BA, Roos KL, Scheld WM, et al. Practice guidelines for the management of bacterial meningitis. Clin Infect Dis. 2004 Nov 1;39(0):1267–84.
6. Aronin SI, Peduzzi P, Quagliarello VJ. Community-acquired bacterial meningitis: risk stratification for adverse clinical outcome and effect of antibiotic timing. Ann Intern Med. 1998;129(11):862–9.
7. Lucas MJ, Brouwer MC, van de Beek D. Delayed cerebral thrombosis in bacterial meningitis: a prospective cohort study. Intensive Care Med. 2013;39(5):866–71.
8. Workowski KA, Bolan GA. Sexually transmitted diseases treatment guidelines, 2015. MMWR Recomm Rep. 2015;64(Rr-03):1–137.
9. Schwartz S, Kontoyiannis DP, Harrison T, Ruhnke M. Advances in the diagnosis and treatment of fungal infections of the CNS. Lancet Neurol. 2018;17(4):362–72.
10. Parpia AS, Li Y, Chen C, Dhar B, Crowcroft NS. Encephalitis, Ontario, Canada, 2002–2013. Emerg Infect Dis. 2016;22(3):426–32.

11. Solomon T, Michael BD, Smith PE, Sanderson F, Davies NW, Hart IJ, et al. Management of suspected viral encephalitis in adults—Association of British Neurologists and British Infection Association National Guidelines. J Infect. 2012;64(4):347–73.
12. Granerod J, Davies NW, Mukonoweshuro W, Mehta A, Das K, Lim M, et al. Neuroimaging in encephalitis: analysis of imaging findings and interobserver agreement. Clin Radiol. 2016;71(10):1050–8.
13. Singh TD, Fugate JE, Hocker S, Wijdicks EFM, Aksamit AJ Jr, Rabinstein AA. Predictors of outcome in HSV encephalitis. J Neurol. 2016;263(2):277–89.
14. Armague T, Spatola M, Vlagea A, Mattozi S, et al. Frequency, symptoms, risk factors, and outcomes of autoimmune encephalitis after herpes simplex encephalitis: a prospective observational study and retrospective analysis. Lancet Neurol. 2018 Sep; 17(9):760–772.
15. Fujimoto H, Asaoka K, Imaizumi T, Ayabe M, Shoji H, Kaji M. Epstein-Barr virus infections of the central nervous system. Intern Med. 2003;42(1):33–40.
16. Dubey D, Pittock SJ, Kelly CR, McKeon A, Lopez-Chiriboga AS, Lennon VA, et al. Autoimmune encephalitis epidemiology and a comparison to infectious encephalitis. Ann Neurol. 2018;83(1):166–77.
17. Steiner I, Budka H, Chaudhuri A, Koskiniemi M, Sainio K, Salonen O, et al. Viral meningoencephalitis: a review of diagnostic methods and guidelines for management. Eur J Neurol. 2010;17(8):999–e57.
18. Davis LE, DeBiasi R, Goade DE, Haaland KY, Harrington JA, Harnar JB, et al. West Nile virus neuroinvasive disease. Ann Neurol. 2006;60(3):286–300.
19. Hawkes MA, Carabenciov ID, Wijdicks EFM, Rabinstein AA. Critical West Nile Neuroinvasive Disease. Neurocrit Care. 2018 Aug;29(1):47–53.
20. Crapp S, Harrar D, Strother M, Wushensky C, Pruthi S. Rocky Mountain spotted fever: 'starry sky' appearance with diffusion-weighted imaging in a child. Pediatr Radiol. 2012;42(4):499–502.
21. Savoldi F, Kaufmann TJ, Flanagan EP, Toledano M, Weinshenker BG. Elsberg syndrome: a rarely recognized cause of cauda equina syndrome and lower thoracic myelitis. Neurol Neuroimmunol Neuroinflamm. 2017;4(4):e355.
22. Brook I. Microbiology and treatment of brain abscess. J Clin Neurosci. 2017;38:8–12.
23. Katlama C, De Wit S, O'Doherty E, Van Glabeke M, Clumeck N. Pyrimethamine-clindamycin vs. pyrimethamine-sulfadiazine as acute and long-term therapy for toxoplasmic encephalitis in patients with AIDS. Clin Infect Dis. 1996;22(2):268–75.
24. Bowen L, Nath A, Smith B. CNS immune reconstitution inflammatory syndrome. Handb Clin Neurol. 2018;152:167–76.

Chapter 8
Acute Neuromuscular Respiratory Failure

Katherine Schwartz and Christopher L. Kramer

Diagnostic Keys
- The pathophysiology of neuromuscular respiratory failure begins with a loss of tidal volume that is initially compensated by recruiting accessory muscles and increasing respiratory rate, but which ultimately progresses to hypoxemic hypercapnic respiratory failure when these compensatory mechanisms become exhausted.
- A normal arterial blood gas is not necessarily reassuring in patients with neuromuscular respiratory failure and is, in fact, abnormal in a tachypneic patient.
- Oropharyngeal weakness can predispose patients to aspiration and thus exacerbate the respiratory compromise.
- Interrupted speech, a sensation of "air hunger," and, especially, paradoxical respiration are late signs of neuromuscular respiratory failure and should prompt consideration of intubation.
- Guillain-Barré syndrome (GBS) and myasthenia gravis (MG) are the most common causes of primary neuromuscular respiratory failure, while critical illness neuromyopathy (CINM) is the most common cause of secondary neuromuscular respiratory failure.

K. Schwartz · C. L. Kramer (✉)
Department of Neurology, University of Chicago, Chicago, IL, USA
e-mail: ckramer1@neurology.bsd.uchicago.edu

Treatment Priorities
- Severe or rapidly developing appendicular weakness, severe oropharyngeal weakness, an abnormal chest X-ray, dysautonomia, and respiratory insufficiency are reasons to admit or transfer a patient to the ICU for close monitoring.
- Patients with oropharyngeal weakness require pulmonary hygiene, including suctioning, chest physiotherapy, humidified air, and mucolytics.
- Employ ventilatory support commiserate with the degree of neuromuscular respiratory failure; non-emergent intubation may reduce complications.
- Non-invasive ventilation can be attempted in patients without an acute respiratory acidosis, relatively stable disease, and in whom rapid improvement is anticipated with treatment, such as MG.
- Disease-modifying immune therapy should be initiated as early as possible in GBS and MG.

Prognosis at a Glance
- The prognosis of patients with neuromuscular respiratory failure depends on the underlying cause.
- Patients in whom the underlying cause of neuromuscular respiratory failure remains elusive generally have a poor prognosis.
- Patients with severe GBS often have a protracted hospital course; providing encouragement and hope is necessary and justified, as many patients ultimately can achieve a good quality of life and the mortality is generally low.
- While some patients may require invasive ventilation and a prolonged ICU stay, many improve rapidly with immunotherapy and the prognosis is generally good.
- While full recovery from CINM is possible, residual physical disability is not uncommon.

Introduction

Patients with acute progressive neuromuscular weakness are encountered by the neurologist or neurointensivist in the emergency department, in other ICUs as consultations, or on the general ward if the patient's condition worsens to cause respiratory insufficiency or difficulty managing secretions. Recognition of the severity of acute respiratory failure and timely intervention matching the degree impairment is the initial step in managing these patients. However, in patients requiring invasive or non-invasive respiratory support, ventilation should be initiated prior to overt signs of impending respiratory collapse. Assessment of the severity of neuromuscular respiratory failure requires knowledge of the pathophysiology, the signs and symptoms of the condition, and the tests that can be employed to support clinical decision making regarding the need for ICU admission or ventilatory support. Assuring cardiopulmonary stability with the appropriate measures and close monitoring for clinical worsening are just the beginning; further management should be focused on the underlying diagnosis. This chapter will review the information needed for the clinician to critically assess and manage acute neuromuscular disorders leading to respiratory failure, including Guillain-Barré syndrome (GBS), myasthenia gravis (MG), and critical illness neuromyopathy (CINM).

Pathophysiology of Neuromuscular Respiratory Failure

Normal Respiratory Mechanics

Knowledge of basic respiratory mechanics and its relationship to the nervous system is fundamental to understanding neuromuscular respiratory failure. Inhalation is achieved primarily by work of the diaphragm, a fatigue-resistant muscle that descends into the abdomen as it contracts, increasing the vertical dimension of the lungs. The diaphragm is innervated by the phrenic nerves, which consists of fibers from the C3 to the C5 nerve roots. Additionally, the accessory respiratory muscles, including the external intercostals, scalenes, pectorals, latissimus dorsi, and sternocleidomastoid muscles, supplement inspiratory effort by further increasing the volume of the chest cavity in the dorsal-ventral direction by lifting the rib cage up and out, particularly during exertion, or when the diaphragm fails. Contraction of the inspiratory muscles generates a negative force that overcomes the respiratory load (comprised of the resistance to inspiratory flow, the elasticity of the lungs and chest wall, and positive pressure at peak inspiration), allowing for air to flow in [1]. Expiration is achieved mostly through passive recoil of the thoracic cage, but some recruitment of the internal intercostal muscles also occurs. However, forced expiration, which is essential to coughing and protecting the airway from aspiration, is achieved primarily by contraction of the abdominal muscles. Equally important to protect the airway are the oropharyngeal muscles, which maintain the patency of the upper airway and handle secretions [1–3].

Neuromuscular Respiratory Failure Mechanics

Because respiratory muscles have substantial reserve, the signs of neuromuscular respiratory failure do not begin in patients without lung pathology until the diaphragm strength drops below 30% (though it may begin sooner in those that do, including patients with aspiration) [3, 4]. First, as the diaphragm begins to fail, accessory muscles are increasingly recruited to maintain adequate tidal volumes. Further progression of weakness results in a drop in tidal volume, though minute ventilation can be maintained through an increase in respiratory rate. However, atelectasis ultimately develops in the setting of reduced tidal volumes, resulting in shunting and hypoxia, that initially is mild and may only be detected by measuring the alveolar-arterial gradient [3]. Eventually, without intervention, further decreases in tidal volume and fatigue, which limits compensation with tachypnea, result in hypoxemic hypercarbic respiratory failure (Fig. 8.1).

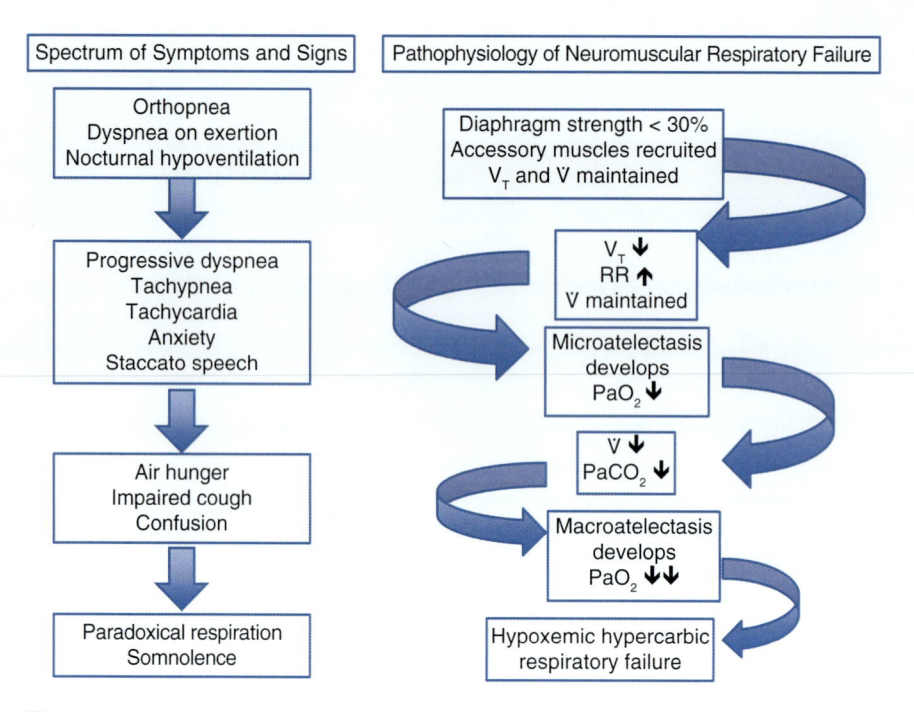

Fig. 8.1 The Downward Spiral pathophysiology of neuromuscular respiratory failure and associated spectrum of symptoms and signs. Rapidity of progression is variable and not all patients will experience all the listed symptoms and signs. Clinical presentation may also vary depending on the stage of neuromuscular respiratory failure when the patient presents. Proper and timely intervention may reverse the course. VT - tidal volume, V̇ - minute ventilation, RR - respiratory rate, PaO_2 - partial pressure of oxygen, $PaCO_2$ - partial pressure of carbon dioxide

Oropharyngeal weakness can be a major factor in the development of neuromuscular respiratory failure by exposing the patient to aspiration, particularly when combined with respiratory muscle weakness. The presence of an impaired cough due to weak abdominal muscles impedes clearance of aspirated materials and may further increase the risk of aspiration [1–4].

Initial Evaluation of Neuromuscular Respiratory Failure

Clinical Features

The early symptoms of neuromuscular respiratory failure are subtle and include dyspnea on exertion, orthopnea, and changes in vocal tone and volume. Nocturnal hypoventilation may also occur, particularly in patients with concomitant pharyngeal weakness or with anatomical predisposition; patients may complain of frequent nocturnal awakenings, daytime sleepiness, cognitive complaints, and morning

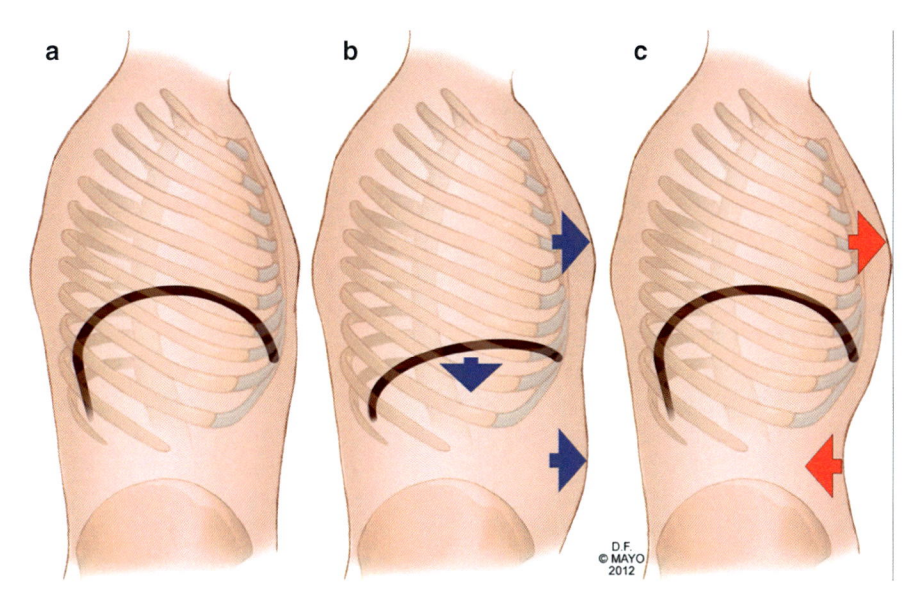

Fig. 8.2 Graphic illustration of paradoxical breathing pattern. (**a**) Diaphragm at rest. (**b**) Normal diaphragm movement during inspiration resulting in expansion of the chest and abdomen. (**c**) Paradoxical breathing pattern (inward abdominal movement during inspiration) because of diaphragmatic weakness. (Used with permission of the Mayo Foundation for Medical Education and Research. All rights reserved)

headaches [5]. When gathering the history, it is essential to determine the rapidity of symptom progression. Patients with rapidly worsening symptoms are at higher risk of more severe disease progression during hospitalization and should be monitored closely.

As neuromuscular respiratory weakness worsens and tidal volumes decrease, patients become anxious, restless, tachycardic, tachypneic, and diaphoretic. Accessory respiratory muscle use becomes more prominent to compensate for the failing diaphragm. Interrupted (or "staccato") speech, a sensation of "air hunger" (indicating stimulation of chemoreceptors by hypercapnia) and, especially, paradoxical respiration are late signs and may indicate the need for intubation [1–3]. Paradoxical respiration becomes apparent only with severe diaphragm weakness or paralysis. It is characterized by inward movement of the abdomen with inspiration and can be best appreciated by placing one hand on the chest and one on the abdomen with the patient in the supine position (Fig. 8.2). Finally, the inability of the patient to count in 1 second intervals up to 20 can also indicate marked reduction in vital capacity. Very late findings associated with hypercapnia, include hypotension, cardiac arrhythmias, and encephalopathy, ranging in severity from somnolence to coma.

Difficulty clearing secretions, flaccid dysarthria, drooling, and inability to smile or frown are signs of oropharyngeal weakness. These findings, in addition to a weak or absent cough, indicate compromised airway protection and increased risk of aspiration.

Diagnostic Evaluation

While not devoid of limitations, arterial blood gas (ABG), chest X-ray, oximetry, and bedside spirometry can be useful adjuncts to the initial management of patients with acute neuromuscular weakness, i.e., ascertainment of the presence and degree of airway or respiratory compromise and the need for invasive or noninvasive ventilation. The ABG can supplement the clinical exam in estimating the stage of neuromuscular respiratory failure. Microatelectases can cause a decrease in the arterial partial pressure of oxygen (PaO_2) or an increase in the alveolar-arterial gradient during the initial phase of neuromuscular respiratory failure and these changes may occur without a noticeable drop in oxygen saturation. In fact, continuous pulse oximetry may be falsely reassuring if normal; frank desaturation is a late finding and often indicates the need for intubation. The respiratory rate must be considered when interpreting the arterial partial pressure of carbon dioxide ($PaCO_2$). A "normal" $PaCO_2$ in a tachypneic patient is actually abnormal and indicates that the patient's minute ventilation is being maintained by an increase in the respiratory rate to compensate for a reduced tidal volume caused by the respiratory muscle weakness [3]. Respiratory acidosis is a late finding and indicates failure of compensatory mechanisms to maintain minute ventilation [1, 2]. Evidence of chronic respiratory acidosis (low or normal pH, high $PaCO_2$, and high bicarbonate) in a patient presenting with acute neuromuscular respiratory failure is associated with worse outcome and higher in hospital mortality [6].

Chest X-ray may disclose atelectasis, which can indicate a reduction in tidal volume, or aspiration from compromised airway protection. Importantly, any pre-existing or acute lung pathology may reduce the patient's pulmonary reserve.

On bedside spirometry, forced vital capacity (FVC), maximal inspiratory pressure (MIP), and maximal expiratory pressure (MEP) are useful to evaluate neuromuscular respiratory weakness. FVC < 20 mL/kg, MIP > −30 mm H_2O, MEP < 40 mm H_2O (the "20/30/40 rule"), or a decrease in any of these variables by >30% is associated with the need for intubation and invasive ventilation in GBS [7]. Trends are more useful in other neuromuscular conditions as cutoffs have not been validated—a drop in FVC of 20% or greater is suggestive of diaphragmatic weakness [1, 2]. The MEP is a particularly important parameter, as it is associated with the patient's ability to effectively cough and clear secretions from the airway. However, bedside spirometry has important limitations, which are summarized in Table 8.1 [8, 9]. To prevent aspiration, testing should be preceded by good pulmonary hygiene [1, 2].

Finally, measurement of diaphragm thickness and contractility using bedside ultrasound can provide dynamic assessment of diaphragmatic function, though further research is needed with regard to its ability to predict the need for ventilatory support [10].

Table 8.1 Common causes of erroneous spirometry values and possible solutions

Cause	Solution
Poor seal due to oropharyngeal weakness	Use of sniff nasal inspiratory pressures (SNIP) or mask spirometry
Variable patient positioning	Ensure consistent degree of supine positioning in serial assessments
Poor effort	Coaching by an experienced respiratory therapist and use of the best of three measurements
Pre-existing lung pathology	Compare bedside spirometry to prior pulmonary function tests (if available) and ensure adequate treatment of lung condition
Fluctuating nature of underlying illness (e.g., myasthenia gravis)	Assess trend over repeated testing, allow for adequate rest between attempts, consider timing of last dose of pyridostigmine

Initial Management and Disposition

Patients with neuromuscular respiratory failure may require mechanical ventilation due to respiratory muscle weakness, for airway protection, and/or dysautonomia (in GBS). Ideally, intubation should be performed electively to avoid complications with emergent intubations, such as exacerbation of dysautonomia in GBS. The decision to intubate so should be made using the clinical exam and diagnostic studies; examples of factors associated with the need for intubation in patients with neuromuscular respiratory failure are summarized in Table 8.2 [3]. Succinylcholine should be avoided during intubation to prevent a dangerous rise in potassium and care should be taken when using vasoactive and cardiotropic medications in patients with dysautonomia. A trial of non-invasive bi-level positive airway pressure (BiPAP) can be effective in patient without an acute respiratory acidosis, relatively stable disease course, and in whom a more rapid improvement is anticipated with treatment, such as MG [11]. Pulmonary hygiene, including suctioning, chest physiotherapy, humidified air, and mucolytics are essential in nearly all intubated patients with those with oropharyngeal weakness and/or impaired cough. Yet, anticholinergics should be avoided in patients with GBS and dysautonomia, as they can provoke dangerous tachyarrhythmias. Additionally anticholinergics can worsen MG.

Patients with acute neuromuscular weakness often present to the emergency department before reaching the stage of requiring ventilatory assistance. Patients with severe or rapidly progressive appendicular weakness, severe bulbar weakness, abnormal chest X-ray, dysautonomia, or respiratory insufficiency should be admitted to the ICU for monitoring (Figs. 8.3 and 8.4).

The duration of intubation depends on the underlying pathology. Generally, MG patients are intubated for days, GBS patients are intubated for weeks, and ALS patients may never be extubated. Factors associated with extubation success are listed in Table 8.3. Patients with GBS who cannot lift their arms off the bed or have electrophysiologic evidence of axonal degeneration 1 week after intubation or who have little improvement in spirometry at 2 weeks will very likely require a tracheostomy [12, 13].

Table 8.2 Factors associated with the need for intubation in patients with neuromuscular respiratory failure

	Determinant factors	Contributing factors
Clinical	Rapid clinical decline[a]	Nocturnal hypoventilation
	Paradoxical respiration	Dyspnea with or without exertion
	Severe bulbar weakness	Shallow breathing
	Absent cough	Interrupted (staccato speech)
	Decreased level of consciousness	Orthopnea
	Severe dysautonomia	Accessory muscle use
		Inability to count to 20 with a single breath
		Cough after swallowing
		Mild to moderate bulbar weakness
		Weak cough
		Neck flexion weakness
		Diaphoresis
		Tachypnea
		Tachycardia
Diagnostic studies	Hypercapnia	Normal $PaCO_2$ in a tachypneic patient
	Oxygen desaturation	Decrease in PaO_2 without desaturation
	Aspiration pneumonia on chest X-ray	Atelectasis on chest X-ray
	Complete diaphragm paralysis on ultrasound	Progressive decline in spirometry values over time
	Vital capacity <1 L or 20 mL/kg, or 30% decrease in VC in one day[a]	
	Maximum inspiratory pressure > 30 cm H2O[a]	
	Maximum expiratory pressure < 40 cm H2O[a]	

[a]Strongest association with Guillain-Barré syndrome

Causes of Neuromuscular Respiratory

While ensuring that the patient is capable of ventilating and protecting the airway remains the first priority, investigation into the cause of the neuromuscular weakness to provide targeted therapy ensues concomitantly or after stabilization. A thorough history can assist not only in discerning the diagnosis, which can include an acute exacerbation or progression of a previously diagnosed neuromuscular condition, but can also aid in estimating the disease course, as rapid progression can predict a more severe nadir and can assist in elucidating the pattern of weakness (i.e., proximal vs. distal and ascending vs. descending) [1–3]. Ascertaining whether the patient's symptoms began while they were hospitalized for a non-neurological condition can narrow the diagnosis to secondary causes of neuromuscular respiratory failure, which includes CINM and prolonged neuromuscular blockade. In contrast, primary neuromuscular respiratory includes patients with a new or exacerbation of a chronic neuromuscular condition, the most common of which are GBS, MG, and ALS.

8 Acute Neuromuscular Respiratory Failure

Check out thiamine and diabetes

Fig. 8.3 Algorithm for the triage and management of patients with Guillain-Barré syndrome

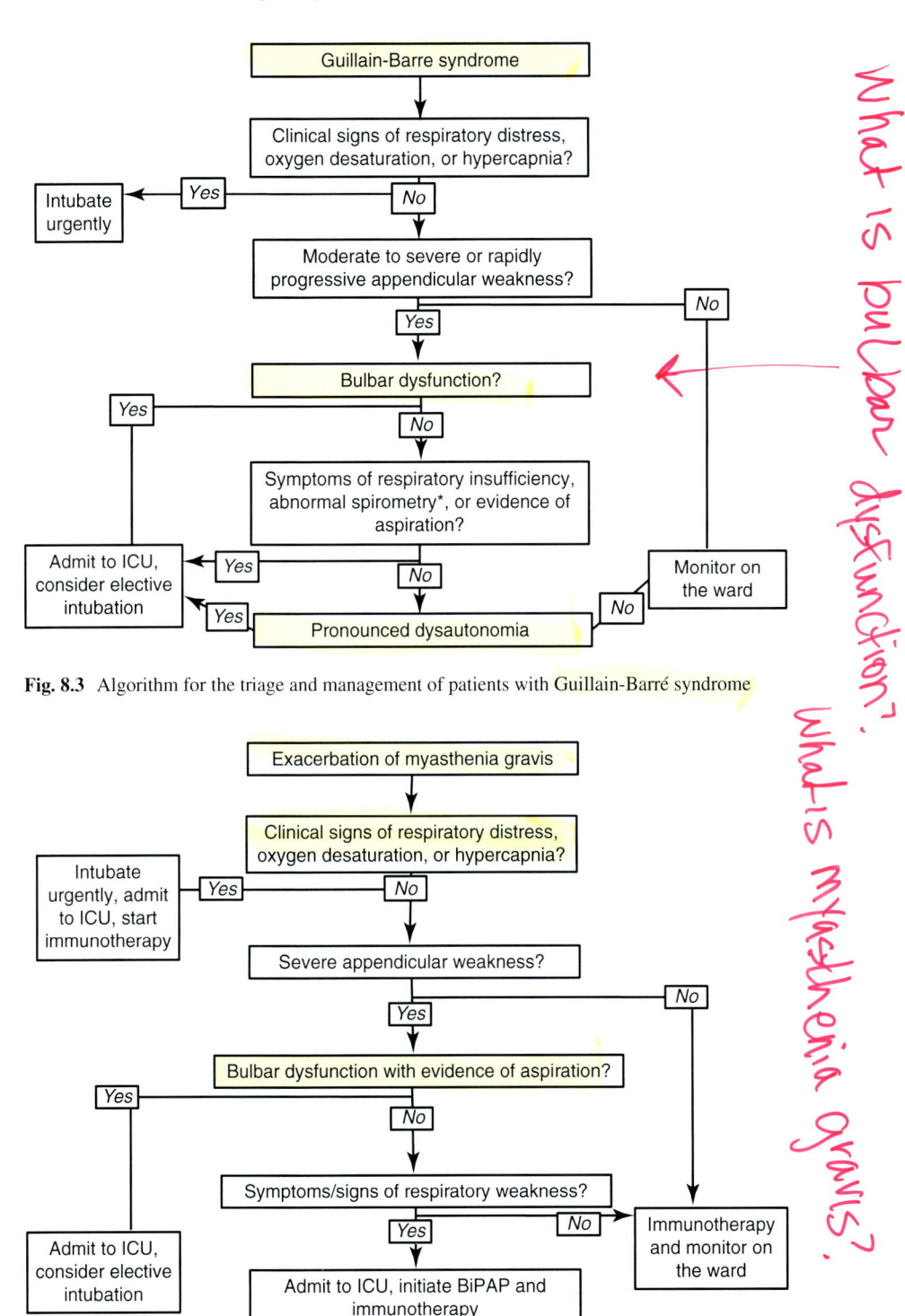

What is bulbar dysfunction?

Fig. 8.4 Algorithm for the triage and management of patients with exacerbation of myasthenia gravis. BiPAP bilevel positive airway pressure

What is myasthenia gravis?

Table 8.3 Factors associated with extubation success in patients with neuromuscular respiratory failure[a]

Improvement in extremity weakness with disease-modifying therapy[b]
Improvement in spirometry values with disease-modifying therapy
Low volume or respiratory secretions
Normal chest X-ray
Tolerates T-piece trial
MIP exceeding − 50 cm H_2O and VC improvement by 4 mL/kg from pre-intubation to pre-extubation
High MEP value, ability to cough up secretions
Low oxygen requirements ($FiO_2 < 40\%$)
Absence of fatigue, hypoxemia or hypercapnia with spontaneous breathing trials using low-pressure support (e.g., 5 mmHg)

MIP - maximal inspiratory pressure, *VC* - vital capacity, *MEP* - maximal expiratory pressure
[a]No single factor guarantees extubation success
[b]Some patients, particularly in GBS, will have improvement in respiratory weakness before extremity weakness and therefore improvement in extremity weakness should not be the sole criteria for extubation

Localization of the pathology can also narrow the differential diagnosis and is formulated using the physical exam. Distribution, severity, and fatigability of weakness, muscle tone, reflexes, presence and pattern of sensory abnormalities, presence of atrophy and fasciculations, and vital sign abnormalities (which may indicate dysautonomia) should be noted and utilized to localize the patient's symptoms within the neuraxis. Examples of etiologies of acute neuromuscular weakness are listed in Table 8.4 according to their localization [14]. Finally, a comprehensive review of systems and general physical exam can elucidate clues to the underlying etiology as well. Distinctive clinical features suggestive of specific conditions causing neuromuscular respiratory failure are summarized in Table 8.5 Diagnostic tests to confirm the diagnosis commonly include nerve conduction studies (NCS) and electromyography (EMG) with or without phrenic nerve and diaphragm evaluation, a basic metabolic panel, muscle enzymes, MG and GBS antibody testing in selected cases, lumbar puncture, brain and/or spine imaging, and nerve and/or muscle biopsy. The fact that patients in whom the underlying cause of the neuromuscular respiratory failure remains elusive generally have a poor prognosis provides justification for an exhaustive workup when the initial workup is unrevealing [15]. Summarized below are the most common causes of neuromuscular respiratory failure: GBS, MG, and CINM.

Guillain-Barré Syndrome

GBS is a monophasic acute inflammatory polyradiculoneuropathy characterized by ascending weakness and areflexia. It is thought to be caused by a humorally mediated autoimmune response against the myelin sheath and Schwann cells in acute inflammatory demyelinating polyneuropathy (AIDP) and the Miller-Fisher variants,

Table 8.4 Differential diagnosis for acute neuromuscular respiratory failure by localization within the peripheral nervous system

Anterior horn cell	ALS
	West Nile virus
	Polio and post-polio syndrome
	Kennedy disease
Peripheral nerve	Guillain-Barré syndrome
	Acute onset CIDP
	Vasculitic neuropathy
	Paraneoplastic neuropathy
	Malignant infiltration
	Critical illness polyneuropathy
	Porphyria
	Amyloid infiltration
	Phrenic nerve injury
	Toxins (e.g., tetrodotoxin)
Neuromuscular junction	Myasthenia gravis
	Prolonged neuromuscular junction blockade
	Botulism
	Organophosphate poisoning
	Lambert-Eaton myasthenic syndrome
	Tick paralysis
	Envenomation
Muscle	Critical illness myopathy
	Rhabdomyolysis
	Acid maltase deficiency
	Inflammatory myopathies
	Metabolic myopathies[a]
	Toxic necrotizing myopathies[b]
	Muscular dystrophy

[a]Hyperthyroidism, hypophosphatemia, hyperkalemia, hypokalemia, and hypernatremia
[b]Statins, colchicine

and against axolemmal surface antigens in acute motor (AMAN) and acute motor and sensory axonal polyneuropathy (AMSAN) variants. Molecular mimicry is implicated in the formation of autoantibodies and up to two-thirds of patients report a preceding infection, with the Zika virus being the most recently associated (see Table 8.6) [16]. The association of preceding diarrhea by *Campylobacter jejuni* with the development of AMAN is particularly well established.

Initial symptoms may be non-specific symmetric distal lower extremity dysesthesias or back pain that are typically followed by lower extremity weakness that often ultimately progresses to involve the upper extremities. This ascending pattern of weakness is characteristic, but neither pathognomonic nor necessary to make the diagnosis of GBS. Oropharyngeal weakness is seen in 50% of cases [1, 2]. Reflexes initially may be normal or increased, but then become depressed or absent. Ophthalmoplegia is more commonly present in the Miller-Fisher variant, along with ataxia. Neuropathic pain is present in most patients and may be severe.

Table 8.5 Key historical and exam features suggestive of a particular cause of neuromuscular respiratory failure

Guillain-Barré	Ascending weakness
	Dysautonomia
	Areflexia
	Recent infection, diarrhea, vaccination, travel to Zika-endemic area
	Acral paresthesia, neuropathic pain
	Ataxia (Miller-Fisher variant)
Myasthenia gravis	Fatiguable and fluctuating symptoms/signs
Vasculitis	Cutaneous manifestations (palpable purpura, petechiae, urticaria, ulcers, livedo reticularis, and nodules)
	Fever, arthralgias, hemoptysis
Malignant infiltration/paraneoplastic	"B symptoms" (i.e., fever, night sweats, sudden unintended weight loss),
	Known presence of malignancy
	Lymphadenopathy
Amyotrophic lateral sclerosis	Combination of upper and lower motor neuron findings
	Atrophy, fasciculations
Botulism	Descending weakness
	Dysautonomia
	Contaminated food product
West Nile virus	Exposure to endemic area
	Meningoencephalitis
	Lack of sensory nerve involvement
Porphyria	Gastrointestinal symptoms
	Dysautonomia
	Red urine
	Periodic "attacks"
Critical illness neuromyopathy	Multiorgan failure
	Sepsis
	Hyperglycemia
	Prolonged ventilation/vasopressor use
Prolonged neuromuscular blockade	Use of paralytic agents in the setting of renal and/or hepatic impairment
	No response on train of four testing
Organophosphate poisoning	History of exposure
	Hypersecretion
	Diarrhea, emesis
	Bronchospasm
	Bradycardia
	Miosis
Tick paralysis	Ascending paralysis
	History of tick exposure
Acid maltase deficiency	Progressive limb-girdle weakness
	Elevated creatinine kinase
	Family history (autosomal recessive inheritance)
Inflammatory/toxic necrotizing myopathy	Severely elevated creatinine kinase
	Cutaneous manifestations (dermatomyositis)
	Exposure to precipitating medications

Table 8.6 Common precipitants of Guillain-Barré syndrome[a]

Infections
Influenza
Campylobacter jejuni
Cytomegalovirus
Epstein-Barr virus
Mycoplasma pneumoniae
Zika virus
Hepatitis E
Human immunodeficiency virus
Vaccinations
Surgery
Thymectomy
Post-transplant
Malignancy
Lymphoma

[a]Despite the triggers listed, approximately one-third of GBS cases do not have an identifiable precipitant

Respiratory failure occurs in about 20–30% of patients and usually presents within a week of the onset of symptoms, though it is very rare in the Miller-Fisher variant [1]. Dysautonomia is present in up to two-thirds of patients and may result in variety of complications. Table 8.7 displays a list of systemic complications and those related to dysautonomia with their respective management. The diagnosis of GBS is clinical, but is supported by electrophysiology and cerebrospinal fluid analysis; the diagnostic findings consistent with the diagnosis of GBS are summarized in Table 8.8.

Recognition of signs of respiratory failure in patients with GBS should prompt intubation, especially in the presence of concomitant dysautonomia. Emergency intubation can be extremely dangerous in dysautonomic patients. Non-invasive ventilation is not a safe alternative in patients with GBS.

Immunomodulatory therapy with intravenous immunoglobulin(IVIG) or plasma exchange (PLEX) constitutes the standard of care for the treatment of GBS [3]. While the beneficial effect of IVIG and PLEX in GBS has been demonstrated when administered within 2 weeks of the onset of symptoms, it is imperative to initiate therapy as early as possible to minimize nerve damage. The choice of agent should be based on hospital and physician experience and side effect profile; Table 8.9 lists the recommend treatment regimens and side effects of IVIG and PLEX. However, despite treatment with IVIG or PLEX, approximately 10% of patients will experience treatment-related fluctuations (TRFs), defined as clinical worsening after initial improvement or stabilization secondary to a prolonged autoimmune response. Anecdotal evidence suggests that these patients may respond to additional courses of IVIG. Approximately half of the patients with TRFs will ultimately be diagnosed with chronic demyelinating polyneuropathy (CIDP), a steroid-responsive condition; two TRFs within 8 weeks of initial therapy or disease progression beyond 8 weeks is suggestive of this entity.

Systemic compilations are very common in GBS patients admitted to the ICU and stem from prolonged immobilization and mechanical ventilation, dysautono-

Table 8.7 Complications associated with Guillain-Barré syndrome by system and associated preventative measures and treatment

System	Complication	Prevention/treatment
Neuropsychiatric	Depression Anxiety Delirium Post-traumatic stress disorder Insomnia Neuropathic pain/dysesthesia	Encouragement Antidepressants (consider SNRI if concomitant neuropathic pain) Pharmacologic and non-pharmacologic sleep aids (avoid benzodiazepines) Gabapentin, pregabalin
Pulmonary	Ventilatory failure Pneumonia Aspiration Atelectasis Mucous plugging Tracheitis Need for tracheostomy with associated complications Pulmonary embolus	Monitoring for and treatment of neuromuscular respiratory failure Proper precautions during intubation if dysautonomia present Elective intubation, avoidance of emergent intubation Adequate tidal volume and PEEP Antibiotics Good pulmonary hygiene Monitoring for change in secretions DVT prophylaxis/anticoagulation
Cardiac	Hypertension Hypotension Blood pressure lability Tachycardia Tachyarrhythmia Bradycardia Atrioventricular block Asystole	Telemetry monitoring Arterial line placement for blood pressure monitoring Cautious treatment of blood pressure extremes with short-acting agents and/or conservative measures Low dose and careful titration of vasopressors Avoidance of nodal blocking agents Atropine at bedside Identification and avoidance of symptomatic vagal maneuvers Pacemaker implantation
Gastrointestinal	Gastroparesis Adynamic ileus Diarrhea Need for nasogastric/PEG tube placement/associated complications Gastric ulcers	Monitoring gastric residuals, frequency of bowel movements, and abdominal distention Aggressive bowel regimen Avoidance of metoclopramide and neostigmine if dysautonomia Minimize use of opiates (can worsen ileus) Gastric and/or rectal tube suctioning for ileus Parenteral nutrition if protracted intolerance of gastric feeding Identification and treatment of pathogen responsible for diarrhea Loperamide for diarrhea Stress ulcer prophylaxis

Table 8.7 (continued)

System	Complication	Prevention/treatment
Genitourinary	Urinary retention Incontinence	Intermittent or continuous bladder catheterization
Endocrinological	Hyponatremia/SIADH	Fluid restriction Hypertonic saline
Integumentary	Deep venous thrombosis (DVT) Pressure ulcers	DVT prophylaxis Mobilization/turning

SIADH syndrome of inappropriate secretion of antidiuretic hormone, *SNRI* serotonin-norepinephrine reuptake inhibitor

Table 8.8 Neuromuscular diseases and their key diagnostic findings

GBS	CSF:
	  Elevated protein without pleocytosis (i.e., albuminocytologic dissociation), though CSF may be normal early. Pleocytosis > 50 cells/microliter suggests alternative diagnosis
	Electrophysiology:
	  AIDP: Prolonged CMAP/SNAP conduction velocity and distal latencies, conduction block, temporal dispersion, and prolonged F waves, normal sural nerve testing
	  AMAN/AMSAN: Decreased CMAP amplitude (and SNAP amplitudes in AMSAN) without demyelinating features, absent F waves, reversible conduction block
	  May be normal early in disease course, abnormalities most pronounced at 2 weeks

MG	Serum antibody testing:
	  85% patients have antibodies to AChR
	  MuSK, LRP-4, and agrin testing can be positive in AChR seronegative patients
	Electrophysiology:
	  CMAP decrement > 10% on repetitive nerve stimulation
	  Increased jitter and blocking on single-fiber EMG (95% sensitive)

CINM	Electrophysiology
	  CIP: Reduced amplitude CMAP and SNAP without demyelinating features, neuropathic changes on EMG
	  CIM: Reduced amplitude CMAPs with prolonged durations, myopathic changes on EMG
	  Peroneal nerve test: two standard deviation drop in CMAP amplitude 100% sensitive but not specific for the diagnosis
	Direct muscle stimulation
	  Used to differentiate CIM and CIP (muscle contracts when stimulated in CIP but not in CIM)
	Muscle ultrasound:
	  Muscle atrophy and loss of muscle architecture
	Biopsy:
	  Muscle: myosin loss, loss of ATPase activity
	  Nerve: axonal degeneration

GBS Guillain-Barré syndrome, *MG* myasthenia gravis, *CINM* critical illness neuromyopathy, *CSF* cerebrospinal fluid, *CMAP* compound muscle action potential, *SNAP* sensory nerve action potential, *AIDP* acute inflammatory demyelinating polyneuropathy, *AMAN* acute motor axonal neuropathy, *AMSAN* acute motor and sensory axonal polyneuropathy, *AChR* acetylcholine receptor, *MuSK* muscle specific tyrosine kinase, *LRP-4* low-density lipoprotein receptor-related protein 4, *EMG* electromyography

Table 8.9 Comparison of possible adverse events with IV immunoglobulin and plasma exchange

IV immunoglobulin Dose: 2 g/kg divided into 5 doses of 0.4 g/kg or 2 doses of 1 g/kg	Plasma exchange Dose: 5 exchanges performed on alternating days

Infusion reaction
  Headache
  Shivering
  Myalgia
	Central venous catheter-related complications
	  Local hematoma
	  Pneumothorax
	  Line-related infection

Chest pain	Hypotension, possibly causing hemodynamic instability in setting of dysautonomia
Hyperviscosity with risk of arterial and venous thrombosis	Hemoconcentration from volume depletion
Aseptic meningitis	Mild coagulopathy
Acute kidney injury	Hypocalcemia
Anaphylaxis (if IgA deficient)	Removal of highly protein-bound medications
Transfusion reaction (including transfusion-related acute lung injury)	Transfusion reaction (including transfusion-related acute lung injury)

IgA immunoglobulin A, *IV* intravenous

mia, neuropathic pain, and depression. Pulmonary complications are most frequent, though diligent supportive care including pulmonary hygiene, nutrition, body rotation and mobilization, gastric and deep venous thrombosis prophylaxis, pain control with neuropathic agents (such as gabapentin, pregabalin, and duloxetine), and monitoring and treatment of depression can mitigate most of these issues (see Table 8.7).

Long-term disability with severe GBS is experienced by 20% of patients and 5% will die. Poor prognosis is associated with older age, evidence of axonal degeneration on electrophysiology, diarrhea at onset (related axonal GBS variants), and functional status at 2 weeks. However, hope for patients and families exists, as clinical improvement can occur for up to 3 years after the diagnosis and even patients with severe disease can make a full recovery.

Myasthenia Gravis

Myasthenia gravis (MG) is an autoimmune disease characterized by fatigable weakness secondary to disrupted neuromuscular junction transmission caused by antibodies against acetylcholine receptors (AChR) or muscle-specific tyrosine kinase (MuSK). MG is more commonly diagnosed in young adults and the elderly [3]. It is a chronic condition punctuated by acute and subacute exacerbations.

Proximal greater than distal limb, oropharyngeal, and/or respiratory weakness is seen in MG, though the hallmark clinical feature is fatigability, which can be revealed by repeated testing or clinical worsening at the end of the day. Superimposed signs of cholinergic toxicity are common in patients presenting with MG exacerbation, either because of prescribed changes or self-escalation of pyridostigmine dose and they are characteristically manifested by increased oral and respiratory secretions, lacrimation, diarrhea, and vomiting [1, 2]. Electrophysiology and serum antibody testing should be used to confirm the diagnosis of MG (Table 8.8). In addition, all newly diagnosed patients should have a CT of the chest to rule out associated thymus abnormalities. Thymectomy can improve the prognosis of the disease [17].

Myasthenic crisis is defined by the presence of neuromuscular respiratory failure. Timely initiation of non-invasive ventilator support with BiPAP – before the establishment of hypercapnia – can avert tracheal intubation with its inherent complications and reduce the duration of ICU and hospital stays [18]. When the patient is already frankly hypercapneic or a BiPAP trial fails to improve the respiratory failure, intubation is indicated.

Immunotherapy with IVIG or PLEX should be administered as soon as possible. Concomitant corticosteroid administration is also standard of care (such as prednisone 1mg/kg of ideal body weight, though ideal dose is not established), however, caution must be exercised when starting or escalating corticosteroid dosing in non-intubated patients as steroids can provoke transient exacerbation of the muscle weakness [19, 20], in addition to other medications (Table 8.10). Rituximab may be an effective option in refractory cases, especially among patients with MuSK antibodies [21]. Cholinesterase inhibitors should be held in intubated patients until ventilator weaning begins, but should be continued in patients on non-invasive ventilation. Steroid sparing agents, such as mycophenolate mofetil and azathioprine are often initiated prior to discharge to prevent recurrent crises.

Many patients with MG improve rapidly after initiation of therapy; however, some patients (particularly elderly individuals) may require more prolonged intubation. Fortunately, mortality in myasthenic crisis has declined from 30% to ≤5% over the last few decades, in great part thanks to advances in critical care.

Table 8.10 Medications that may exacerbate myasthenia gravis

Anesthetic agents	Erythromycin	Class 1a antiarrhythmics
Isoflurane	Aminoglycosides	Quinidine
Halothane	Gentamycin	Procainamide
Bupivacaine	Tobramycin	Disopyramide
Lidocaine	Amikacin	Glucocorticoids
Procaine	Nitrofurantoin	Neuromuscular blockers
Interferon	Anticonvulsants	Depolarizing: succinylcholine
D-Penicillamine	Carbamazepine	Nondepolarizing: Vecuronium, rocuronium
Tetracyclines	Ethosuximide	Checkpoint inhibitors
Doxycycline	Gabapentin	Pembrolizumab
Tetracycline	Phenobarbital	Nivolumab
Macrolides	Phenytoin	Ipilimumab
Azithromycin	Psychiatric drugs	
Clarithromycin	Haloperidol	
Ketolide	Chlorpromazine	
Telithromycin	Prochlorpromazine	
Fluoroquinolones	Lithium	
Ciprofloxacin	Magnesium	
Levofloxacin	Atorvastatin	

Critical Illness Neuromyopathy

Despite substantial improvements in mortality for patients with sepsis and critical illness over the last decade, up to 70% of critically ill patients will have lingering disability, in large part due to ICU acquired weakness (ICUAW). While muscle atrophy from deconditioning may play a role in the development of ICUAW, critical illness myopathy (CIM), critical illness polyneuropathy (CIP), and the common co-occurrence of both conditions, termed critical illness neuromyopathy (CINM), are most commonly the cause. CINM is speculated to result from the downstream effects of systemic inflammation. The most prominently associated risk factors are sepsis and multiorgan failure.

CIP is a length-dependent sensorimotor axonal polyneuropathy. CIM is characterized by preferential loss of myosin filaments, reduced ATPase activity, and muscle inexcitability secondary to a sodium channelopathy. CINM most commonly presents as flaccid quadriparesis with failure to wean from mechanical ventilation, though the pattern of weakness, reflexes, and sensory symptoms vary depending on the proportion and severity of CIP and CIM [22]. ICUAW is a clinical diagnosis, but diagnostic studies can be used for confirmation (Table 8.8).

Currently, there are no specific therapies for CINM. A bundle of interventions that include minimizing sedation, spontaneous breathing trials, and early rehabilitation (started as soon as possible in the ICU) has been associated with increased rates of functional independence, shorter length of stay, and lower mortality [23]. In patients who cannot be mobilized, active and passive cycle ergometry and muscle stimulation show promise for improving disability, though further study is necessary. Intensive insulin therapy (blood glucose target 80–110mg/dL) reduces the incidence of CINM, but is offset by the associated higher incidence of dangerous hypoglycemic events [22].

CINM is independently associated with higher short- and long-term mortality and with greater physical disability and poorer quality of life in survivors. Elderly patients and CIP-predominant cases have a less favorable outcome, though younger patients and less severe patients can enjoy a full recovery.

Cardinal Messages
- Normal ventilation depends on the ability to maintain adequate tidal volume and respiratory rate with the diaphragm and accessory muscles, manage secretions with the oropharyngeal muscles, and clear secretions with the abdominal and internal intercostal muscles.
- Neuromuscular respiratory failure can result from any disease that causes weakness of bulbar and respiratory muscles.
- Patients with neuromuscular respiratory failure typically develop progressive atelectasis and decreased tidal volume; once compensatory mechanisms (recruitment of accessory muscles, increased respiratory rate) are overwhelmed, hypoxemic and hypercapnic respiratory failure ensues.

- The diagnosis of neuromuscular respiratory failure is primarily clinical, but arterial blood gases, chest films, bedside spirometry, and diaphragmatic ultrasound can be valuable tools in the early assessment of these patients.
- Aggressive pulmonary hygiene to prevent aspiration and consideration of the need for ventilatory support with invasive or non-invasive ventilation, deployed in accordance with the degree of neuromuscular weakness and ability to manage secretions are essential in the initial management of patients with neuromuscular respiratory failure.
- ICU admission or transfer should be considered for patients with severe oropharyngeal or rapidly progressing appendicular weakness, dysautonomia, signs of respiratory insufficiency, or abnormal chest X-ray.
- Ideally, intubation should be performed electively in patients with neuromuscular respiratory failure, particularly those with dysautonomia, to prevent complications associated with emergent intubation.
- GBS and MG are the two most common causes of primary neuromuscular respiratory failure and disease-modifying immunotherapy should be initiated as soon as possible in both conditions.
- CINM is the most common cause of secondary neuromuscular respiratory therapy; while it does not have any specific treatment, sedation holidays with spontaneous breathing trials and early physical therapy can improve prognosis.
- While the ultimate prognosis in patients with neuromuscular respiratory failure depends on the underlying etiology, patients with an identified and treatable cause have the potential to regain functional independence with appropriate therapy and meticulous ICU care.

References

1. Wijdicks EFM. The neurology of acutely failing respiratory mechanics. Ann Neurol. 2017;81:485–94.
2. Wijdicks EFM. Management of acute neuromuscular disorders. Handb Clin Neurol. 2017;140(3):229–37.
3. Rabinstein AA. Acute neuromuscular respiratory failure. Continuum. 2015;21(5):1324–45.
4. Howard RS. Respiratory failure because of neuromuscular disease. Curr Opin Neurol. 2016;29(5):592–601.
5. Irfan M, Selim B, Rabinstein AA, St. Louis EK. Neuromuscular disorders and sleep in critically ill patients. Crit Care Clin. 2015;31(3):533–50.
6. Cabrera Serrano M, Rabinstein AA. Usefulness of pulmonary function tests and blood gases in acute neuromuscular respiratory failure. Eur J Neurol. 2012;19(3):452–6.
7. Lawn ND, Fletcher DD, Henderson RD, Wolter TD, Wijdicks EF. Anticipating mechanical ventilation in Guillain-Barre syndrome. Arch Neurol. 2001;58(6):893–8.
8. Walterspacher S, Kirchberger A, Lambeck J, et al. Respiratory muscle assessment in acute Guillain-Barre syndrome. Lung. 2016;194:821–8.
9. Kramer CL, McCullough M, Wijdicks EF. Teaching video neuroimages: how to unmask respiratory strength confounded by facial diplegia. Neurology. 2015;84:e57–8.

10. Boon AJ, O'Gorman C. Ultrasound in the assessment of respiration. J Clin Neurophysiol. 2016;33:112–9.
11. Rabinstein AA. Non-invasive ventilation for neuromuscular respiratory failure: when to use and when to avoid. Curr Opin Crit Care. 2016;22(2):94–9.
12. Walgaard C, Lingsma HF, van Doorn PA, et al. Tracheostomy or not: prediction of prolonged mechanical ventilation in Guillain-Barre syndrome. Neurocrit Care. 2017;26:6–13.
13. Lawn ND, Wijdicks EF. Post-intubation pulmonary function test in Guillain-Barre syndrome. Muscle Nerve. 2000;23:613–6.
14. Caulfield AF, Flower O, Pineda JA, Uddin S. Emergency neurological life support: acute non-traumatic weakness. Neurocrit Care. 2017;27(Suppl 1):29–50.
15. Cabrera Serrano M, Rabinstein AA. Causes and outcomes of acute neuromuscular respiratory failure. Arch Neurol. 2010;67(9):1089–94.
16. Mier-Y-Teran-Romero L, Delorey MJ, Sejvar JJ, Johansson MA. Guillain–Barré syndrome risk among individuals infected with Zika virus: a multi-country assessment. BMC Med. 2018;16(1):67.
17. Wolfe GI, Kaminski HJ, Aban IB, Minisman G, Kuo HC, et al; MGTX Study Group. Randomized trial of thymectomy in myasthenia gravis. N Engl J Med. 2016;375(6):511–22.
18. Seneviratne J, Mandrekar J, Wijdicks EF, Rabinstein AA. Predictors of extubation failure in myasthenic crisis. Arch Neurol. 2008;65(7):929–33.
19. Sanders DB, Wolfe GI, Benatar M, et al. International consensus guidance for management of myasthenia gravis: executive summary. Neurology. 2016;87(4):419–25.
20. Farmakidis C, Pasnoor M, Dimachkia MM, Barohn RJ. Treatment of myasthenia gravis. Neurol Clin. 2018;36:311–37.
21. Iorio R, Damato V, Alboini PE, Evoli A. Efficacy and safety of rituximab for myasthenia gravis: a systematic review and meta-analysis. J Neurol. 2015;262(5):1115–9.
22. Kramer CL. Intensive care unit-acquired weakness. Neurol Clin. 2017;35(4):723–36.
23. Pun BT, Balas MC, Barnes-Daly MA, Thompson JL, Aldrich JM, Barr J, et al. Caring for critically ill patients with the ABCDEF bundle: results of the ICU liberation collaborative in over 15,000 adults. Crit Care Med. 2019;47(1):3–14.

Chapter 9
Acute Ischemic Stroke

Maximiliano A. Hawkes and Alejandro A. Rabinstein

Diagnostic Keys
- Assessment of time of symptom onset and stroke severity.
- Exclusion of brain hemorrhage and assessment of irreversible brain damage with emergency CT scan.
- CT angiography to identify candidates for endovascular treatment in the early time window (6 hours).
- CT perfusion (or MRI diffusion/perfusion) to identify candidates for endovascular treatment in the extended time window (6–24 hours).

Treatment Priorities
- Rapid reperfusion of the ischemic brain tissue.
- Prevention of secondary brain injury and early diagnosis of potential complications.
- Early initiation of the appropriate secondary prevention treatment.

M. A. Hawkes (✉)
Departments of Neurology and Internal Medicine, FLENI, Buenos Aires, Argentina
e-mail: mhawkes@fleni.org

A. A. Rabinstein
Department of Neurology, Mayo Clinic, Neuroscience ICU, Rochester, MN, USA

> **Prognosis at a Glance**
> - Stroke is a leading cause of death and disability worldwide.
> - Prognosis mainly depends on timely reperfusion of the ischemic brain.
> - Prevention of secondary brain injury and early stroke recurrence in a dedicated stroke unit also improve outcomes.

Introduction

Since the approval of intravenous thrombolysis (IVT) in 1995, the treatment of acute ischemic stroke has dramatically changed. More recently, the development of more effective endovascular reperfusion devices has allowed to effectively treat patients with occlusions of proximal intracranial vessels. Advanced imaging (CT perfusion and MR diffusion/perfusion) allows to identify who may benefit from reperfusion therapies up to 24 hours after symptoms onset. Following treatment with reperfusion therapies, patients should be carefully monitored in a dedicated stroke unit for the prevention, early detection and treatment of potential complications. After the hyperacute phase, the identification of the underlying stroke mechanism should guide the institution of an appropriate secondary stroke prevention regimen. Modern evaluation and management of stroke patients have become a complex task that requires a multidisciplinary team needs under constant training. In this chapter, we provide an evidence-based, yet practical approach, to the initial evaluation and treatment of acute stroke patients.

Pathophysiology of Acute Stroke

The understanding of three basic pathophysiologic concepts is essential to optimize the evaluation and treatment of patients with acute ischemic stroke.

Ischemic Core and Penumbra

The immediate consequences of an arterial occlusion in the downstream brain tissue are heterogeneous. There is an area of irreversible brain damage (core) surrounded by hypoperfused and non-functioning but salvageable tissue (penumbra). Advanced brain imaging (CTP perfusion or MRI diffusion/perfusion) can delineate core and penumbra. The penumbra has a variable outcome; transition to irreversible brain damage is mainly determined by the severity and duration of ischemia and the quality of collateral blood flow [1]. Thus, early recanalization and enhancement of collateral circulation are high priorities of acute stroke treatment.

Collateral Circulation

Collateral circulation is a subsidiary network of vascular channels that may provide enough flow to the affected tissue to prevent critical ischemia when the main artery is compromised [2]. In other words, collateral flow supports the viability of the ischemic penumbra. Collateral status differs across patients; it is often tenuous and can sustain brain viability only for a limited period of time. Collateral flow can be supported by avoiding blood pressure drops, and possibly, by administering intravenous fluids. Hemodynamic augmentation with vasopressors may be beneficial in well-selected cases (such as patients with cervical internal carotid artery occlusion without tandem intracranial occlusion), but the safety and efficacy of this strategy remain largely unknown [3]. Keeping the head of the bed flat in an attempt to improve collateral flow and patients' outcomes was not beneficial in the head position in Stroke Trial (HeadPoST) [4] and this intervention may increase the risk of aspiration, especially in patients with decreased level of consciousness and dysphagia. Yet, lowering the head of the bed may be helpful as a bridging alternative in selected patients with critical cerebral ischemia.

Secondary Brain Damage

Several neuroprotective treatments have failed to improve outcomes in acute stroke patients. However, secondary brain insults such as hypoglycemia, hypoxemia, and fever worsen stroke patients' outcomes by exacerbating the biochemical disturbances of the ischemic brain. Hence, avoiding them can be considered neuroprotection. Hypoglycemia exacerbates energy failure and should be avoided. Hyperglycemia also worsens stroke patients' outcomes. Current guidelines recommend to maintain a glycemia between 140 and 180 mg/dL [5]. Tighter glycemic control (80–130 mg/dL) proved ineffective to improve functional outcomes in the Stroke Hyperglycemia Insulin Network Effort (SHINE) trial [6]. Fever is also associated with poorer outcomes. Underlying mechanisms include increased brain metabolic demand, excitotoxicity, free-radical production, blood–brain barrier breakdown, and proteolysis. The routine administration of paracetamol to acute stroke patients does not improve outcomes, but treating fevers showed some benefits in the Paracetamol (Acetaminophen) Stroke (PAIS) trial [7]. A trial evaluating a higher dose of paracetamol is ongoing. The rate of oxygen extraction is increased in the area of penumbra, thus, providing adequate oxygen to avoid hypoxemia is recommended.

Evaluation in the Emergency Department

Sudden onset focal neurological symptoms should be regarded as secondary to ischemic stroke until proven otherwise. This situation should be considered a "brain code" and patients must be evaluated in the emergency department with maximal priority. After ruling out hemorrhage with neuroimaging, establishing the time of symptoms onset allows to decide whether the patient is a candidate for any reperfusion treatment: IVT, mechanical thrombectomy (typically with a retrievable stent) or both.

The effectiveness of reperfusion treatments decrease and the risk of serious side effects increase over time. Thus, a speedy response of the stroke team is crucial. The main metrics are the door-to-needle time for IVT and door-to-groin time for endovascular procedures. IVT within 60 minutes of arrival is associated with lower in-hospital mortality and lower rates of symptomatic intracranial hemorrhage. For every 15-minute reduction in door-to-needle time, there is a 5% reduction in in-hospital mortality [8].

Practical Steps for Initial Evaluation

Secure Airway, Breathing, and Circulation (ABC)

- Insert two peripheral lines. At least one 16G line is recommended for IV contrast studies.
- Supplementary oxygen to ensure an oxygen saturation >94%.
- Cardiac and blood pressure monitoring. Blood pressure should be stable below 185/110 mm/Hg in order to start IVT. Avoid hypotension.

A Brief Questionnaire Focusing on

- *Time of symptoms onset.* If the exact time is not known, the last known normal time should be recorded.
- *Past medical history of potential stroke mimickers*, e.g., epilepsy, migraine with aura, use of insulin or oral hypoglycemic drugs, psychiatric diseases, brain tumors, etc.
- *Vascular risk factors:* when present they increase the likelihood of stroke as a cause of symptoms.
- *Current medications* with especial focus on anticoagulants. If the patient was on an anticoagulant, the dose, indication, and time of last dose should be recorded.
- *Contraindications for intravenous thrombolysis* (Table 9.1). The exclusion criteria originally used in the NINDS trial have changed over time in light of safety data from stroke registries which demonstrated the safety of alteplase (recombinant tissue plasminogen activator or rtPA) in patients originally excluded from clinical trials. Currently, there are only a few absolute contraindications. The decision of giving alteplase should be based on the risk/benefit equation in individualized patients.

9 Acute Ischemic Stroke

Table 9.1 Contraindications for intravenous thrombolysis [5]

Acute head trauma or severe head trauma within 3 months	Extensive hypoattenuation or hemorrhage on head CT
Ischemic stroke within 3 months (if large)	SBP > 185 mm Hg or DBP > 110 mm Hg and cannot be lowered safely
Previous ICH	Known bleeding diathesis
Suspected SAH	INR >1.7
Intracerebral tumor	Heparin within 48 hours with abnormal activated partial thromboplastin time or therapeutic dose of low molecular weight heparin within 24 hours
Intracranial or intraspinal surgery within 3 months	Platelets <100,000/mm³
Active internal bleeding	Current use of direct thrombin inhibitor or factor Xa inhibitor (unless not received for >48 hours or appropriate coagulation tests exclude ongoing anticoagulation)
GI malignancy or serious GI bleeding within 3 months	
Aortic dissection	
Infective endocarditis	

SBP systolic blood pressure, *DBP* diastolic blood pressure, *INR* international normalized ratio, *AVM* arteriovenous malformation, *ICH* intracranial hemorrhage, *SAH* subarachnoid hemorrhage

Physical Examination

The examination should be rapid and focused. The National Institute of Health Stroke Scale (NIHSS) is a validated tool developed for this purpose (http://www.nihstrokescale.org). Beyond calculating a number, the neurologist should decide if the symptoms are disabling for the individual patient. A rapid general examination is useful to find signs of head trauma, infectious endocarditis and coagulopathies, especially in those cases in which no reliable history can be obtained.

Additional Tests

After ruling out a history of coagulopathy with the anamnesis, hypoglycemia and hemorrhagic stroke on brain CT, the initiation of IV alteplase should not be delayed while waiting for the result of additional testing.

- Brain CT: Non-contrast brain CT is necessary to differentiate between ischemic and hemorrhagic stroke. Once hemorrhage has been excluded, this scan also allows to identify patients with a low chance for recovery and a high chance for hemorrhagic complications with IVT (e.g., hypodensity of more than one-third of the MCA) and to find alternative diagnoses (e.g., brain tumor). In patients with a NIHSS of 6 or greater (or a high suspicion for proximal artery occlusion), the intracranial arteries should be studied with CT angiogram, MR angiogram, or catheter angiography in order to select candidates for mechanical thrombectomy.

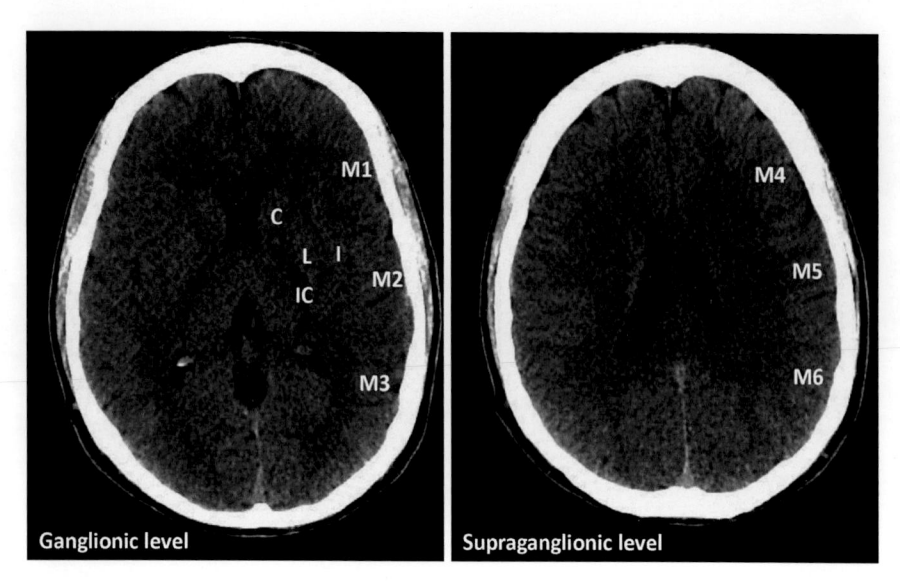

Fig. 9.1 The Alberta Stroke Program Early CT Score (ASPECTS)

Early ischemic changes can be quantified using the Alberta Stroke Program Early CT Score (ASPECTS) [9]. An ASPECTS of 10 corresponds to a normal CT scan. In patients with acute stroke, 1 point should be subtracted for each one of 10 predefined regions when early ischemic change exists (Fig. 9.1). Lower ASPECTS correlates with larger ischemic damage.
- Capillary glycemia: Hypoglycemia is a potential stroke mimicker and should be corrected before deciding to proceed with any reperfusion therapy.
- Coagulation and platelets: It is highly unlikely to find abnormal laboratory tests values in patients with no history of hemorrhagic diathesis. Thus, if the past medical history is negative for coagulation disorders, the initiation of IV alteplase should not be delayed while waiting laboratory results. Yet, it is prudent to wait for these results in those patients in whom a history cannot be appropriately obtained. Patients receiving warfarin can receive IV rtPA within 3 hours of symptom onset if the international normalized ratio (INR) is 1.7 or less. Per current guidelines, IV alteplase should be held in patients receiving warfarin who present within the 3–4.5 hours window. Patients with platelet count lower than 100,000 per mm^3 should not receive alteplase. Neither adequate safety data nor reliable laboratory studies to quantify the degree of anticoagulation are available for patients on direct oral anticoagulants (DOACs, dabigatran, rivaroxaban, apixaban, and edoxaban). Thus, it is most prudent to withhold thrombolysis in these patients. However, anticoagulated patients with proximal intracranial artery occlusion may benefit from mechanical thrombectomy regardless of whether they are on warfarin or DOACs.

With all these data the clinician should be able to decide on the most appropriate reperfusion therapy. Figure 9.2 provides an algorithm for guidance.

9 Acute Ischemic Stroke

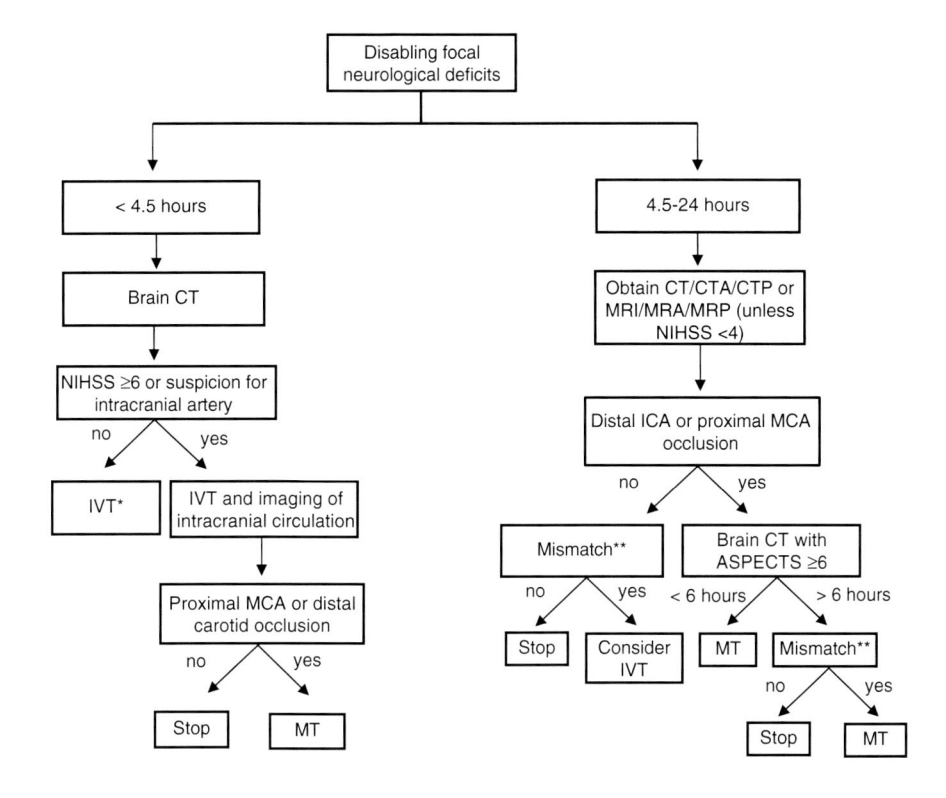

Fig. 9.2 Selecting candidates for reperfusion therapies in acute ischemic stroke

IVT, intravenous thrombolysis; MT, mechanical thrombectomy

*Additional restrictions apply for the 3-4.5 hour window

** Candidates for IVT in the extended window should be selected according to the following criteria:
WAKE-UP trial criteria (4.5-24-hour window): Infarct in DWI with no FLAIR correlation.
EXTEND trial criteria (4.5-9-hour window): Ischemic core mismatch was defined as a ratio greater than 1.2 between the volume of penumbra/core > 1.2, penumbra at least 10 ml greater than the core and ischemic ischemic-core volume < 70 ml.

*** Candidates for MT in the extended window should be selected according to on othe two following criteria:
DAWN trial criteria : >80 year-old if NIHSS ≥10 and core < 20 cc; < 80 year-old if NIHSS ≥10 and core < 30 cc or if NIHSS ≥20 and core 31-50 cc.
DEFUSE 3: core < 70 cc, core/penumbra >1.8, mismatch volume >15 cc.

Intravenous Thrombolysis

In 1995, the NINDS study showed that IV alteplase administered within 3 hours of stroke symptom onset increases the chances of functional independence at 3 months by one-third [10]. A second landmark was the publication of the ECASS 3 trial in 2009 [11]. With its results, the therapeutic window for IV alteplase was expanded up to 4.5 hours. The number necessary to treat to help one more patient achieve functional independence increases from 3.6 within the first 90 minutes to 4.3 between 91 and 180 minutes and to 5.9 from 181 to 270 minutes, highlighting the time-dependent benefit of brain reperfusion ("time is brain") [12] Thereafter, numerous data from stroke registries have expanded our knowledge on the efficacy and safety profile of IV alteplase.

Patients with Mild or Improving Symptoms and Relative Contraindications: A Judgment Call

Deciding whether to administer IVT in patients with mild or improving symptoms and those with relative contraindications is challenging. Observational data have shown that one-third of patients with mild or rapidly improving symptoms in whom thrombolysis was held were eventually disabled at 3 months [13]. Recently, the Effect of Alteplase vs Aspirin on Functional Outcome for Patients With Acute Ischemic Stroke and Minor Nondisabling Neurologic Deficits (PRISMS) trial randomized 313 patients with nondisabling acute ischemic stroke to receive alteplase vs. aspirin. There was no increase in the likelihood of a favorable functional outcome at 90 days with IVT. However, the study was stopped early because of slow recruitment and this precludes any definitive conclusions [14]. Until more conclusive data are available, the decision of whether to proceed with IVT in these situations should be individualized. Yet, if symptoms are causing disability at the time of the evaluation in the emergency department, we favor treatment with IV alteplase even if the symptoms are relatively mild or appear to be getting better.

IV Alteplase Administration

The total dose of IV alteplase is 0.9 mg/kg (do not exceed 90 mg); 10% as a 1-minute bolus and 90% as a 60-minute infusion. Subsequently, the patient should be monitored in a stroke unit or neuroscience ICU for at least 24 hours. IVT should not be delayed until the patient is transferred to such environments. Moreover, hospitals with no stroke capabilities can start the treatment while transfering the patient to a primary or comprehensive stroke center with stroke capabilities (drip-and-ship strategy). When not available, a stroke neurologist can assist with the therapeutic decision via telemedicine.

A lower dose of IV alteplase (0.6 mg/kg) administered within 4.5 hours of stroke onset did not meet the endpoint of non-inferiority when compared to standard dose alteplase in the ENCHANTED trial [15]. Tenecteplase has a longer life than alteplase which allows its administration as a single bolus. Tenecteplase at a dose of 0.4 mg/kg failed to prove superiority over alteplase 0.9 mg/kg in patients with mild stroke, though both drugs had a similar safety profile [16]. Yet, the efficacy and safety profile of tenecteplase still needs to be confirmed in patients with mild stroke and better studied in patients with more severe strokes.

Complications of IV Alteplase Infusion

The most feared complication of IVT is intracranial hemorrhage. The original studies that supported the approval of this therapy showed a total rate of intracranial hemorrhage of 6%, being symptomatic (causing deterioration of at least 4 points in the NIHSS) in about 4% [10]. Data from stroke registries and newer clinical trials showed that this number is probably lower (as low as 1.9% in some studies, depending on the definition of symptomatic ICH) [17].

When sudden neurologic decline, severe hypertension or vomiting occurs during alteplase infusion, the infusion should be immediately stopped and a CT scan should be emergently obtained. The treatment of symptomatic intracranial hemorrhage post IVT consists of control of hypertension (systolic target 140–160 mm Hg) and reversal of the fibrinolytic effect (Fig. 9.3). Orolingual angioedema occurs in 1.3–5% of patients who receive alteplase. It usually presents as a transient and self-limited swelling of the lips and tongue contralateral to the stroke. It is more common in patients with strokes affecting the insula and in those taking angiotensin-converting enzyme inhibitors. The most severe cases can compromise airway patency; thus, careful monitoring is indispensable. Treatment consists of a combination of diphenhydramine (50 mg IV), ranitidine (50 mg IV), and dexamethasone (10 mg IV). Emergent intubation and epinephrine may be needed in serious cases.

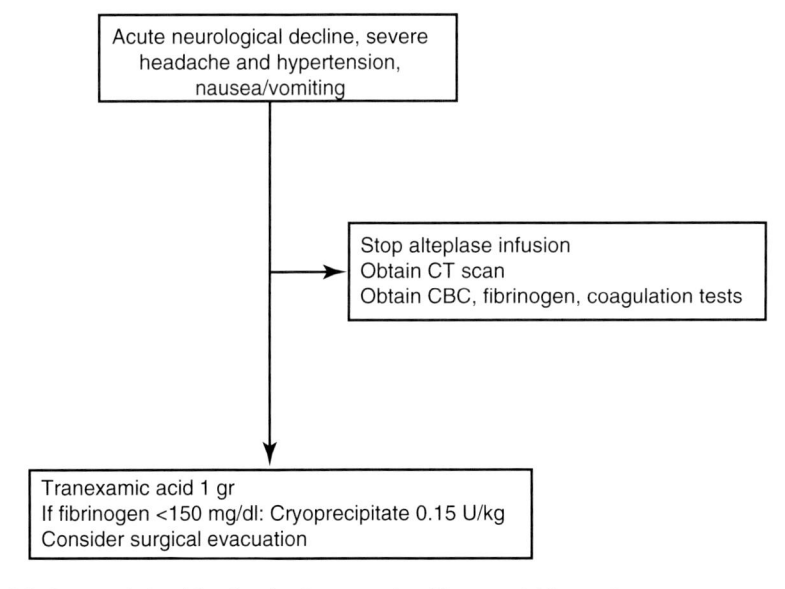

Fig. 9.3 Proposed algorithm for alteplase-associated intracranial hemorrhage

Mechanical Thrombectomy

Intravenous thrombolysis is poorly effective to open proximal occlusions of the major intracranial arteries and carotid bifurcation by large clots. These cases represent up to one-third of anterior circulation strokes and are associated with a poor prognosis. Detailed meta-analysis of multiple randomized controlled trials demonstrate that mechanical opening of the occluded vessel, generally with stent retrievers and in addition to IVT when indicated, allow 46% of treated patients to regain functional independence (relative benefit of 19%; odds ratio 2.35 [95% confidence intervals 1.85–2.98]; number necessary to treat of 2.8–3) [18]. The clinical trials that demonstrated the effectiveness of mechanical thrombectomy used different inclusion criteria and have been extensively reviewed elsewhere, but most of the patients enrolled in the initial trials of endovascular stroke therapy were treated within 6 hours of symptom onset [3]. Selection criteria proposed by the American Heart Association guidelines are presented in (Table 9.2) [5].

The fact that a patient is a candidate for endovascular treatment should not delay the infusion of alteplase when there are no contraindications. In one trial of patients with stroke symptoms from proximal artery occlusions, tenecteplase (0.25 mg/kg) was superior to alteplase in achieving recanalization of the occluded vessel and it was also associated with better functional outcomes at 3 months [19]. Yet, further studies are necessary to support the use of tenecteplase rather than alteplase in these cases before a change in practice can be broadly recommended.

Patients with basilar artery occlusion have been systematically excluded from randomized controlled trials testing IVT or mechanical thrombectomy. However, given the very poor prognosis of this type of stroke when reperfusion is not achieved, IVT and mechanical thrombectomy should be strongly considered.

Table 9.2 Criteria for mechanical thrombectomy

Candidates for acute endovascular stroke therapy
Age ≥ 18 years
NIHSS score ≥ 6
Good pre-stroke functional status (mRS 0–1)
ASPECTS score ≥ 6 on baseline CT scan
Presence of proximal intracranial artery occlusion (proximal MCA or distal ICA)
Time from symptom onset to groin puncture <6 hours (up to 24 hours if large mismatch between core and penumbra documented by neuroimaging)

ASPECTS Alberta Stroke Program Early CT Score, *CT* computed tomography, *NIHSS* National Institutes of Health Stroke Scale, *mRS* modified Rankin Scale, *MCA* middle cerebral artery, *ICA* internal carotid artery

Patients with Unknown Time of Onset and Extended Window Beyond 6 Hours

Two clinical trials have demonstrated that a subgroup of patients with proximal intracranial artery occlusion with unknown time of onset or symptoms for more than 6 hours may benefit from mechanical thrombectomy when carefully selected by advanced imaging (see Fig. 9.2 for specific selection criteria). An illustrative example of CT perfusion is displayed in Fig. 9.4.

The DAWN trial enrolled patients with terminal carotid or proximal MCA occlusion and a mismatch between clinical deficits and brain infarct (assessed by DWI or CT perfusion) who were last known normal 6–24 hours before presentation. The rate of functional independence at 90 days among patients randomized to mechanical thrombectomy was 49% compared to 13% in the standard medical therapy alone [20].

Similarly, the DEFUSE 3 trial randomized patients presenting between 6 and 16 hours from symptom onset (or last known normal time) with proximal intracranial artery occlusion and salvageable brain tissue assessed by CT perfusion or MRI DWI/perfusion to undergo mechanical thrombectomy vs. standard therapy alone. Patients in the mechanical thrombectomy group were more likely to be functionally independent at 90 days (45% vs. 17%) and also had a trend toward a lower mortality (14% vs. 26%) [21].

Intravenous alteplase may also have a role in patients with unknown time of onset. The MRI-Guided Thrombolysis for Stroke with Unknown Time of Onset (WAKE UP) trial randomized patients who had an unknown time of stroke onset with an ischemic lesion visible on DWI but no parenchymal hyperintensity on

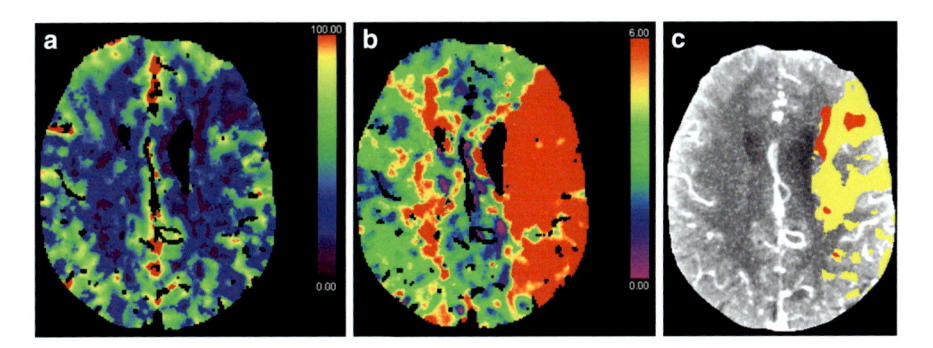

Fig. 9.4 Patient who awoke with aphasia and right hemiparesis. CT perfusion showed a mismatch between (**a**) the area of reduced cerebral blood flow (less than 30% than the contralateral region representing the ischemic core) and (**b**) the area with delayed arrival of contrast (time to maximum of the residue function [Tmax] greater than 6 seconds representing the region affected by hypoperfusion) as illustrated by the combined map (**c**) were the ischemic core is depicted in red and hypoperfusion is shown in yellow

FLAIR to receive alteplase or placebo. Those patients who received alteplase were more likely to have no disability at 90 days compared to those who did not (53.3% vs. 41.8%). There were no statistical differences in the rate of symptomatic ICH or death between the two groups [22].

More recently, the EXTEND trial randomized patients with salvageable brain tissue between 4.5 and 9 hours after stroke symptoms onset or wake-up stroke (if within 9 hours from the midpoint of sleep) to receive alteplase or placebo. Salvageable brain tissue could be measured by DWI-weighted MRI-MR perfusion or CT perfusion (Fig. 9.2). Additional inclusion criteria were minimal previous disability (mRS <2) and a stroke severity between 4 and 26 points in the NIHSS. The trial was terminated with 72% of the planned recruitment because of a loss of equipoise after the publication of the WAKE-UP trial. The primary outcome (no disability with or without residual symptoms [mRS 0–1] at 90 days) occurred in 35.4% and 29.5% of patients in the alteplase and placebo groups, respectively. Symptomatic ICH was more frequent in the alteplase group (6.2% vs 0.9%) [23]. These results, along with those of the ECASS4 and EPITHET trials, were included in a meta-analysis of individual patient data. Again, patients who received alteplase were more likely to have no disability (mRS 0–1) at 90 days (36% vs 29%) with an excess of symptomatic ICH (5% vs <1%). Yet, this excess did not negate the benefit of IVT [24].

Care After Reperfusion Therapy

- *Admission to a stroke unit* reduces mortality by 13%, mortality or institutionalization by 22% and mortality or dependency by 21%, without increasing hospital length of stay [25].
- *Continuous cardiac monitoring* allows to diagnose paroxysmal atrial fibrillation and other arrhythmic complications. Atrial fibrillation is a leading cause of stroke, especially in older patients.
- Keeping the head of the bed flat may improve collateral flow in selected patients as explained above. Patients with dysphagia, decreased level of consciousness or early brain edema may benefit with the head of the bed at 30° to prevent aspiration and intracranial hypertension.
- *Avoid unnecessary urinary and nasogastric catheters*, at least for the first few hours, if the patient received IV alteplase.
- *Serial neurological examination and blood pressure checks* every 15 minutes during alteplase infusion and for 2 hours after its finalization. Later, measurements can be spaced out as per guidelines. To avoid unwanted hypotension, it is prudent to hold antihypertensive drugs the patient was previously taking. However, in order to avoid rebound tachycardia, home beta-blockers should be cut down in half rather than fully stopped. If blood pressure increases beyond safe limits it should be treated with IV drugs. Hypovolemia should be strictly avoided by providing IV saline in patients unable to tolerate oral intake.

- *Avoid hyperthermia.* A third of patients with acute stroke have body temperatures greater than 37.5 °C within the first hours after onset and this is associated with poorer outcomes. Treating fever may be beneficial. [7]
- *Correct electrolyte disturbances*, especially hyponatremia in patients with large strokes at risk of brain edema.
- *Prevention of deep venous thrombosis.* Prophylaxis with heparin or low molecular weight heparin should be held in the first 24 hours after the reperfusion attempt due to the potential stroke hemorrhagic transformation. Sequential compression devices should be used during this timeframe.
- *Swallowing assessment to prevent aspiration pneumonia.* This is necessary in patients with dysarthria, aphasia, and facial paresis.
- *Control neuroimaging within 24–36 hours of reperfusion therapy.* It allows to assess the location and extension of the established stroke and to rule out hemorrhagic transformation. This will guide the timing of DVT prophylaxis and secondary stroke prevention strategy initiation. While a CT scan is enough in most cases, in selected patients, a brain MRI may be useful to clarify the mechanism of the stroke and to evaluate the long-term risk of bleeding on antithrombotics, which is higher in patients with cerebral micro-bleeds.

Transient Ischemic Attack, Stroke with Transient Symptoms, and Stroke with no Reperfusion Treatment

Many patients with transient symptoms, especially those lasting more than 60 minutes have an established infarct when assessed with MRI. These patients and those with transient ischemic attacks (symptoms lasting <24 hours without infarcts in DWI) [26] may benefit from hospital admission for an expedited work-up in order to diagnose stroke etiologies with a high risk of recurrence (e.g., carotid artery stenosis >70%) [27].

Patients who are not candidates for reperfusion therapies because symptoms are nondisabling, they have an established stroke and are beyond the time window for reperfusion or have other contraindications for reperfusion therapies, should be admitted for stroke work-up and receive the above-mentioned care. This will help to sustain the ischemic penumbra, prevent medical complications, diagnose the underlying stroke mechanism, and start rehabilitation. All stroke patients should receive treatment with antiplatelets and statins within the first 48 hours unless they have contraindications for those medications. Dual antiplatelet drugs for 3 weeks help to prevent early recurrences among patients presenting with mild strokes or transient ischemic attack [28]. In cases with a demonstrated cardioembolic source, anticoagulation should be started as soon as deemed safe. The size of the stroke is the main consideration when deciding on the timing of initiation of anticoagulation.

Classification and Secondary Prevention

After the hyperacute phase, all stroke patients should be evaluated to find the underlying mechanism of the ischemia. This will allow to tailor the most appropriate secondary prevention regimen. Classifying the mechanism of the stroke also has prognostic implications. There are many classification systems but we continue to prefer the classic TOAST system because it is practical and has been broadly validated [29].

Large Vessel Disease

Large vessel disease strokes are caused by an atheromatous obstruction greater that 50% of the cervical or intracranial artery perfusing the infarcted area. Symptoms at presentation generally produce cortical dysfunction (e.g., aphasia, neglect, hemianopia, etc.) but also can cause brainstem and cerebellar dysfunction. A careful questioning may reveal multiple TIAs in the affected vascular territory. Intermittent claudication, diminished peripheral pulses, and carotid bruits are additional findings of systemic atheromatosis. Brain imaging usually shows cortical or cerebellar infarcts. When producing subcortical infarcts, they are greater than 1.5 cm (macrolacunes); the greater size differentiates them from strokes caused by small vessel disease. Patients with ipsilateral carotid stenosis greater than 70% have the highest recurrence rate of ischemic stroke, and most recurrences occur within 2 weeks of the initial event. In these cases, the treatment choice is carotid revascularization: endarterectomy, or stenting. When the stenosis ranges from 50 to 70% the benefit of revascularization is less clear. Patients with a good functional status and more than 5 years of expected life may benefit from surgical intervention. Patients with intracranial stenosis were included in the SAMMPRIS trial that compared medical treatment (dual antiplatelet regimen with aspirin and clopidogrel for 3 months, high-dose statin, and strict blood pressure control) with a surgical approach (stenting). Patients in the medical treatment arm had fewer stroke recurrences [30].

Small Vessel Disease

Small vessel disease is also known as lacunar infarcts or lacunes. These patients present with lacunar syndromes (pure motor, pure sensory, motor-sensory, dysarthria clumsy hand, and ataxia-hemiparesis). Brain imaging show infarcts in the deep white or grey matter (including brainstem) smaller than 1.5 cm. However, in this context, it is prudent to exclude large artery disease and cardiac embolism. These patients will benefit from control of vascular risk factors, antiplatelets, and stains.

Cardiac Embolism

Clinical and imaging findings may be similar to large vessel disease stroke because they share the embolic mechanism. Strokes affecting multiple vascular territories are highly suggestive of a cardioembolic mechanism. Additionally, these patients may have a past medical history of systemic embolism. To be classified as cardioembolic, a cardioembolic source should be conclusively identified, and large vessel stenosis ruled out. The most common cause of cardioembolic stroke by far is atrial fibrillation. The treatment choice is anticoagulation. Other rarer cardioembolic sources (e.g., cardiac myxoma) may need specific treatments.

Other Causes

Cervical dissections are especially frequent in young patients, causing approximately 20% of ischemic strokes in this age group. The culprit mechanism is a tear in the intimal layer of the vessel, which creates a false lumen and subsequently stenosis and thrombosis with a high-risk of distal embolism. It should be suspected in patients with a history of trauma, which can be mild (e.g., massage or chiropractic maneuvers in the neck), who present with headache and neck pain. *Patent foramen ovale* (PFO) is the persistence of the embrionary foramen ovale in adulthood. This foramen communicates right and left atria, and may allow the passage of venous thrombi to the arterial circulation or produce local thrombosis due to turbulent flow. A PFO is present in 25% of the general population and 40% of patients with cryptogenic strokes. The ROPE score is a tool that can help to differentiate whether the finding of a PFO is pathogenic or an incidental finding [31]. Recent trials have shown that closing the PFO in selected patients decreases the rate of recurrent stroke [32]. This category also includes unusual etiologies such as hypercoagulable states and vasculitis. Given that this group is heterogeneous, clinical presentation and imaging findings vary. It should be suspected in young patients, without classic vascular risk factors, signs, and symptoms of systemic affection and signs of systemic inflammation (such as sedimentation rate or C reactive protein).

Undetermined

A patient can be classified in this group when:
- There are two or more probable causes.
- Negative work up.
- Incomplete work up.

When patients have undetermined strokes due to a negative workup, antiplatelets are the mainstay for secondary prevention. If the infarct has an embolic appearance and clinical suspicion is high, covert atrial fibrillation should be ruled out with serial Holter monitoring or implantable recording devices. Vulnerable carotid plaques (i.e., with signs of inflammation, intramural hemorrhage, ulcerations) may be the culprit mechanism in some of these patients even if they do not produce major luminal stenosis. In such cases, control of vascular risk factors, statins, and antiplatelets should be optimized.

Cardinal Messages
- The ischemic penumbra is an area of potentially salvageable brain that benefits from maximal therapeutic efforts.
- Arterial recanalization, optimization of collateral flow, and avoidance of secondary brain injury determine the outcome of the ischemic penumbra.
- Arterial recanalization can be achieved by intravenous thrombolysis and/or mechanical thrombectomy.
- The severity of initial deficits and timely reperfusion are the main determinants of acute stroke outcome.
- A minority of patients with proximal artery occlusion, small core, and large penumbra benefit from mechanical thrombectomy up to 24 hours from symptoms onset.
- Organized inpatient care in a dedicated stroke unit improves mortality and functional outcomes.
- Secondary stoke prevention treatments should be individually tailored based on the mechanism of ischemia.

References

1. Kaufmann AM, Firlik AD, Fukui MB, Wechsler LR, Jungries CA, Yonas H. Ischemic core and penumbra in human stroke. Stroke. 1999;30:93–9.
2. Bang OY, Goyal M, Liebeskind DS. Collateral circulation in ischemic stroke. Stroke [online serial]; 2015;46:3302–3309.
3. Rabinstein AA. Treatment of acute ischemic stroke. Continuum (Minneap Minn). 2017;23:62–81.
4. Anderson CS, Arima H, Lavados P, et al. Cluster-randomized, crossover trial of head positioning in acute stroke. N Engl J Med [online serial]. 2017;376:2437–47.
5. Powers WJ, Rabinstein AA, Ackerson T, et al. 2018 Guidelines for the early management of patients with acute ischemic stroke: a guideline for healthcare professionals from the American Heart Association/American Stroke Association. Stroke [online serial]. 2018;49:e46–110. Accessed at: http://www.ncbi.nlm.nih.gov/pubmed/29367334.
6. Johnston KC, Bruno A, Pauls Q, et al Intensive vs Standard Treatment of Hyperglycemia and Functional Outcome in Patients With Acute Ischemic Stroke The SHINE RandomizedClinical TrialJAMA. 2019;322(4):326–335.

7. den Hertog HM, van der Worp HB, van Gemert HMA, et al. The Paracetamol (Acetaminophen) In Stroke (PAIS) trial: a multicentre, randomised, placebo-controlled, phase III trial. Lancet Neurol. 2009;8:434–40.
8. Fonarow GC, Smith EE, Saver JL, et al. Improving door-to-needle times in acute ischemic stroke: the design and rationale for the American Heart Association/American Stroke Association's target: stroke initiative. Stroke. 2011;42:2983–9.
9. Barber PA, Demchuk AM, Zhang J, Buchan AM. Validity and reliability of a quantitative computed tomography score in predicting outcome of hyperacute stroke before thrombolytic therapy. ASPECTS Study Group. Alberta Stroke Programme Early CT Score. Lancet [online serial]. 2000;355:1670–4. Accessed at: http://www.ncbi.nlm.nih.gov/pubmed/10905241.
10. The National Institute Of Neurological Disorders and Stroke rt-PA Stroke Study Group. Tissue plasminogen activator for acute ischemic stroke. N Engl J Med. 1995;333:1581–7.
11. Hacke W, Kaste M, Bluhmki E, et al. Thrombolysis with alteplase 3 to 4.5 hours after acute ischemic stroke. N Engl J Med [online serial]. 2008;359:1317–1329. Accessed at: http://www.ncbi.nlm.nih.gov/pubmed/18815396. Accessed 4 April 2016.
12. Lansberg MG, Schrooten M, Bluhmki E, Thijs VN, Saver JL. Treatment time-specific number needed to treat estimates for tissue plasminogen activator therapy in acute stroke based on shifts over the entire range of the modified Rankin Scale. Stroke. 2009;40:2079–84.
13. Khatri P, Conaway MR, Johnston KC. Ninety-day outcome rates of a prospective cohort of consecutive patients with mild ischemic stroke. Stroke. 2012;43:560–2.
14. Khatri P, Kleindorfer DO, Devlin T, et al. Effect of alteplase vs aspirin on functional outcome for patients with acute ischemic stroke and minor nondisabling neurologic deficits: the PRISMS randomized clinical trial. JAMA. 2018;320:156–66.
15. Anderson CS, Robinson T, Lindley RI, et al. Low-dose versus standard-dose intravenous alteplase in acute ischemic stroke. N Engl J Med. 2016;374:2313–23.
16. Logallo N, Novotny V, Assmus J, et al. Tenecteplase versus alteplase for management of acute ischaemic stroke (NOR-TEST): a phase 3, randomised, open-label, blinded endpoint trial. Lancet Neurol. 2017;16:781–8.
17. Seet RCS, Rabinstein AA. Symptomatic intracranial hemorrhage following intravenous thrombolysis for acute ischemic stroke: a critical review of case definitions. Cerebrovasc Dis [online serial]. 2012;34:106–114. Accessed at: https://www.karger.com/Article/FullText/339675.
18. Goyal M, Menon BK, van Zwam WH, et al. Endovascular thrombectomy after large-vessel ischaemic stroke: a meta-analysis of individual patient data from five randomised trials. Lancet. 2016;387:1723–31.
19. Campbell BCV, Mitchell PJ, Churilov L, et al. Tenecteplase versus alteplase before thrombectomy for ischemic stroke. N Engl J Med [online serial]. 2018;378:1573–82.
20. Nogueira RG, Jadhav AP, Haussen DC, et al. Thrombectomy 6 to 24 hours after stroke with a mismatch between deficit and infarct. N Engl J Med [online serial]. Massachusetts Medical Society; 2017;378:11–21.
21. Albers GW, Marks MP, Kemp S, et al. Thrombectomy for stroke at 6 to 16 hours with selection by perfusion imaging. N Engl J Med [online serial]. Massachusetts Medical Society; 2018;378:708–18.
22. Thomalla G, Simonsen CZ, Boutitie F, et al. MRI-guided thrombolysis for stroke with unknown time of onset. N Engl J Med [online serial]. Massachusetts Medical Society; 2018;379:611–22.
23. Ma H, Campbell BCV, Parsons MW, et al. Thrombolysis guided by perfusion imaging up to 9 hours after onset of stroke. N Engl J Med. 2019;380:1795–803.
24. Campbell BCV, Ma H, Ringleb PA, et al. Extending thrombolysis to 4.5–9 h and wake-up stroke using perfusion imaging: a systematic review and meta-analysis of individual patient data. Lancet. 2019;394(10193):139–47.
25. Stroke Unit Trialists' Collaboration. Organised inpatient (stroke unit) care for stroke. Cochrane Database Syst Rev. 2013;(9):CD000197.
26. Easton JD, Saver JL, Albers GW, et al. Definition and evaluation of transient ischemic attack: a scientific statement for healthcare professionals from the American Heart Association/

American Stroke Association Stroke Council; Council on Cardiovascular Surgery and Anesthesia; Council on Cardio. Stroke [online serial]. 2009;40:2276–93.
27. Lavallee PC, Meseguer E, Abboud H, et al. A transient ischaemic attack clinic with round-the-clock access (SOS-TIA): feasibility and effects. Lancet Neurol. 2007;6:953–60.
28. Johnston SC, Easton JD, Farrant M, et al. Clopidogrel and aspirin in acute ischemic stroke and high-risk TIA. N Engl J Med [online serial]. Massachusetts Medical Society; 2018;379:215–25.
29. Adams HP, Bendixen BH, Kappelle LJ, et al. Classification of subtype of acute ischemic stroke. Definitions for use in a multicenter clinical trial. TOAST. Trial of Org 10172 in Acute Stroke Treatment. Stroke [online serial]. 1993;24:35–41. Accessed at: http://www.ncbi.nlm.nih.gov/pubmed/7678184. Accessed 10 June 2016.
30. Chimowitz MI, Lynn MJ, Derdeyn CP, et al. Stenting versus aggressive medical therapy for intracranial arterial stenosis. N Engl J Med. 2011;365:993–1003.
31. Thaler DE, Ruthazer R, Weimar C, et al. Recurrent stroke predictors differ in medically treated patients with pathogenic vs. other PFOs. Neurology. 2014;83:221–6.
32. Søndergaard L, Kasner SE, Rhodes JF, et al. Patent foramen ovale closure or antiplatelet therapy for cryptogenic stroke. N Engl J Med [online serial]. Massachusetts Medical Society; 2017;377:1033–42.

Chapter 10
Acute Cerebral Venous Stroke

Catherine Arnold Fiebelkorn and Sherri A. Braksick

Diagnostic Keys
- Patients with cerebral venous thrombosis often present with nonspecific symptoms, the most common being headache.
- Presentations of cerebral venous thrombosis can be classified into four major categories: (1) increased intracranial pressure, (2) focal neurologic deficits, (3) seizures, and (4) encephalopathy.
- MRI and MRV are the diagnostic imaging modalities of choice.

Treatment Priorities
- Management of cerebral venous thrombosis includes anticoagulation and monitoring for secondary complications.
- Unfractionated heparin or low-molecular-weight heparin are first-line therapies for initial treatment.
- Oral anticoagulation with vitamin K antagonists is preferred for long-term therapy; duration of therapy is specific to each individual and dependent on the underlying cause.

C. A. Fiebelkorn (✉) · S. A. Braksick
Department of Neurology, Mayo Clinic, Rochester, MN, USA
e-mail: arnold.catherine@mayo.edu

> **Prognosis at a Glance**
> - Prognosis is generally favorable due to increased clinical awareness, advanced neuroimaging, and improved treatment.
> - With prompt diagnosis and treatment, the majority of patients have resolution of their symptoms.
> - Mortality rate and rate of moderate to severe disability are both approximately 10%.

Introduction

Acute thrombosis of the cerebral sinuses or veins (i.e., cerebral venous thrombosis or CVT) is an uncommon, likely under-recognized, form of cerebrovascular disease, accounting for 0.5% of all strokes. It may occur at any age, but predominately affects young adults, especially women [1]. Historically, CVT portended a poor prognosis, but now is regarded as a treatable condition with a generally favorable outcome. This shift is largely due to increased clinical awareness and advanced diagnostic imaging allowing for earlier diagnosis and treatment. This chapter will review the basic pathophysiology, clinical manifestations, diagnostic evaluations, and treatment of this uncommon, but important, cerebrovascular condition.

Pathophysiology

The venous system of the brain consists of two interconnected systems: the superficial cortical venous system and the inner (deep) cerebral venous system. The superficial cortical veins are anastomosed in a vascular network which results in collateralization and drainage into the dural sinuses. There is great anatomical variability in the superficial venous system. The inner cerebral veins provide drainage from the deeper, subcortical structures and have a relatively consistent anatomy [2, 3].

The underlying pathophysiology of cerebral venous infarction secondary to CVT is incompletely understood. Studies have shown venous occlusive disease causes increased intracranial pressure and cerebral blood volume, which ultimately results in decreased cerebral blood flow. More specifically, as venous pressure increases because of the occlusion, capillary perfusion pressure decreases. This leads to a "back pressure" and disruption of the blood-brain barrier, causing vasogenic edema. Further, due to diminished arterial cerebral blood flow and the subsequent decrease in nutrient delivery, there is dysfunction of the Na+-K+ ATPase pumps, which leads to intracellular water entry and cytotoxic edema. Tissue damage or infarction occurs in about 50% of cases of CVT, clearly less often than in arterial occlusive disease. This is largely due to the collateralization of the venous system which allows for reverse venous flow through alternative routes, resulting in

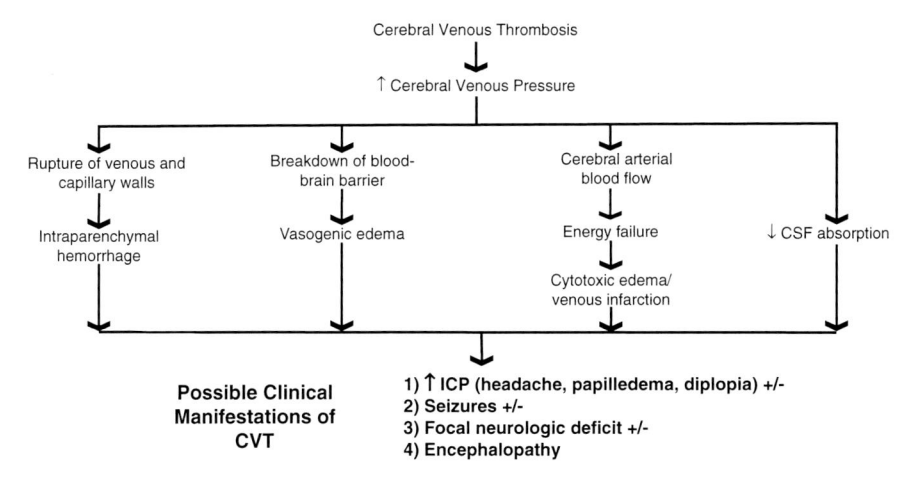

Fig. 10.1 Pathophysiology of cerebral venous thrombosis: CVT causes increased cerebral venous pressure. This may lead to several pathophysiologic processes which can result in vasogenic edema, cytotoxic edema with or without venous infarction, and/or intraparenchymal hemorrhage. It is from these cerebral insults that the clinical manifestations of CVT arise. ↓ Increased; ↑ Decreased; +/− with or without

decreased venous pressure and adequate arterial perfusion of the brain tissue. However, cerebral infarction may occur if collateral flow is limited. Thus, the outcome of CVT depends largely upon the structure of the collateral network and the ability to maintain sufficient venous flow [2].

When CVT occurs, as pressure increases further within the deep or superficial venous system, blood may extravasate into the cerebral parenchyma or subarachnoid space resulting in intraparenchymal or subarachnoid hemorrhages, respectively. In addition, hydrocephalus may also occur secondary to increased venous pressure and impaired CSF absorption by the arachnoid granulations. In cases of deep cerebral vein occlusion, parenchymal edema from tissue damage may obstruct CSF outflow pathways [4] (Fig. 10.1).

Clinical Presentation

Cerebral infarction secondary to venous thrombosis represents approximately 0.5% of all strokes and affects five people per million annually [1, 5]. In a large majority of cases, an underlying risk factor can be identified (Table 10.1). Risk factors are classically linked to the Virchow's triad: hemodynamic changes (blood stasis), endothelial injury or dysfunction, and hypercoagulability [1]. Affected individuals are typically younger compared to those with arterial occlusion or infarction, with a mean age of 39 years [6]. Rarely, CVT may occur in patients older than 65 years of age [3]. CVT also occurs more commonly in females

Table 10.1 Risk factors of cerebral venous thrombosis [1, 3, 5, 6, 7, 10]

Category	Conditions
Thrombophilia	Factor V Leiden mutation Protein C, protein S or antithrombin III deficiency Prothrombin gene mutation Antiphospholipid antibodies Hyperhomocysteinemia
Reproductive conditions	Pregnancy Post-partum period
Inflammatory disorders	Systemic inflammatory disorders CNS vasculitis Systemic vasculitis Inflammatory bowel disease
Trauma/invasive procedures	Head trauma Local injury to sinuses/veins Lumbar puncture Neurosurgical procedures
Infections	Focal infection (e.g., otitis, mastoiditis) Meningitis Sinusitis Systemic infection
Malignancy/tumor	Local compression/mass effect Secondary hypercoagulable state
Hematologic disorders	Polycythemia vera Thrombocytopenia Paroxysmal nocturnal hemoglobinuria
Medications	IV immunoglobulin (IVIG) Oral contraceptives Hormone replacement therapy Lithium Vitamin A Antineoplastic drugs (e.g., tamoxifen)
Other	Severe dehydration Cardiac failure

Table 10.2 Clinical manifestations of cerebral venous thrombosis [5, 8, 10]

Category of presentation	Signs/symptoms
Intracranial hypertension	Headache Nausea Papilledema Visual obscurations Cranial nerve VI palsy
Focal neurologic deficit	Hemiparesis Aphasia Sensory disturbance Visual field deficit or diplopia
Seizure	Focal seizure with semiology correlating to area of thrombosis/tissue damage Generalized seizure
Encephalopathy	Confusion Obtundation Stupor Coma Psychosis

compared to males which is thought due to sex-related factors including puerperium, and the use of oral contraceptives or hormonal replacement therapy [7]. The highest risk of CVT in women of reproductive age occurs during the first 6 weeks post-partum [8]. Both inherited (i.e., genetic thrombophilia or autoimmune disease) and acquired conditions (i.e., head trauma, infection, malignancy) can be risk factors for CVT, and often CVT occurs in the setting of innate individual risk factors and acquired precipitants [3].

The clinical presentation of CVT can be quite variable, and may mimic numerous other disorders, making diagnosis difficult. Each individual presentation depends on several factors, including sex and age of the patient, location and extent of the occlusion, and time from thrombus formation to presentation for medical evaluation [9]. Despite the vast number of potential signs and symptoms, the presentations can typically be classified into four main categories: (1) isolated intracranial hypertension, (2) focal neurologic deficits, (3) seizures, and (4) encephalopathy [5, 9] (Table 10.2). These categories are obviously nonspecific with many potential causes for each, which only further illustrates the importance of considering CVT or venous infarction within the differential diagnosis in each of these clinical scenarios.

Headache is the most common symptom, occurring in upwards of 90% of individuals with CVT [6]. The headache is often described as diffuse and progressive over the course of several days. Isolated headache without associated neurologic signs or symptoms occurs in the minority of cases (25%) [10]. More often, the headache is associated with other signs or symptoms, such as papilledema or diplopia (primarily due to cranial nerve VI palsy), suggestive of increased intracranial pressure. Focal signs and symptoms occur when CVT results in neurologic injury due to edema, venous ischemia, or hemorrhage [9]. Despite the potentially nonspecific presentation, a few clinical features can help distinguish CVT from other CNS pathologies. First, patients often present with progressive symptoms. The average time from symptom onset to medical attention is 4 days [6]. Additionally, seizures (both focal and generalized) are more common in patients with CVT compared to other cerebrovascular pathologies. Further, bilateral brain involvement is not uncommon. For example, paraparesis may result due to thrombosis of the sagittal sinus and encephalopathy may be present in cases of bithalamic involvement due to thrombosis of the deep venous system [1].

Diagnostic Evaluation

Once clinical suspicion is raised, neuroimaging is essential in confirming the diagnosis. CT (computed tomography) scan, CT venogram (CTV), MRI, and MRV, as well as conventional angiogram, are all potential imaging modalities used to evaluate CVT. MRI and MRV have been recommended as the preferred studies given their higher combined sensitivity [1, 11].

Imaging: Venous and Sinus Abnormalities

Because of its wide availability and rapid image acquisition, head CT is frequently used to assess patients with acute neurological symptoms. Non-contrast CT is frequently unremarkable in cases of CVT, but 30% of scans may demonstrate abnormalities [7]. When present, a thrombosed cortical vein or sinus appears as an elongated, homogenous hyperdensity [12]. The "filled delta sign" or "dense triangle" may be seen in cases of posterior superior sagittal or transverse sinus thrombosis [1] (Fig. 10.2). On contrast-enhanced CT, this appears as the classic "empty delta" sign due to slow or absent flow within the sinus and surrounding enhancement of the sinus dura [1]. Notably, contrast-enhanced CT improves the sensitivity of CVT detection almost threefold as compared to non-contrast CT [7]. Indirect signs of CVT such as brain edema or intracerebral hemorrhage can be seen on CT scan [6]. CTV may be used to detect thrombosis involving the sinuses and jugular veins (Figs. 10.3 and 10.4), but has limited ability to detect cortical thromboses due to the obscuration by bone artifact from the skull [9].

As previously mentioned, MRI and MRV are the preferred imaging studies, and are considered the gold standard in the evaluation of CVT. MRI findings suggestive of CVT include the absence of flow void signal and abnormal flow signal within the venous sinuses or veins. As a thrombus ages, MRI findings change due to the shift in the biochemical status of hemoglobin [9, 11] (Table 10.3). In the acute state, the

Fig. 10.2 CT head with high attenuation and slight expansion of the posterior superior sagittal sinus suggestive of cerebral venous sinus thrombosis (filled delta sign or dense triangle sign indicated with the arrow)

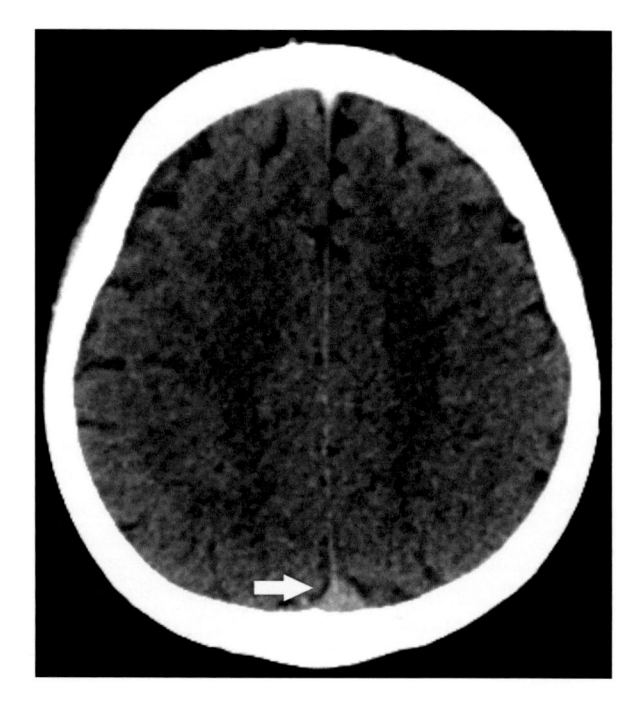

Fig. 10.3 CT Venogram demonstrating the absence of flow within the right transverse sinus consistent with right transverse sinus thrombosis (arrows)

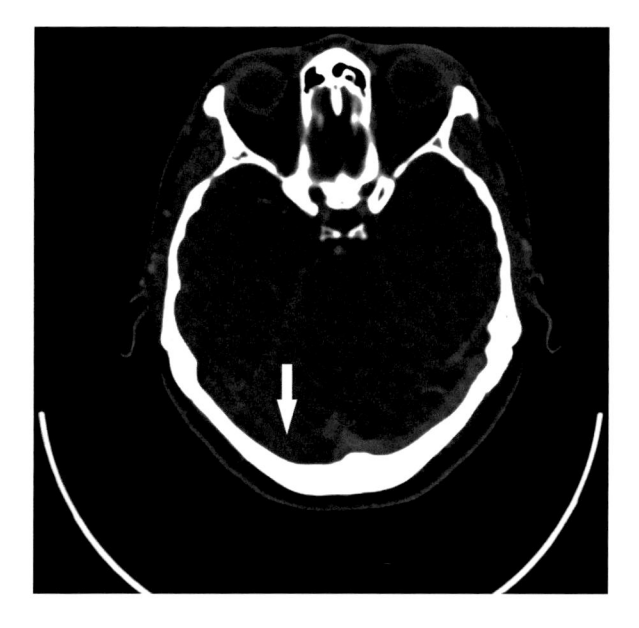

Fig. 10.4 CT Venogram showing an expansile thrombus within the superior sagittal sinus overlying the frontal and parietal lobes (arrows)

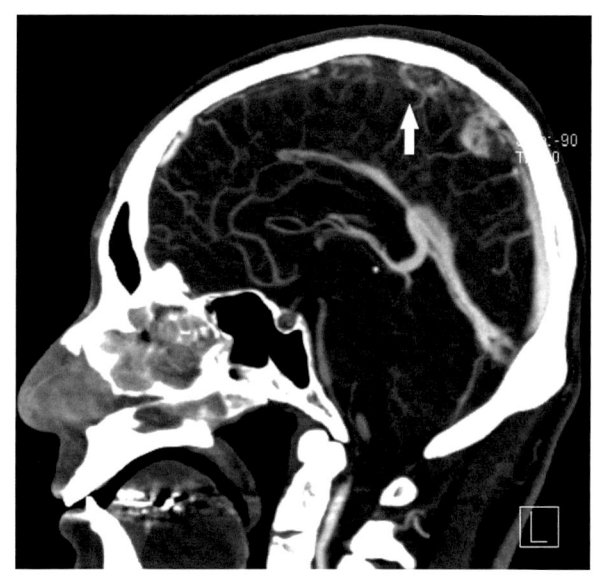

Table 10.3 MRI signal changes over time [9, 12, 13]

Age of thrombus	T1-weighted signal	T2-weighted signal
Acute (day 1–5)	↔	↓
Subacute (day 6–15)	↑	↑
Chronic (>16 days)	↔	↔ to ↑

↔ = isointense signal; ↑ = hyperintense signal; ↓ = hypointense signal

thrombus appears isointense on T1-weighted images and hypointense on T2-weighted images (Fig. 10.5a–c). The thrombus is often easier to appreciate several days after initial thrombus formation as it becomes hyperintense on T1- and T2-weighted images [1, 9, 13]. Gradient-echo (GRE) and susceptibility-weighted imaging (SWI) MRI sequences are also of significant value in detecting CVT given their ability to amplify signal drop-out at the site of the thrombus, which can help detect CVT that may be otherwise difficult to visualize on T1 or T2 imaging (Figs. 10.5d and 10.6). Often, blooming artifact allows for more accurate localization of the thrombus as well [13]. MRV can be performed with gadolinium contrast or without a contrast agent using the time of flight (TOF) technique (Figs. 10.5e–f, 10.7, and 10.8). Gadolinium-enhanced MRV improves the diagnostic yield of CVT detection, including the detection of small cortical vein thromboses, when compared to TOF images [9].

Conventional angiogram is most often used in cases of indeterminate diagnoses despite neuroimaging or when alternative imaging modalities are unavailable [3, 9, 14].

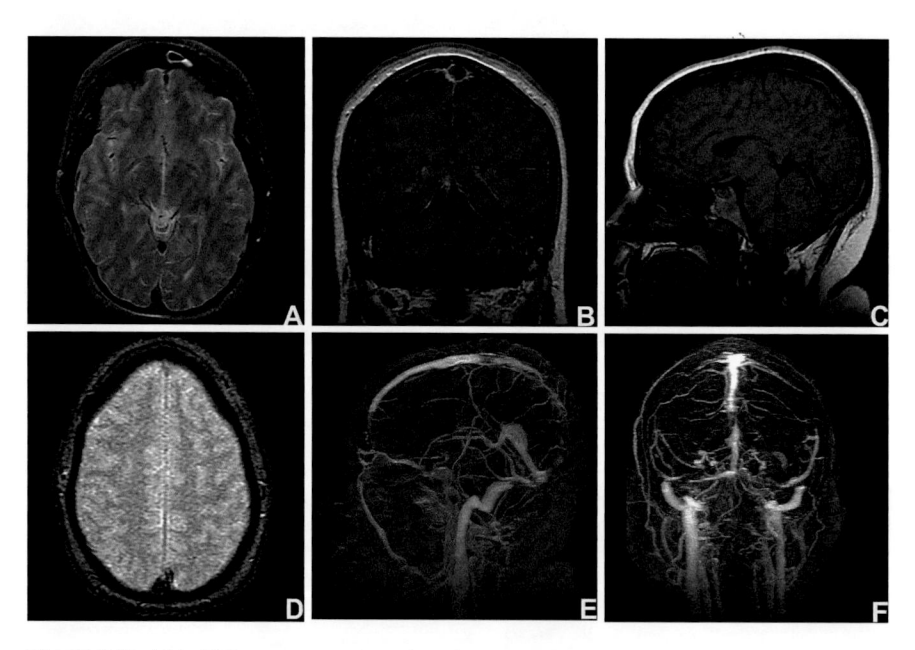

Fig. 10.5 Variable MRI sequences suggestive of an acute thrombus involving the posterior superior sagittal sinus and proximal bilateral transverse sinuses. (**a**) Axial T2 sequence demonstrating hypointensity of the posterior superior sagittal sinus. (**b**) Contrast-enhanced coronal T1 and (**c**) sagittal T1 sequences demonstrating isointense signal of the posterior superior sagittal sinus. (**d**) Axial GRE sequence demonstrating an area of hemosiderin deposition within the posterior superior sagittal sinus. (**e**) Contrast-enhanced MRV demonstrating thrombus within the posterior superior sagittal sinus. The thrombus within the bilateral transverse sinuses is better appreciated on coronal view (**f**)

Fig. 10.6 GRE sequence demonstrating a linear area of hypointensity in the left posterior frontal lobe which correlates to incomplete contrast opacification on MRV (not pictured) suggestive of a small, thrombosed vein. The thrombosed vein is secondary to compression by an overlying meningioma which is not appreciated on this view

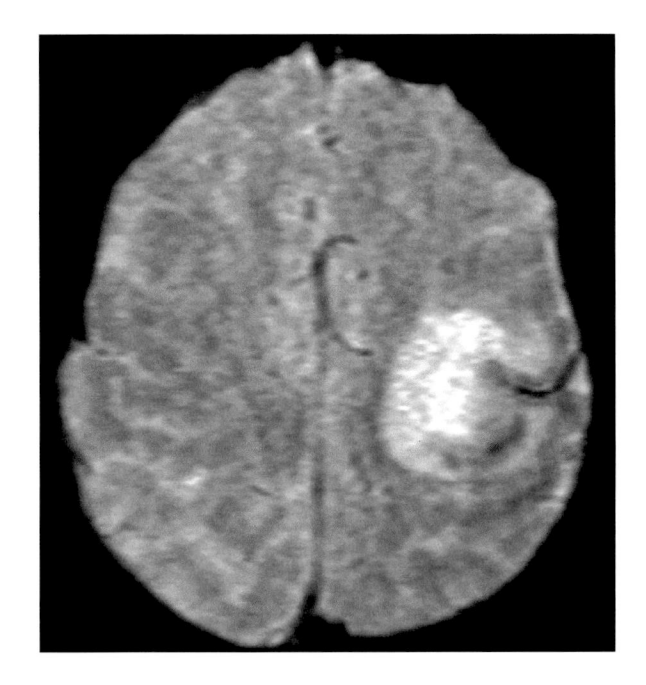

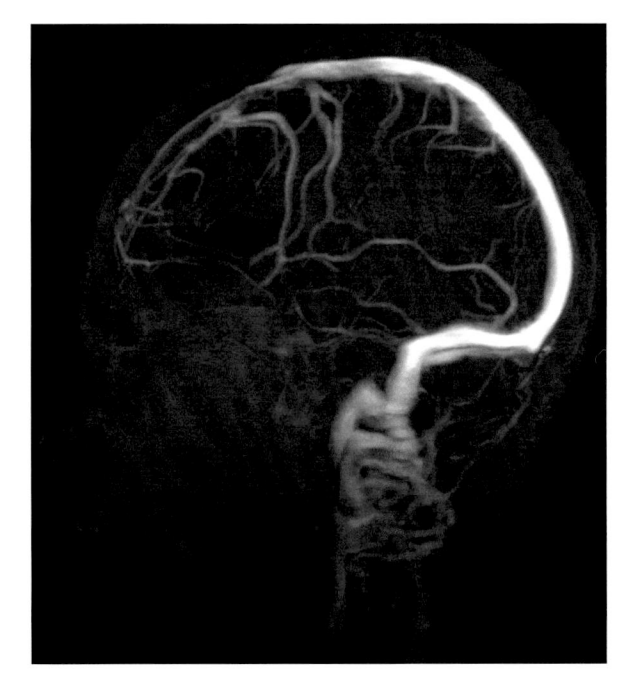

Fig. 10.7 Contrast-enhanced MRV demonstrating thrombosis of the deep venous system including the internal cerebral veins, the vein of Galen, the straight sinus, and the inferior sagittal sinus

Fig. 10.8 Contrast-enhanced MRV demonstrating thrombosis of the right transverse and sigmoid sinuses

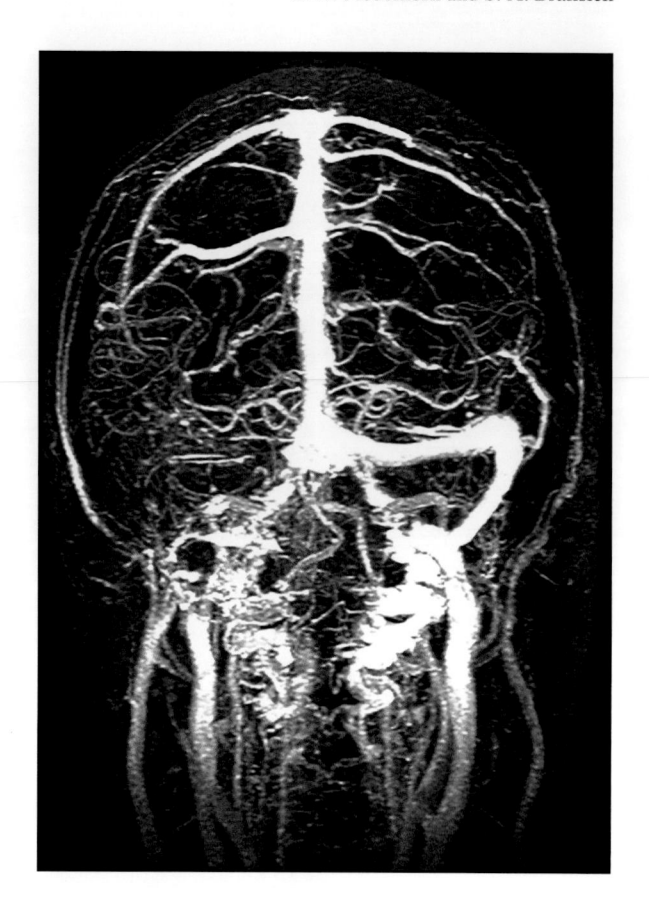

Imaging: Focal Parenchymal and Other Abnormalities

Focal brain abnormalities are present in the majority of patients with CVT and are often better appreciated on MRI than CT [12, 15]. Edema is a relatively common finding, occurring in up to half of the cases [3]. Diffusion-weighted imaging (DWI) is useful to discriminate between vasogenic and cytotoxic edema. In the former, the increased DWI signal is associated with a correlating increase in apparent diffusion coefficient (ADC) signal. In the latter, the increased DWI signal correlates to a similar area of decreased ADC signal, suggesting cellular energy disruption and infarction [15] (Fig. 10.9). In general, when an infarction extends beyond a typical arterial boundary, especially if there is an associated hemorrhagic component, or if an infarction is near a venous sinus, CVT should be strongly considered [1].

Parenchymal hemorrhages are present in approximately 30–40% of cases [15]. The location of the hemorrhage can help determine the location of CVT. Flame-shaped hemorrhages in the parasagittal frontal and parietal lobes are typically found

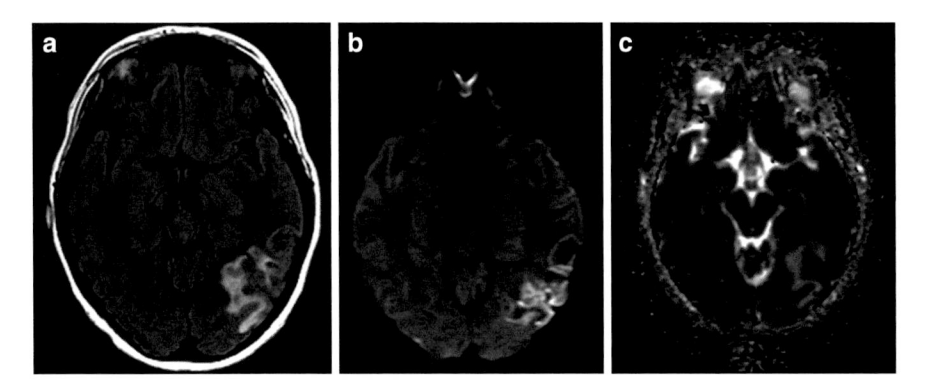

Fig. 10.9 A left temporal-occipital infarction with internal hemorrhage in a patient with an occlusive thrombus of the left transverse sinus, sigmoid sinus, and superior internal jugular vein. Note the hyperintensity on DWI sequence and hypointense ADC correlate, suggestive of infarction. (**a**) T2 FLAIR sequence, (**b**) DWI sequence, and (**c**) ADC sequence

Fig. 10.10 CT demonstrating intraparenchymal hemorrhage with the left parietal lobe in a patient with a superior sagittal sinus thrombosis

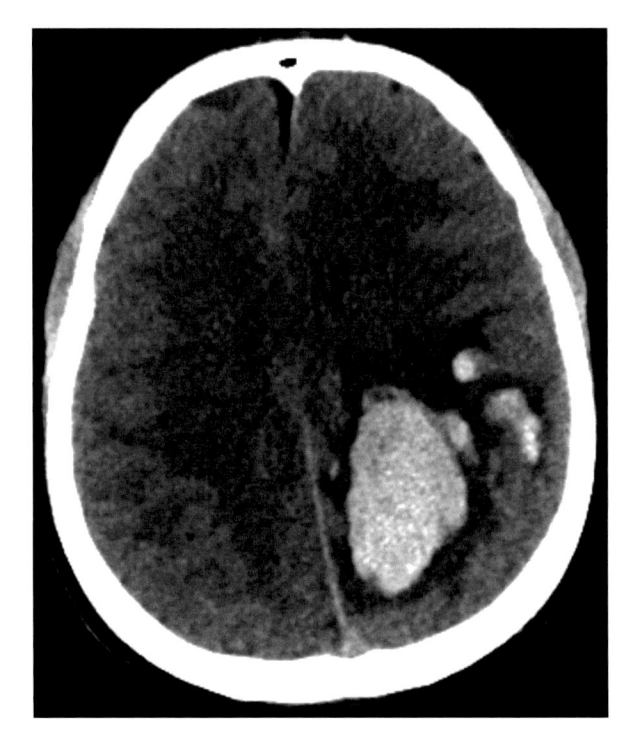

in patients with superior sagittal sinus thrombosis whereas hemorrhages in the temporal or occipital lobes more often correlate with thrombus in the transverse sinus [14] (Figs. 10.10, 10.11, and 10.12). Less commonly, isolated subarachnoid hemorrhage may be seen (Fig. 10.13).

Fig. 10.11 MRI demonstrating an intraparenchymal hemorrhage within the right parietal lobe as well as an area of edema in the anterior left frontal lobe in a patient with a superior sagittal sinus thrombosis

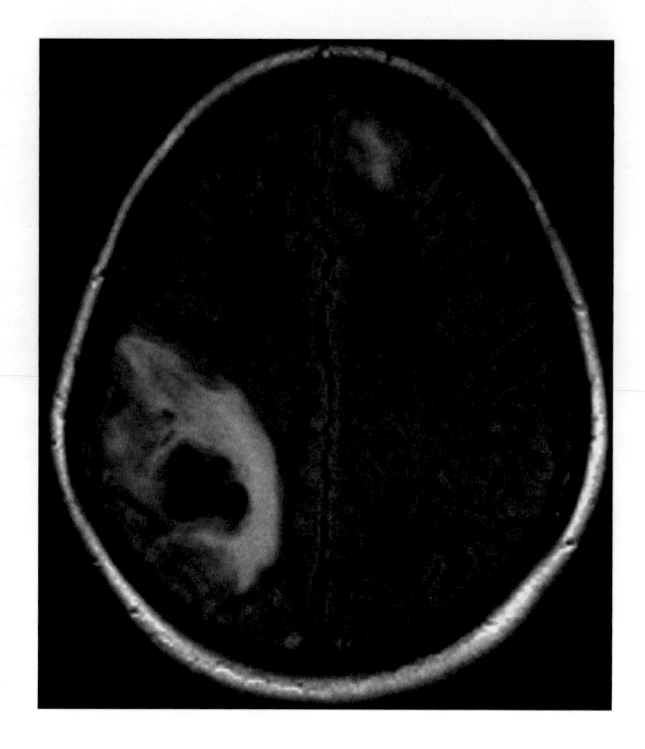

Parenchymal enhancement occurs in up to 30% of cases of CVT and is typically located within the gyri with extension into the white matter. Pachymeningeal enhancement may also be present, indicating disruption of the blood-brain barrier [14] (Fig. 10.12c).

Additional Investigations

Most patients with an acute CVT have a D-dimer level greater than 500 ug/L [1]. In one meta-analysis, D-dimer had a mean sensitivity of almost 94% and a specificity of almost 90% [16]. However, it should be noted that D-dimer may be falsely low in cases of lesser clot burden and, because levels decrease over time, may also be falsely low in cases of subacute or chronic CVT. In general, the use of D-dimer does not definitely exclude or confirm the presence of CVT.

Once the diagnosis is confirmed, testing for underlying thrombophilias including protein C, protein S, and antithrombin III deficiencies; antiphospholipid syndrome; factor V Leiden mutation; and prothrombin G20210A mutation may be useful in determining the underlying cause of CVT in individuals without known

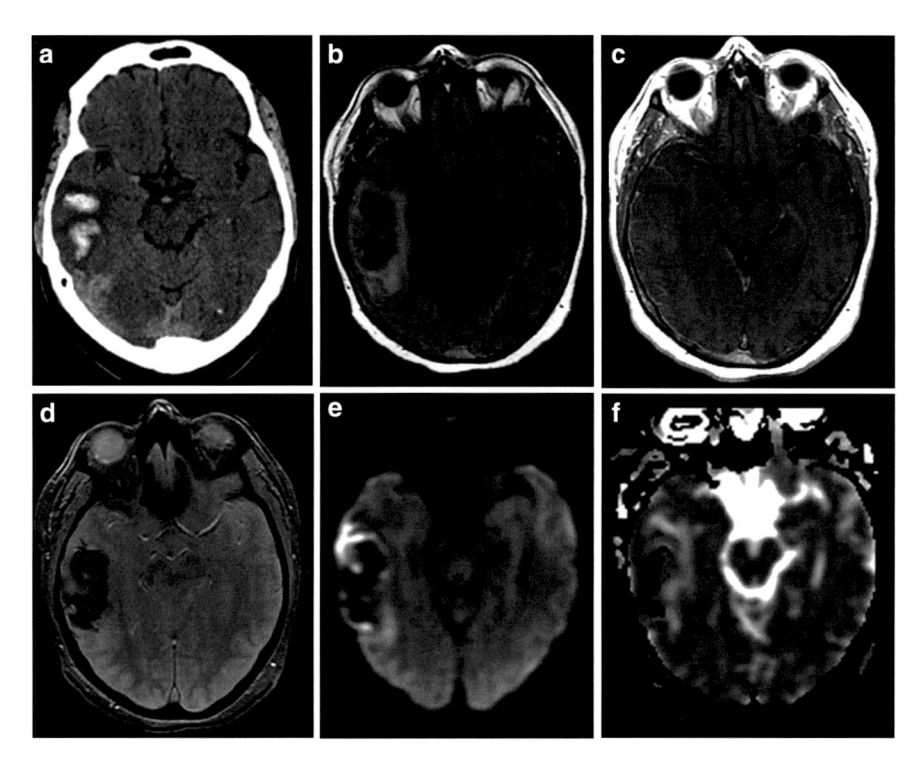

Fig. 10.12 Variable imaging sequences demonstrating a large right temporal-occipital intraparenchymal hemorrhage in a patient with a right transverse sinus and jugular vein thrombosis. (**a**) CT head. In addition to the intraparenchymal hemorrhage, a small amount of subarachnoid hemorrhage is also noted posteriorly. (**b**) MRI T2 FLAIR sequence demonstrating the hypointense region of hemorrhage surrounded by a hyperintense region of edema. (**c**) MRI contrast-enhanced T1 sequence showing increased vascularity and enhancement in the region of the hemorrhage (**d**) MRI GRE sequence demonstrating hemosiderin staining in the region of the hemorrhage (**e**) MRI DWI sequence demonstrating areas of hyperintensity with correlating areas of (**f**) ADC hypointensity and hyperintensity consistent with cytotoxic and vasogenic edema, respectively

risk factors. This information is helpful to direct long-term management; however, these tests are best performed before or several weeks after treatment with anticoagulation [1, 11].

Acute Management

The management of CVT includes treating the thrombosis, preventing and treating potential secondary complications, and developing a long-term individualized treatment plan (Fig. 10.14). In general, patients with acute CVT should be admitted

Fig. 10.13 Bilateral frontal and parietal subarachnoid hemorrhage (arrows) in a patient with thrombosis of the superior sagittal sinus, the right transverse sinus, and the right internal jugular vein

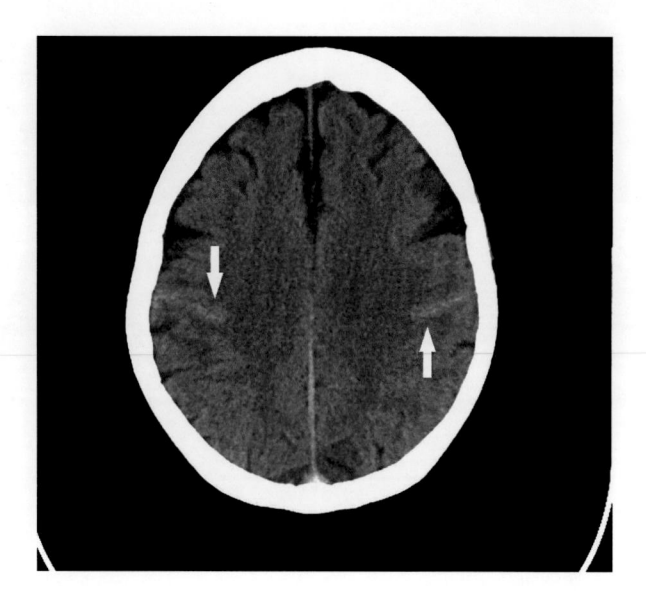

to a stroke unit for treatment and close monitoring for neurological deterioration and complications, and later transition to outpatient management with close follow-up.

Anticoagulation, Thrombolysis, and Endovascular Therapy

Anticoagulation is the recommended therapy in the initial phase of treatment, although it may seem counterintuitive in cases where venous infarction with hemorrhagic transformation is present. Despite the presence of hemorrhage, anticoagulation is often necessary to treat the underlying thrombus and to relieve retrograde pressure from venous occlusion. Unfractionated heparin or weight-based low-molecular-weight heparin are typically used as the initial therapy. Available studies have shown that the benefit outweighs the potential risk even in patients with hemorrhage on neuroimaging [1]. Benefits of anticoagulation include preventing growth of the thrombus, facilitating recanalization, and preventing further thrombotic events [1, 7, 11].

Unlike treatment of acute arterial stroke, systemic or catheter-directed thrombolysis and endovascular intervention with mechanical thrombectomy are not currently recommended as first-line therapy. Only in severe presentations or in cases of neurologic deterioration despite intensive anticoagulation are these interventions considered [1].

Several other supportive measures can also improve outcomes. Dehydration is a known precipitant and risk factor for worsening clinical status in CVT [9]. Therefore, adequate hydration with intravenous fluids is critical. Typically, normal saline is recommended. Hypotonic fluids should be avoided due to the potential for worsening

10 Acute Cerebral Venous Stroke

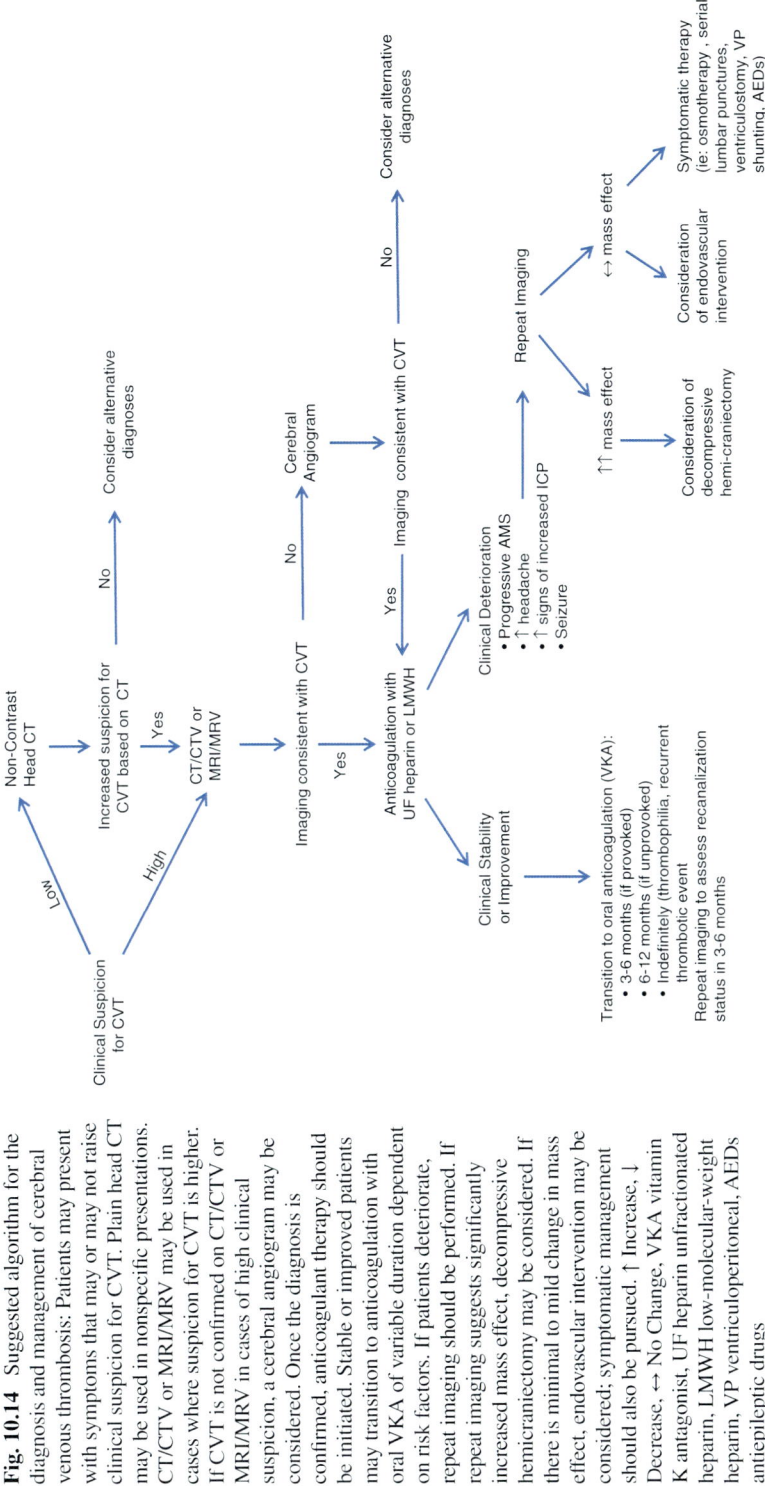

Fig. 10.14 Suggested algorithm for the diagnosis and management of cerebral venous thrombosis: Patients may present with symptoms that may or may not raise clinical suspicion for CVT. Plain head CT may be used in nonspecific presentations. CT/CTV or MRI/MRV may be used in cases where suspicion for CVT is higher. If CVT is not confirmed on CT/CTV or MRI/MRV in cases of high clinical suspicion, a cerebral angiogram may be considered. Once the diagnosis is confirmed, anticoagulant therapy should be initiated. Stable or improved patients may transition to anticoagulation with oral VKA of variable duration dependent on risk factors. If patients deteriorate, repeat imaging should be performed. If repeat imaging suggests significantly increased mass effect, decompressive hemicraniectomy may be considered. If there is minimal to mild change in mass effect, endovascular intervention may be considered; symptomatic management should also be pursued. ↑ Increase, ↓ Decrease, ↔ No Change, VKA vitamin K antagonist, UF heparin unfractionated heparin, LMWH low-molecular-weight heparin, VP ventriculoperitoneal, AEDs antiepileptic drugs

brain edema and thus increasing intracranial pressure. Additionally, although there is no specific data to suggest strict blood pressure control has significant benefit on clinical outcome, systolic blood pressure less than 160 mmHg is generally recommended, especially in the cases with intracerebral hemorrhage.

Management of Medical Complications

Seizures occur in one-third of adults with CVT and happen more frequently in patients with supratentorial parenchymal lesions (i.e., venous infarction or intraparenchymal hemorrhage) as well as in patients with intracranial hypertension [1, 7, 9]. Despite this, the routine use of prophylactic antiepileptic therapy is not recommended [1]. However, early treatment with antiepileptic drug therapy is clearly warranted in patients who have suffered seizures [1].

Communicating hydrocephalus may occur in patients with CVT when the major sinuses are involved (i.e., superior sagittal or transverse sinuses) and disruption of CSF absorption by the arachnoid granulations occurs. Obstructive hydrocephalus may also occur but is less common and is typically associated with internal cerebral venous thromboses causing abnormality of the adjacent parenchyma, and consequent obstruction of normal CSF flow. Hydrocephalus is associated with a threefold higher risk of death [7]. Therefore, patients should be closely monitored and quickly treated for this complication. Initial management includes decreasing CSF production (i.e., acetazolamide therapy) and treatment of the underlying thrombosis. Neurosurgical consultation should also be sought early in the event that ventriculostomy or ventriculoperitoneal shunting is necessary [4].

Intracranial hypertension can be seen in up to 40% of patients due to venous congestion, increased blood volume, decreased CSF resorption, and/or mass effect. Treatment is largely targeted to symptom management with the use of acetazolamide, osmotherapy, and serial lumbar punctures in the absence of significant mass effect. If symptoms persist despite therapy, CSF diversion may be required. Additionally, if there is severe mass effect or otherwise intractable intracranial hypertension, decompressive hemicraniectomy may also be considered, especially in younger patients [9].

Permanent vision loss can also occur due to increased intracranial hypertension. Ophthalmologic consultation may be useful in this setting, though treatment of the underlying thrombus is the most effective strategy to preserve vision.

Chronic Management

After the initial phase of treatment, the patient is transitioned to oral anticoagulation. Typically, a vitamin K antagonist (VAK) is the anticoagulant of choice with a goal INR of 2.0–3.0 except in the setting of pregnancy during which weight-based LMWH is recommended due to the teratogenic potential of VKAs [7].

Direct oral anticoagulants (DOACs) have been shown to have a similar efficacy and an improved safety profile compared to VKAs in patients with pulmonary embolic or deep vein thromboses, but patients with CVT were excluded from these particular trials, and therefore, the potential value of these medications in the setting of CVT is currently unknown [1, 7, 11].

The duration of treatment should be determined on a patient-by-patient basis, weighing individual potential risks versus benefits of continued therapy. In general, the duration of anticoagulation varies depending on whether the patient has persistent and unmodifiable risk factors and whether the event was provoked or unprovoked. Patients with a transient risk factor or who are considered to have a provoked event (i.e., pregnancy/post-partum, surgical procedure, medication-induced) should receive anticoagulation for 3 to 6 months. For those without a known or identifiable risk factor (i.e., unprovoked CVT), anticoagulation is recommended for 6–12 months. In patients with recurrent CVT or CVT associated with severe thrombophilia (i.e., antiphospholipid syndrome, protein C, S, and antithrombin deficiency, homozygous prothrombin G20210A mutation, homozygous factor V Leiden; deficiencies of protein C, protein S, or antithrombin III, or combined thrombophilia defects), indefinite anticoagulation is recommended [1, 11].

Recanalization occurs with treatment over a period of months [17, 18]. Repeat imaging with either CT/CTV or MRI/MRV is recommended 3–6 months from the time of the initial event to assess recanalization status as this, too, can impact the duration of therapy [7].

Prognosis and Risk of Recurrence

Previously, CVT was a potentially devastating and life-threatening condition, but due to improved clinical awareness, advanced neuroimaging, and improved treatment, current prognosis after CVT is generally favorable [7]. With contemporary management, the majority of patients improve, with 79% having complete resolution of their symptoms within 16 months [6]. However, mortality rate and the rate of moderate to severe functional disability have both been reported at almost 10% [6, 19]. Certain clinical and radiographic characteristics have been associated with worse clinical outcomes as shown in Table 10.4 [1].

Table 10.4 Factors associated with poor outcome [1]

Patient characteristics	Clinical presentations	Imaging findings
Male sex	Encephalopathy	Intracerebral hemorrhage
>37 years of age	Severe NIHSS	Venous infarct
Diagnosis of malignancy	Seizures	Involvement of the straight sinus or deep venous system
Diagnosis of inherited thrombophilia	Hemiparesis	Hydrocephalus
Diagnosis of CNS infection	Depressed level of consciousness/coma	

Recurrence largely depends on the underlying cause of the CVT, with the presence of thrombophilia understandably increasing the risk [1, 5]. Those with transient or provoked risk factors have lower risk of recurrence if the risk factor is appropriately addressed.

Conclusion

Cerebral venous thrombosis of the dural sinuses and/or cerebral veins represents a rare cause of acute cerebrovascular disease that occurs most often in young adults, particularly women. Patients often present with nonspecific symptoms, with headache being most common, sometimes associated with focal neurologic signs. Neuroimaging is critical in confirming the diagnosis. With the initiation of anticoagulation therapy, and rarely, the use of angiographic thrombectomy or catheter-directed thrombolysis, prognosis is generally favorable.

Cardinal Messages
- Cerebral venous thrombosis most commonly affects young women.
- Headache is the most common presenting symptom.
- Because presenting symptoms and signs are often nonspecific, a low threshold for suspecting this diagnosis is critical to avoid delayed recognition.
- MRI and MRV are the recommended diagnostic imaging modalities of choice.
- Initial anticoagulation therapy consists of unfractionated heparin or weight-based low-molecular-weight heparin, and long-term management typically includes anticoagulation with oral vitamin K antagonists.
- Secondary complications are possible and include seizures, hydrocephalus, and increased intracranial pressure.
- In a majority of cases, prognosis is favorable with prompt diagnosis and treatment.

References

1. Saposnik G, Barinagarrementeria F, Brown RD, Bushnell CD, Cucchiara B, Cushman M, et al. Diagnosis and management of cerebral venous thrombosis a statement for healthcare professionals from the American Heart Association/American Stroke Association. Stroke. 2011;42(4):1158–92.
2. Schaller B, Graf R. Cerebral venous infarction: the pathophysiological concept. Cerebrovasc Dis. 2004;18(3):179–88.
3. Dmytriw AA, Song JSA, Yu E, Poon CS. Cerebral venous thrombosis: state of the art diagnosis and management. Neuroradiology. 2018;60:669.
4. Zuurbier SM, van den Berg R, Troost D, Majoie CB, Stam J, Coutinho JM. Hydrocephalus in cerebral venous thrombosis. J Neurol. 2015;262(4):931–7.

5. Bousser MG, Ferro JM. Cerebral venous thrombosis: an update. Lancet Neurol. 2007;6(2):162–70.
6. Ferro JM, Canhao P, Stam J, Bousser MG, Barinagarrementeria F, Investigators I. Prognosis of cerebral vein and dural sinus thrombosis: results of the International Study on Cerebral Vein and Dural Sinus Thrombosis (ISCVT). Stroke. 2004;35(3):664–70.
7. Capecchi M, Abbattista M, Martinelli I. Cerebral venous sinus thrombosis. J Thromb Haemost. 2018;16(10):1918–31.
8. Silvis SM, Lindgren E, Hiltunen S, Devasagayam S, Scheres LJ, Jood K, Zuurbier SM, Kleinig TJ, Silver FL, Mandell DM, Middeldorp S, Putaala J, Cannegieter SC, Tatlisumak T, Coutinho JM. Postpartum period is a risk factor for cerebral venous thrombosis. Stroke. 2019;50(2):501–3.
9. Bushnell C, Saposnik G. Evaluation and management of cerebral venous thrombosis. Continuum (Minneap Minn). 2014;20(2 Cerebrovascular Disease):335–51.
10. Coutinho JM. Cerebral venous thrombosis. J Thromb Haemost. 2015;13(Suppl 1):S238–44.
11. Ferro JM, Bousser MG, Canhao P, Coutinho JM, Crassard I, Dentali F, et al. European Stroke Organization guideline for the diagnosis and treatment of cerebral venous thrombosis—endorsed by the European Academy of Neurology. Eur J Neurol. 2017;24(10):1203–13.
12. Lee SK, terBrugge KG. Cerebral venous thrombosis in adults: the role of imaging evaluation and management. Neuroimaging Clin N Am. 2003;13(1):139.
13. Diacinti D, Cartocci G, Colonnese C. Cerebral venous thrombosis: a case series and a neuroimaging review of the literature. J Clin Neurosci. 2018;58:142.
14. Leach JL, Fortuna RB, Jones BV, Gaskill-Shipley MF. Imaging of cerebral venous thrombosis: current techniques, spectrum of findings, and diagnostic pitfalls. Radiographics. 2006;26 Suppl 1:S19–41; discussion S2–3.
15. Mullins ME, Grant PE, Wang B, Gonzalez RG, Schaefer PW. Parenchymal abnormalities associated with cerebral venous sinus thrombosis: assessment with diffusion-weighted MR imaging. AJNR Am J Neuroradiol. 2004;25(10):1666–75.
16. Dentali F, Squizzato A, Marchesi C, Bonzini M, Ferro JM, Ageno W. D-dimer testing in the diagnosis of cerebral vein thrombosis: a systematic review and a meta-analysis of the literature. J Thromb Haemost. 2012;10(4):582–9.
17. Arauz A, Vargas-Gonzalez JC, Arguelles-Morales N, Barboza MA, Calleja J, Martinez-Jurado E, et al. Time to recanalisation in patients with cerebral venous thrombosis under anticoagulation therapy. J Neurol Neurosurg Psychiatry. 2016;87(3):247–51.
18. Herweh C, Griebe M, Geisbusch C, Szabo K, Neumaier-Probst E, Hennerici MG, et al. Frequency and temporal profile of recanalization after cerebral vein and sinus thrombosis. Eur J Neurol. 2016;23(4):681–7.
19. Hiltunen S, Putaala J, Haapaniemi E, Tatlisumak T. Long-term outcome after cerebral venous thrombosis: analysis of functional and vocational outcome, residual symptoms, and adverse events in 161 patients. J Neurol. 2016;263(3):477–84.

Chapter 11
Intraparenchymal Hemorrhage (Cerebral and Cerebellar)

David P. Lerner, Anil Ramineni, and Joseph D. Burns

Diagnostic Keys
- There is no clinically sensitive and specific means of discriminating ICH from acute ischemic stroke. All patients presenting with acute neurologic symptoms that are consistent with a vascular territory must undergo rapid CT imaging to determine next most appropriate treatment.
- Concise clinical and radiographic assessment of ICH should include determination of level of consciousness, severity of deficits, hemorrhage volume and location, and radiographic findings of elevated intracranial pressure and/or intraventricular hemorrhage.
- Although primary and secondary ICH have the same initial treatment (correction of coagulopathy, treatment of hypertension, and treatment of mass effect and elevated ICP), determination of underlying etiology is crucial. Secondary causes of ICH require additional, etiology-specific interventions to prevent recurrent hemorrhage and secondary neurologic injury.

D. P. Lerner · A. Ramineni
Department of Neurology, Lahey Hospital and Medical Center, Burlington, MA, USA

Department of Neurology, Tufts University School of Medicine, Boston, MA, USA

J. D. Burns (✉)
Department of Neurology, Lahey Hospital and Medical Center, Burlington, MA, USA

Department of Neurology, Tufts University School of Medicine, Boston, MA, USA

Department of Neurosurgery, Tufts University School of Medicine, Boston, MA, USA
e-mail: joseph.d.burns@lahey.org

Treatment Priorities
- Ensuring adequate circulation, airway, and breathing constitute the initial priorities in the field and in the Emergency Department.
- Rapid assessment for correctable coagulopathy and/or thrombocytopenia is essential. Medication history and laboratory assessment of the complete blood count, activated partial thromboplastin time, and prothrombin time should be completed. Reversal of coagulopathy is determined by the underlying cause and should be rapidly pursued in all patients (Fig. 11.1).
- Hypertension is common in patients with ICH. A systolic blood pressure goal of 140–160 mmHg is reasonable, with a goal of achieving it within 1 hour of presentation. Intravenous nicardipine, clevidipine, or labetalol work well for this purpose (Fig. 11.1).
- ICH resulting in horizontal displacement of the third ventricle or compression of the fourth ventricle and/or brainstem confers high risk for cerebral herniation and treatment with hyperosmolar therapy should be considered (Fig. 11.1).
- Surgical management of mass effect directly attributable to hematoma and surrounding edema should be considered as lifesaving only and not expected to have beneficial effect on functional outcome. Minimally invasive surgery remains investigational.

Prognosis at a Glance
- Prognostication in ICH is difficult, but nihilism should be avoided especially during the very early stages after the bleeding.
- Excluding exceptionally severe cases, prognosis should not be delivered within at least 24 hours after admission to avoid premature withdrawal of life-sustaining therapy.
- Available scales for outcome prediction provide only gross estimates of the risk for death and disability and should not be used in isolation for individual patients.

Introduction

Intracerebral hemorrhage (ICH) is the second most common type of stroke and is caused by bleeding directly into brain parenchyma. It can be primary (more common, due to hypertensive or cerebral amyloid angiopathy) or secondary (less common, directly related to congenital or acquired macrovascular abnormalities, tumors, and other identifiable etiologies; Table 11.1) In the United States, ICH accounts for 10–15% of all strokes or approximately 80,000 new cases of ICH yearly [1].

11 Intraparenchymal Hemorrhage (Cerebral and Cerebellar)

Intracerebral Hemorrhage (ICH) Emergency Management

Airway/Breathing/Circulation

Monitor neurological status every 15 and vital signs every 10 minutes

---

Blood Pressure Control

** Goal for titration of antihypertensives; SBP <160 mmHg within 1 hour of presentation**

- Check BP every 10 minutes
- If SBP >160 mmHg
  □ Initiate treatment of HTN w/ Nicardipine IV continuous infusion. Start at 5 mg/hr and titrate as needed infusion. Start at 5 mg/hr and titrate as needed to achieve goal by increments of 2.5 mg/hr every 5 min to max dose of 15 mg/hr
  □ For pts w/ concomitant severe tachycardia or MI - consider Labetalol 10 mg IV every 15 min as needed to achieve goal or continous infusion at 0.5-4 mg/min and titrate as needed by increments of 0.5 mg/min every 10 min
  □ Nitroglycerin & nitroprusside should *not* be used in ICH patients
- If SBP <160 mmHg w/out tx
  □ Continue to monitor BP every 10 min and initiate Nicardipine as above if sustained SBP >160 mmHg on 2 consective BP reads

---

Initiate Anticoagulant Reversal Immediately
□ D/C all anticoagulants and antiplatelets

- Vitamin K antagonists (warfarin)
  □ Vitamin K 10 mg IV AND
  □ Kcentra (dose based on weight, and INR) if INR > 1.4 OR
  □ FFP (10-15 mL/kg) if INR > 1.6 and Kcentra not available or contraindicated (1 unit ~250 mL)
- Dabigatran
  □ Activated charcoal 50 g ≤2 hours of ingestion AND
  □ Idarucizumab 5 g IV (given as 2 does of 2.5g/50mL) if dTT prolonged
  □ Consider hemodialysis if Idarucizumab is not available
- Factor Xa inhibitors
  □ Activated charcoal (50 g)≤2 hours of ingestion AND
  □ Consider 4 factor PCC (KCentra) 25-50 units/kg OR
  □ Consider andexanet alfa (dose depends on timing and dose of factor Xa inhibitor)
- Antiplatelet agents
  □ Consider demopressin 0.4 mcg/kg IV x 1.0 mit if hyponatremic
  □ If surgery (including EVD) planned: transfuse platelets (1-2 apheresis units), timing per Neurosurgery

---

ICP Management

□ Maintain HOB 45°
□ Maintain temp < 38.3° φn acetamilophenl

For patient with signs of increased ICP

Consider:
□ Mannitol 0.5-1.5 g/kg IV OR
□ 3% Saline 3-6 mL/kg OR
□ 23.4% Saline 30-60 mL
□ ICP moniter (Camino or EVD) placement
□ STAT Non-contrast Head CT to evaluate hematoma expansion

Witnessed Seizure Managment

□ Phenytoin or Fosphenytoin 20 mg PE/kg load, then phenytoin 100 mg IV every 8 house OR
□ Levetiracetam 20-40 mg/kg IV load, then 500-1000 mg IV every 12 hours
Prophylactic treatment not recomended

Fig. 11.1 Simple algorithm for acute management of intracerebral hemorrhage. Initial evaluation and treatment of ABC's followed by simultaneous evaluation/management of blood pressure, coagulopathy, and intracranial pressure

Table 11.1 Causes of secondary intracerebral hemorrhage

Macrovascular lesions
Arteriovenous malformation
Saccular aneurysm
Cavernous malformation
Dural arteriovenous fistula
Intracranial artery dissection ± pseudoaneurysm
Moyamoya syndrome and disease
Hemorrhagic transformation of infarct
Bland
Septic embolic (endocarditis)
Posterior reversible encephalopathy syndrome
Reversible cerebral vasoconstriction syndrome
Intracranial neoplasm
Primary
Glioblastoma multiforme
Oligodendroglioma
Meningioma
Metastatic
Lung
Melanoma
Breast
Renal cell
Thyroid
Choriocarcinoma
Intracranial venous thrombosis
Cerebral venous sinus thrombosis
Cortical vein thrombosis
Sudden severe hypertension[a]
Sympathomimetic drugs (cocaine, amphetamines)
Pheochromocytoma
Coagulopathy[a]
Anticoagulant therapy
Liver disease
Diffuse intravascular coagulation (DIC)
Immune thrombocytopenic purpura
Thrombotic thrombocytopenic purpura
Congenital bleeding diathesis
Vasculitis
Infectious
Primary central nervous system (CNS)
Systemic vasculitis
Intravascular lymphoma

[a]Acute hypertension and coagulopathy are rarely the sole cause of intracerebral hemorrhage and most often contribute by exacerbating other, more common etiologies

On average ICH is much more severe than ischemic stroke. One-month case fatality is 40%; nearly twice that of ischemic stroke [2]. Only 20% of all ICH patients, or approximately 55% when considering only survivors, achieve functional independence at 1 year [2].

ICH injures the brain in two distinct ways: direct mechanical disruption and distortion due to the bleeding, followed by edema and delayed inflammation triggered by the toxicity of extravasated blood [3]. While bleeding in ICH begins abruptly, it commonly continues to accumulate over many minutes to hours. Hematoma expansion occurs in >70% of patients within 24 hours of symptom onset, most of which occurs in the first 6 hours. Even small amounts of expansion confer an increased risk of death and worse disability [4]. Therefore, interventions to limit hematoma expansion are crucial and must be implemented as soon as the diagnosis of ICH has been made. Delayed, secondary brain injury due to inflammation in response to extravasated blood begins to have important effects a couple of days after the initial bleeding and continues for many days. This process contributes to edema formation and mechanical injury as well as direct brain injury via inflammation-mediated necrosis and apoptosis [3].

Interventions occurring in the first "golden hour" after ICH are crucial for minimizing risks of death and disability. This chapter will describe a pragmatic approach to the emergency care of patients with ICH, focusing on topics most likely to improve outcomes.

Initial Evaluation and Management

Because ICH can only be reliably discriminated from acute ischemic stroke (AIS) by brain imaging, prehospital evaluation and management of ICH is the same as that for ischemic stroke (Table 11.2). Initial diagnostic evaluation and management of patients with ICH has four main aims:

1. Identify and treat immediately life-threatening complications
2. Diagnose ICH and differentiate from other types of stroke

Table 11.2 Prehospital evaluation of stroke patients	Assess and manage airway, breathing, and circulation (ABCs)
	Provide supplemental oxygen to maintain oxygen saturation > 94%
	Initiate cardiac monitoring
	Establish IV access
	Obtain blood glucose level and treat accordingly
	Determine symptoms onset time, last known well time, and family contact information
	Triage and rapidly transport patient to most appropriate stroke capable hospital
	Notify hospital of impending stroke patient

3. Minimize the risk of and secondary brain injury from ICH (hematoma expansion, elevated intracranial pressure, and cerebral herniation)
4. Determine the underlying etiology of the ICH

Identify and Treat Immediately Life-Threatening Complications

As with any medical emergency, initial assessment of circulation, airway, and breathing is paramount—the goal is to ensure adequate oxygen and blood delivery to the brain.

Airway and Breathing

The most common life-threatening complication from ICH is respiratory failure caused by poor airway control from depressed level of consciousness and/or oropharyngeal sensorimotor dysfunction. If there is poor airway control, immediate orotracheal intubation should be pursued. If there is any concern for elevated intracranial pressure (ICP) or herniation, the head of the bed should be lowered for as brief a time as possible, lidocaine can be applied to the vocal cords prior to intubation to blunt potential ICP rise during intubation, and a rapid sequence intubation protocol should be followed. Normal oxygenation saturations should be maintained before, during, and after intubation. The default ventilation goal is eucapnia ($PaCO_2$ 35–45 mmHg) except in patients who have active intracranial hypertension or herniation, in whom hyperventilation to a goal $PaCO_2$ of approximately 30 mmHg is appropriate (see Section "Assess for and Treat Elevated ICP and Herniation").

Initial Hemodynamic Management

Hypertension is common in patients with acute stroke of all types, including ICH. Although hypertension is probably an important contributor to hematoma expansion, until ICH is diagnosed by imaging, a conservative blood pressure goal of <180/105 mmHg balances objectives for ICH and AIS and is an appropriate first step because (1) ICH cannot be differentiated from AIS prior to computerized tomography (CT) and (2) hypertension may be an adaptive response to elevated ICP. Shock is rarely a presenting problem in patients with ICH. When it occurs, the most common cause is drugs used for intubation and subsequent sedation combined with intravascular volume depletion. Much less commonly, shock can occur due to concomitant sepsis, myocardial infarction, neurogenic stress cardiomyopathy, or injury to the vasomotor centers of the brainstem. There are no specific considerations for the treatment of shock in patients with ICH aside from maintaining an adequate cerebral perfusion pressure, and shock should be treated as dictated by the underlying cause.

Assess for and Treat Elevated ICP and Herniation

Elevated ICP and/or brain herniation can be present early in ICH patients depending on size and location of the hematoma, presence of acute hydrocephalus, or both. Cerebral herniation results from regional elevations in ICP and shift of tissue across dural folds with resultant compression of healthy brain (Fig. 11.2) and frequently disastrous consequences. Patients with any of the following findings should be suspected to be herniating: decreased level of consciousness, pupillary dysfunction, or extensor posturing. Acute hydrocephalus in ICH is caused by obstruction of CSF flow due to ventricular compression or intraventricular hemorrhage (IVH) and results in depressed level of consciousness, often accompanied by some combination of the following: bilateral mid-position to large poorly reactive pupils, bilateral abducens palsy, upgaze restriction, sunsetting gaze, extensor posturing, and, when

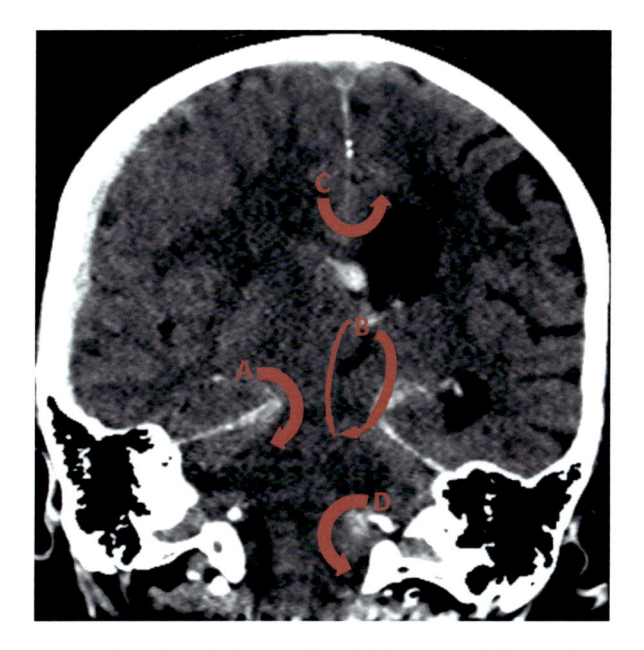

Fig. 11.2 Cartoon depiction of cerebral herniation. (**a**) Transtentorial herniation: medialization of the temporal lobe (uncus) with resultant compression of the ipsilateral cerebral peduncle. Commonly presents with ipsilateral fixed, dilated pupil with impaired adduction, exotropia and depression of the eye, and contralateral hemiparesis. (**b**) Central herniation: bilateral thalamic downward displacement with resultant compression of the midbrain. Commonly presents with coma, fixed and misposition pupils, and extensor posturing. (**c**) Subfalcine herniation: cingulate gyrus displacement inferior to the central falx resulting in compression of the pericallosal cerebral arteries and contralateral cingulate gyrus which can infrequently cause contralateral leg weakness. (**d**) Tonsillar herniation: cerebellar tonsil displacement through the foramen magnum resulting in compression of the cervicomedullary junction. Commonly presents with coma and severe dysautonomia with profound hypertension, irregular respirations, bradycardia

severe, the Cushing reflex (bradycardia, hypertension, and irregular respirations). Patients with any of these signs should be treated with elevation of the head of the bed to at least 45 degrees, sedation, hyperventilation, and bolus-dose osmotherapy. Osmotherapy can be given as mannitol 1 g/kg ideal body weight intravenous (IV) or 3% saline 3–6 mL/kg ideal body weight IV. If central venous access is in place, 23.4% saline 30–60 mL IV can be used. These are all generally administered as boluses over approximately 15 minutes. Surgical treatment may be indicated based on the CT imaging (*see* Section "Intracranial Hypertension, Hydrocephalus, and Herniation").

Diagnose ICH and Differentiate from Other Types of Stroke

Clinical Evaluation

The clinical presentation of ICH holds true to the definition of stroke: abrupt onset of focal brain injury due to a vascular etiology with resultant neurologic deficits attributable to the injured region. Although this does not differentiate ICH from AIS, initial diagnostic evaluation should always begin with a rapid, focused history and physical examination emphasizing the time course of the problem (especially the time the patient was last known to be without stroke symptoms, the "last known well" time), presence of risk factors for primary and secondary ICH (especially a detailed history of antithrombotic medications and other coagulopathies), and defining the neurologic signs and symptoms (Table 11.3). Calculation of the Glasgow Coma Scale (GCS) or the Full Outline of UnResponsiveness (FOUR) score and National Institutes of Health Stroke Scale (NIHSS) scores, when done by clinicians familiar with their use, is an efficient and reliable way to characterize the initial deficits.

Imaging

Although certain general features of the clinical presentation may be more frequent in ICH compared to AIS—including gradually progressive deficits over approximately minutes to hours, decreased level of alertness, seizure, headache, and vomiting—no clinical feature or combination thereof is specific enough to reliably differentiate between these two very different conditions [5]. Therefore CT, nearly 100% sensitive and specific for ICH is required as soon as it is safe to perform. CT is generally preferred over magnetic resonance imaging (MRI) in the emergent setting in most centers because it is faster, more readily available, and generally done in a more controlled setting with easier access to the patient and no difference in diagnostic performance.

Table 11.3 Initial diagnostic evaluation for intracerebral hemorrhage

History
Time of symptom onset or time last seen well
Specifics of the presenting stroke syndrome
Elapsed time from initial manifestations to the peak stroke syndrome
Headache: presence, evolution over time, location, and quality
Recent trauma
Medications, especially antithrombotic drugs and antihypertensive agents
Detailed past medical history focusing on presence or absence of hypertension, malignancy
Personal or family history of stroke and/or abnormal bleeding or clotting
Use of illicit drugs
Physical examination
Vital signs
Detailed neurologic examination
National Institutes of Health Stroke Severity (NIHSS)
Glasgow Coma Score (GCS) or Full Outline of UnResponsiveness (FOUR) Score
General medical examination to detect signs of cardiorespiratory dysfunction
Examination for signs of possibly associated conditions
Head lacerations or contusions, Battle sign, raccoon eyes (recent head trauma)
Meningismus (infectious vasculitis, septic venous thrombosis, aneurysmal subarachnoid hemorrhage)
Cutaneous embolic lesions (endocarditis)
Jaundice, chest spider angiomata, palmar erythema (cirrhosis)
Laboratory
Prothrombin time (PT), international normalized ratio (INR), partial thromboplastin time (PTT)
Complete blood count (CBC)
Serum or capillary glucose
Electrolytes and renal function
Serum troponin concentration
Serum and urine screening tests for drugs of abuse
Human chorionic gonadotrophin (HCG) (women of childbearing age)
Electrocardiogram (ECG)
Imaging
Non-contrast head CT for all patients
Strongly consider CT or MR angiography and venography for patients with any of the following features
Age < 60 years
No significant known history of hypertension or coagulopathy
Pregnant, ≤ 6 months postpartum, or on oral contraceptives
Known thrombophilia
History of deep vein thrombosis (DVT) or pulmonary embolism (PE)
Lobar, infratentorial, parasagittal, or bithalamic location
Multiple acute/subacute hemorrhages
Associated intraventricular or subarachnoid hemorrhage

Treat Causes of Secondary Brain Injury

Hypertension

Acute hypertension has been associated with larger hematoma volumes and worse clinical outcomes. Two large randomized control trials, INTERACT 2 and ATACH 2, showed that aggressive lowering of the systolic blood pressure (SBP) below 140 mm Hg did not definitively lead to less hematoma expansion or better clinical outcomes when compared to a SBP target below 180 mm Hg [6, 7]. Further, in ATACH 2, a post hoc analysis of safety outcomes revealed the possibility of an increased rate of renal complications in <140 mmHg arm [6]. Considered together, these trials indicate that for patients with ICH and acute hypertension, a goal SBP range of 140–160 mmHg is reasonable. This should ideally be reached within 1 hour of presentation. Intravenous infusions of nicardipine or clevidipine or intermittent intravenous labetalol boluses work well for this purpose.

Coagulopathy

Rapid assessment for correctable coagulopathy or thrombocytopenia is essential (Table 11.4). This consists of a history focusing on liver, kidney, or hematologic disease, recent ingestion of anticoagulants or antiplatelet agents, and personal or family history of bleeding diathesis and laboratory assessment of the complete blood count, activated partial thromboplastin time, and prothrombin time with international normalized ratio [8]. When available with rapid turnaround times, the dilute thrombin time (dTT) can be used to screen for coagulopathy due to dabigatran, and anti-factor Xa assays calibrated to either the specific agent or low molecular weight heparin can screen for coagulopathy due to factor Xa inhibitors.

Warfarin Correction of warfarin coagulopathy is best accomplished with 4-factor prothrombin complex concentrate (PCC). A freeze-dried concentrate of vitamin K-dependent coagulation factors, PCC is a specific antidote to warfarin that can be infused much faster and in much smaller volumes than fresh frozen plasma (FFP) [9]. The INCH trial compared PCC to FFP in 50 patients with acute vitamin K antagonist-associated ICH. The trial had to be stopped early because PCC was frankly associated with better outcomes: much faster normalization of the international normalized ratio (INR) (40 vs. 1482 minutes, $p = 0.05$), half the risk of significant hematoma expansion or death (30% PCC vs. 60% FFP, $p = 0.024$), and no increased risk of thromboembolic events [10]. Because half-lives of coagulation factors supplied by PCC (and FFP) are short, administration of these agents should always be immediately followed by 10 mg of intravenous vitamin K to prevent a rebound rise of the INR, and the INR should be monitored every 6 hours for the first 24 hours.

Table 11.4 Antithrombotic reversal

Vitamin K antagonists (warfarin)
Vitamin K 10 mg intravenous (IV)
AND
Prothrombin complex concentrate (dose based on weight, and INR) if INR > 1.4
OR
FFP (10–15 mL/kg) if prothrombin complex concentrate not available or contraindicated
Dabigatran
Activated charcoal 50 g ≤ 2 hours of ingestion
AND
Idarucizumab 5 g IV (given as 2 doses of 2.5 g/50 mL) if dTT is prolonged
Consider hemodialysis or idarucizumab re-dosing for recurrent/refractory bleeding
Factor Xa inhibitors
Activated charcoal (50 g) ≤ 2 hours of ingestion
AND
Andexanet alpha (bolus and up to 2-hour infusion—dose dependent on specific Xa inhibitor being reversed and time of last dose of the Xa inhibitor)
OR
4- factor prothrombin complex concentrate 50 units/kg
OR
Activated prothrombin complex concentrate 50 units/kg IV
Heparinoids
Unfractionated heparin
Protamine sulfate 1 mg per 100 units unfractionated heparin within last 2 hours
Enoxaparin
Protamine sulfate 1 mg per 1 mg enoxaparin within 8 hours of last administration
OR
Protamine sulfate 0.5 mg per 1 mg enoxaparin if re-dosing after first treatment
Protamine sulfate 0.5 mg per 1 mg enoxaparin within 12 hours of last administration

INR international normalized ratio, *dtt* dilute thrombin time

Factor Xa Inhibitors Management of ICH patients taking oral factor Xa (FXa) inhibitors (apixaban, betrixaban, edoxaban, rivaroxaban) is challenging. Determination of the presence of coagulopathy related to these medications is difficult: routine coagulation tests (PT and aPTT) are insensitive to their effect, and the most useful test, anti-Xa assays calibrated to each of the four available Xa inhibitors, is not widely available [8]. In the absence of specifically calibrated anti-Xa assays, one must use history: clinically relevant coagulopathy related to an oral factor Xa inhibitors is likely to be present if the last drug ingestion was within 3–5 terminal half-lives, longer in the presence of hepatic or renal dysfunction [8]. Activated charcoal should be given to patients at low risk of aspiration (including intubated patients with enteral access) if it can be administered within 2 hours of last oral FXa inhibitor ingestion [8]. Indirect evidence from experiments in animal hemorrhage models, healthy human volunteers as well as retrospective case series of patients with ICH, and other major bleeding indicates that PCC, typically at a dose of 50 Units/kilogram (U/kg), can at least partially reverse the effects of oral factor Xa inhibitors [8]. Andexanet alfa was recently approved as a specific antidote to FXa inhibitors apixaban and rivaroxaban. It is an inactivated form of FXa that serves as a decoy target that binds and neutralizes FXa inhibitors. Andexanet alfa was associated with excellent or good hemostasis in 82% of 352 patients treated after a major FXa-related bleeding (including 227 patients with ICH) [11]. Thrombotic complications within 30 days of drug administration were observed in 10% of cases. FDA approval of andexanet is conditional and requires a post-marketing randomized clinical trial of andexanet vs. usual care. The financial cost of andexanet, the durability of its reversal effect (re-emergence of coagulopathy could occur after the infusion of andexanet is stopped), and the lack of comparison with PCC remain concerns for the use of this medication.

Dabigatran Patients taking dabigatran should have a dilute thrombin time (dTT) checked immediately. If this is normal, no significant anticoagulation from dabigatran is present. If the dTT is prolonged, reversal of dabigatran coagulopathy with the specific antidote idarucizumab should be considered. In addition, activated charcoal should be given to patients at low risk of aspiration (including intubated patients with enteral access) if it can be administered within 2 hours of last dabigatran ingestion [8].

Heparin and Low Molecular Weight Heparin (LMWH) Protamine can reverse the effects of unfractionated heparin and may have some benefit in bleeding patients anticoagulated with low molecular weight heparin. Andexanet may prove to be useful for reversal of LMWH in the future, but this remains to be proven.

Antiplatelet Drugs In a single center, prospective, randomized trial, platelet transfusion was beneficial for patients with aspirin-associated ICH for which surgery (including external ventricular drain placement) was planned [12]. In contrast, for ICH patients taking a single antiplatelet agent (mostly aspirin) with no planned surgical treatment, the PATCH trial demonstrated that platelet transfusion was associated with possible harm without reduction in hematoma expansion [13]. The safety and efficacy of platelet transfusion in nonsurgical patients on single drug therapy with agents other than aspirin and combination antiplatelet therapy has not been sufficiently studied and remains undefined. Therefore, the Neurocritical Care Society suggests that for patients with antiplatelet-associated ICH, platelet transfusion should be given only to patients who are planned for a neurosurgical procedure [8]. A single dose of IV desmopressin (DDAVP), typically used for uremic bleeding, can be considered in all ICH patients taking oral antiplatelet medications [8].

Intracranial Hypertension, Hydrocephalus, and Herniation

Careful interpretation of the initial CT can allow for anticipation and prevention of intracranial hypertension and herniation, a much more effective strategy than reacting to these problems when they are already clinically apparent. First, the volume of the hematoma should be estimated using the ABC/2 method (Fig. 11.3). Next, the presence of intraventricular hemorrhage (IVH), hydrocephalus, and mass effect should be sought (Fig. 11.4a). In supratentorial hemorrhages, concerning mass effect is generally considered to be present when the perimesencephalic cisterns are crowded or the third ventricle is horizontally displaced by ≥ 5 mm (Fig. 11.4b). For cerebellar hemorrhages, mass effect is assessed by determining the degree of compression and horizontal displacement of the fourth ventricle and brainstem and the degree of effacement of the prepontine cistern (Fig. 11.5).

As described above, the initial treatment for any patient with manifest or impending intracranial hypertension or herniation should include immediate elevation of the head of bed to at least 45 degrees, sedation, hyperventilation, and bolus-dose osmotherapy.

Fig. 11.3 Non-contrast axial head CT showing acute ICH within the right thalamus and internal capsule with extension into the right lateral ventricle (arrow). The volume of ICH can be estimating using the ABC/2 method with the largest cross-sectional diameters of 3.84 cm (a), 2.63 cm (b), and seen on 6 slices at 0.5 cm thickness 3.0 cm (c). Thus the hematoma volume is $(3.84 \times 2.63 \times 3)/2 = 15.2$ mL

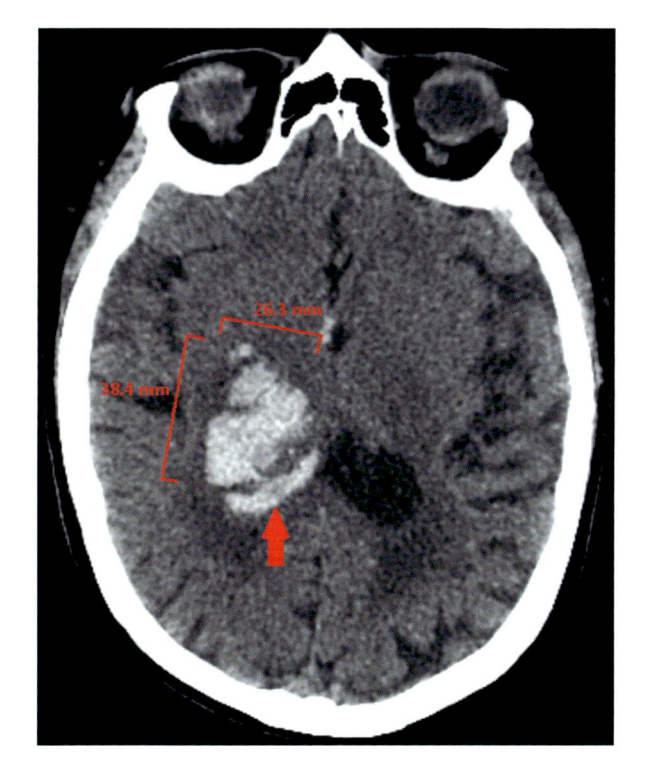

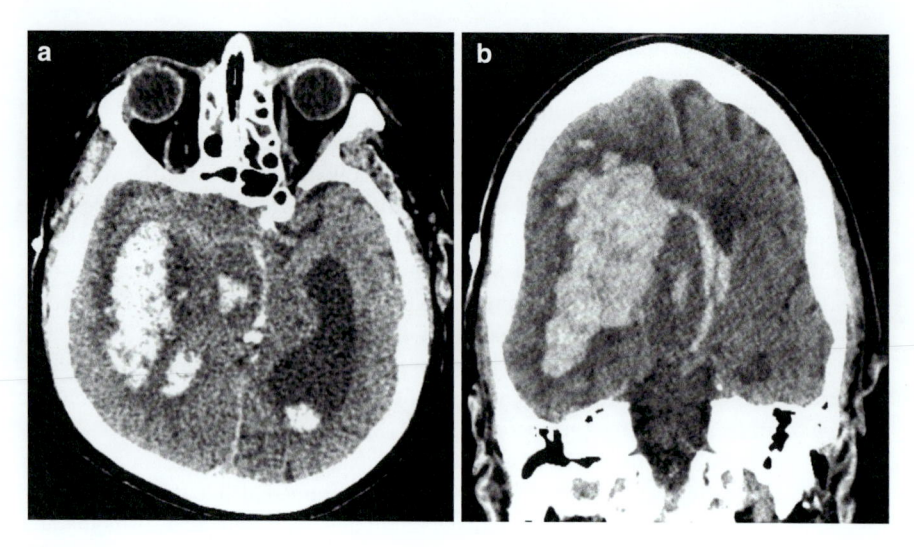

Fig. 11.4 Non-contrast head CT (**a**) axial and (**b**) coronal views. There is a large, acute ICH in the right temporal lobe and thalamus with massive extension into the lateral ventricles. This image depicts two early life-threatening diseases: obstructive hydrocephalus as demonstrated by the dramatically enlarged left lateral ventricle and cerebral herniation (both transtentorial as seen by medialization of the right temporal lobe and compression of the brainstem (**a**) and (**b**) and subfalcine as seen by shift of the right frontal lobe below the falx and compression of the medial left frontal lobe (**b**)

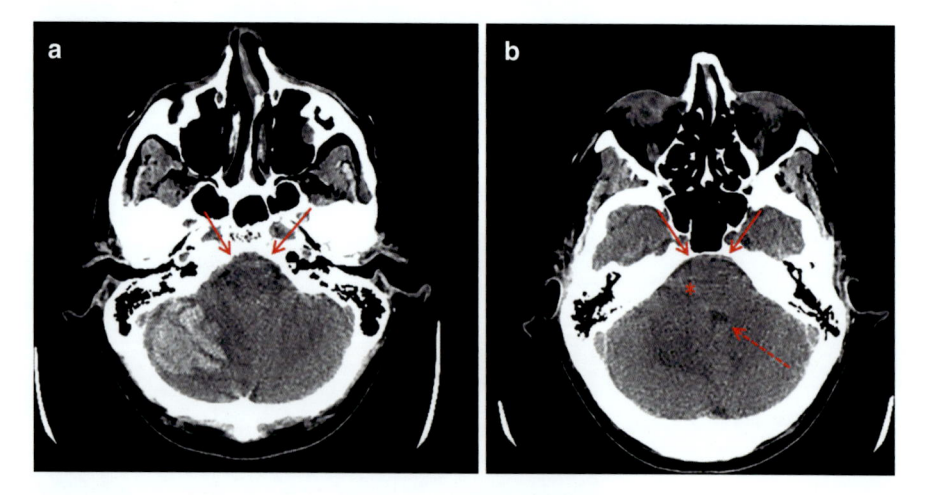

Fig. 11.5 Cerebellar hemorrhage with mass effect. Panel (**a**) demonstrates a large ICH in the inferior R cerebellar hemisphere and effacement of the perimedullary cisterns (arrows). Panel **b** is from the same scan, slightly more rostral, and shows compression and shift of the fourth ventricle (dashed arrow) and pons (asterisk) and effacement of the prepontine cistern (solid arrows)

Corticosteroids should not be used in ICH because of increased complications without benefit [14]. Patients with an abnormal level of consciousness attributable to IVH and/or hydrocephalus should be considered for emergent placement of an external ventricular drain (EVD) [14]. This will allow for immediate cerebrospinal fluid (CSF) drainage, which often rapidly can reduce the ICP; ongoing monitoring of the ICP, most useful in comatose patients in whom the neurologic examination is limited; and more rapid removal of IVH (*see* Section "Intraventricular Hemorrhage").

The utility of surgical treatment for mass effect directly attributable to the hematoma and surrounding edema in supratentorial ICH has been extensively investigated. Two large clinical trials showed that a uniform policy of early surgery (craniotomy and hematoma evacuation) leads to the same outcomes as a strategy of initial medical management with surgery for delayed neurologic deterioration [15, 16]. Surgery, therefore, should be considered a potentially lifesaving treatment for patients deteriorating due to mass effect, but should not be expected to have a beneficial effect on functional outcome. The severity of delayed deterioration that should be used as a trigger for surgery is not well defined, but operating before a decline in level of alertness is probably too early, yet surgery should occur before signs of focal brainstem compression are apparent. Decompressive hemicraniectomy alone for supratentorial ICH has not been thoroughly investigated, but may achieve similar results [17]. Because these disappointing results may be, at least in part, attributable to injury of viable perihematomal brain caused by traditional surgical techniques, the MISTIE III trial investigated the value of stereotactic hematoma evacuation (i.e., minimally invasive surgery) aided by local thrombolysis. However, this large randomized controlled trial did not show improved outcomes in patients who underwent stereotactic hematoma evacuation compared to those who did not [18].

Seizure Treatment

The risk of early seizure following ICH depends on the volume of hemorrhage, etiology, and location but is reported as high as 16% [14]. Routine antiepileptic drug prophylaxis is not recommended in the most recent American Heart and Stroke Association (AHA/ASA) guidelines [14]. Case series have suggested that prophylactic antiepileptic treatment may be associated with increased death and disability. If a seizure occurs, treatment with an appropriate antiepileptic drug should be administered, but the choice of initial drug depends on individual considerations.

Determine ICH Etiology

Although most ICH is primary (caused by chronic hypertension or cerebral amyloid angiopathy), identifying secondary etiologies (Table 11.1) is crucial as many of these necessitate use of unique treatments. Diagnosis of a ruptured arteriovenous malformation, for example, would lead to more aggressive blood pressure lowering and consideration of neurosurgical and/or endovascular treatment while diagnosis of a cerebral venous sinus thrombosis would indicate emergent initiation of anticoagulation despite the presence of acute hemorrhage. This process begins with the history, physical exam, and laboratory evaluation (Table 11.3), the findings of which will inform interpretation of the non-contrast CT and help determine if advanced neuroimaging is indicated. Patients identified as being at risk for having a macrovascular etiology should undergo emergent CT arteriography and CT venography or MR arteriography and MR venography.

Special Considerations

Much of what has been studied in ICH concerns supratentorial hemorrhages, which comprise approximately 80% of all primary ICH. However, this leaves out about 10% of primary ICH which occur in the cerebellum, 5% in the brainstem, and 5% as primary IVH. Further, hemorrhage into the ventricular system can accompany a parenchymal hematoma at any site. When ICH involves the posterior fossa or ventricles, there are important management caveats that must be considered.

Intraventricular Hemorrhage

IVH occurs in approximately 45% of patients with ICH. It is most commonly caused by basal ganglia or thalamic hemorrhages that extend into adjacent ventricles, but "primary" IVH confined to the ventricles is responsible for about 5% of ICH cases. IVH is a strong independent risk factor for death and poor functional outcome, and this risk is proportionate to the amount of IVH and associated hydrocephalus. In patients with IVH and a depressed level of consciousness, placement of an EVD to treat hydrocephalus and/or intracranial hypertension by diverting cerebrospinal fluid diversion and hastening blood clearance should be immediately pursued, yet maintaining drain patency is often a problem. When performed in strict accordance with the CLEAR-III IVH trial protocol, intraventricular administration of recombinant tissue-type plasminogen activator (rtPA) through an EVD can be safely performed in patients with extensive IVH and small or no ICH. However, while this treatment accelerates clearance of IVH, it has not yet been shown to be beneficial in terms of patient outcomes [19]. As outcomes seemed proportional to the degree and rapidity of clearance of ICH, it is hoped that future trials that improve the efficiency of IVH clearance might show clinical benefit.

Cerebellar Hemorrhage

In patients with cerebellar ICH (Fig. 11.5), the small and rigid confines of the posterior fossa confer a high risk for rapid neurologic deterioration due to compression of the adjacent brainstem, hydrocephalus due to compression and obstruction of the fourth ventricle or aqueduct, or both. Thus, cerebellar hemorrhage should always be considered a potential neurosurgical emergency. Suboccipital decompressive craniectomy with hematoma evacuation should be considered if there is a hemorrhage >3 cm in largest diameter, brainstem compression, or hydrocephalus [14]. EVD placement to relieve obstructive hydrocephalus is frequently performed along with surgical the decompression.

Brainstem Hemorrhage

Because numerous critical neurologic structures are contained within a very small region in the brainstem, clinical presentation and prognosis vary depending on the exact location of the hemorrhage. Medullary and midbrain hemorrhages are infrequent and most often caused by underlying lesions such as cavernous malformations, arteriovenous malformation, or severe coagulopathy. Pontine hemorrhages, most often caused by hypertensive vasculopathy, make up at least 75% of all brainstem hemorrhages. Depending on pontine areas involved, clinical manifestations can include decreased level of consciousness (including coma), pupillary changes (often pinpoint but reactive), eye movement abnormalities, dysarthria, sensory loss and paralysis on one or both sides of the face and limbs, extensor posturing, shivering and other non-seizure convulsive movements, and dysautonomia. Prognosis is largely dependent on the level of consciousness, precise location of the hemorrhage, and the presence or absence of IVH. Lesions that involve the pontine tegmentum (the small but crucial region just anterior to the fourth ventricle in which the reticular activating system and multiple cranial nerve nuclei are located) bilaterally are associated with the worst prognosis. Surgical hematoma evacuation does not play a role in management of primary brainstem ICH.

General Medical Management

Optimal prevention and management of medical complications of ICH is crucial, although a thorough discussion of this topic is beyond the scope of this chapter. Care of patients with ICH in a dedicated neurosciences intensive care unit or stroke care unit results in improved outcomes [20].

Hyperglycemia is prevalent in patients with ICH and is associated with increased mortality and morbidity regardless of the presence of premorbid diabetes [21]. *Hypoglycemia* also significantly exacerbates brain injury. To balance these issues, a moderately aggressive plan to keep the blood glucose concentration between 100 and 180 mg/dL is reasonable.

Fever is consistently associated with worse outcomes in neurological injury, including ICH [22]. Induction of hypothermia using external or intravascular cooling devices, however, has yet to be shown to be beneficial and is associated with increased rates of adverse events [17]. Moderately aggressive efforts to maintain body temperature in the normothermic range using acetaminophen for fever and having a low threshold start antibiotics for suspected concomitant infections (most frequently pneumonia) should be a point of emphasis.

Intravascular volume depletion is prevalent in patients with ICH and may compromise cerebral blood supply. Isotonic fluids, most commonly normal saline, should be used to target euvolemia. Hypotonic fluids are contraindicated as they may worsen cerebral edema. Hypervolemia should be avoided given the potential for worsening cerebral edema and non-neurologic complications such as pulmonary edema.

Dysphagia is common after ICH and substantially increases the risk of aspiration [14]. Patients should be maintained strictly nothing by mouth (NPO) unless they pass a dysphagia screening test. Essential enteral medications can be delivered through a nasogastric tube for patients who cannot swallow safely.

Venous thromboembolism is a major complication after ICH, and therefore prevention of deep venous thrombosis in the legs should be consistently offered through the application of intermittent pneumatic compression [23]. In general, chemoprophylaxis with heparin products can be safely added after the first 48 hours.

Prognosis

Prognostication in ICH is difficult. Multiple scoring systems exist that combine simple clinical elements to predict the probability of mortality and poor functional outcome, the most widely used being the ICH Score [24, 25] and the FUNC Score [26, 27]. Although objective, these scales are imprecise and affected by biases and therefore cannot be the relied upon as the primary basis for prognostication in the individual patient. In fact, physicians with considerable experience treating ICH may more accurately predict outcome than these scores [28]. Final formulation of clinical prognosis relies on synthesis of the multiple variables including the ICH and FUNC scores, the scores themselves, hemorrhage location, premorbid condition, clinical "gestalt," and clinical evolution over time. Excluding exceptionally severe cases, prognosis should not be delivered to the family within at least the first 24 hours after admission to avoid premature withdrawal of life-sustaining therapy.

Cardinal Messages
- As with any medical emergency, *initial assessment of circulation, airway, and breathing is paramount*—without adequate oxygen and blood delivery to the brain, subsequent ICH-specific interventions are moot.
- Rapid assessment for correctable coagulopathy and/or thrombocytopenia is essential. Medication history and laboratory assessment of the complete blood count, activated partial thromboplastin time, and prothrombin time should be completed. *Reversal of coagulopathy is determined by the underlying cause and should be rapidly pursued in all patients* (Fig. 11.1).
- Hypertension is common in patients with ICH. A systolic blood pressure goal of 140–160 mmHg should be reached as quickly as possible, with a goal of within 1 hour of presentation. Intravenous nicardipine and labetalol work well for this purpose (Fig. 11.1).
- ICH resulting in horizontal displacement of the third ventricle or compression of the fourth ventricle and/or brainstem confers high risk for cerebral herniation and elevated ICP. Treatment with hyperosmolar therapy should be considered, and neurosurgical consultation is necessary (Fig. 11.1).
- Although primary and secondary ICH have the same initial treatment (correction of coagulopathy, treatment of hypertension, and treatment of mass effect and elevated ICP), *determination of underlying etiology is crucial*. Secondary causes of ICH require additional, etiology-specific interventions to prevent recurrent hemorrhage and neurologic injury.
- Surgical management of mass effect directly attributable to hematoma and surrounding edema should be considered as *lifesaving with no beneficial effect on functional outcome*. Minimally invasive surgery is an exciting possibility that may change this, but it remains investigational.
- Prognostication in ICH is difficult yet necessary. Although there are scales for outcome prediction, these scales provide only gross estimates of risk for death and disability and should not be used in isolation for individual patients. *Excluding exceptionally severe cases, prognosis should not be delivered within at least 24 hours after admission* to avoid premature withdrawal of life-sustaining therapy.

References

1. Mozaffarian D, Benjamin EJ, Go AS, Arnett DK, Blaha MJ, et al. Executive summary: heart disease and stroke statistics-2016 update: a report from the American Heart Association. Circulation. 2016;133:447–54.
2. Van Asch CJ, Luitse MJ, Rinkel GJ, van der Tweel I, Algra A, et al. Incidence, case fatality, and functional outcome of intracerebral haemorrhage over time, according to age, sex, and ethnic origin: a systematic review and meta-analysis. Lancet Neurol. 2010;9:167–76.

3. Aronowski J, Zhao X. Molecular pathophysiology of ierebral hemorrhage: secondary brain injury. Stroke. 2011;42:1781–6.
4. Davis SM, Broderick J, Hennerici M, Brun NC, Diringer MN, et al. Hematoma growth is a determinant of mortality and poor outcome after intracerebral hemorrhage. Neurology. 2006;66:1175–81.
5. Runchey S, McGee S. Does this patient have a hemorrhagic stroke?: clinical findings distinguishing hemorrhagic stroke from ischemic stroke. JAMA. 303:2280–6.
6. The ATACH-2 Trial Investigators. Intensive blood-pressure lowering in patients with cerebral hemorrhage. N Engl J Med. 2016;375:1033–43.
7. The INTERACT2 Investigators. Rapid blood-pressure lowering in patients with acute intracerebral hemorrhage. N Engl J Med. 2013;386:2355–65.
8. Frontera JA, Lewin JJ III, Rabinstein AA, Aisiku IP, Alexandrov AW, et al. Guideline for reversal of antithrombotics in intracranial hemorrhage: a state for healthcare professionals from the neurocritical care society and society of critical care medicine. Neurocrit Care. 2016;24:6–46.
9. Sarode R, Milling TJ Jr, Refaai MA, Mangione A, Schneider A, et al. Efficacy and safety of a 4-factor prothrombin complex concentrate in patients on vitamin K antagonists presenting with major bleeding: a randomized, plasma-controlled, phase IIIb study. Circulation. 2013;128:1234–43.
10. Steiner T, Poli S, Briebe M, Husing J, Hajda J, et al. Fresh frozen plasma versus prothrombin complex concentrate in patients with intracerebral haemorrhage related to vitamin K antagonists (INCH): a randomised trial. Lancet Neurol. 2016;15:566–73.
11. Connolly SJ, Crowther M, Eikelboom JW, Gibson CM, Curnutte JT, Lawrence JH, et al. ANNEXA-4 Investigators. Full study report of andexanet alfa for bleeding associated with factor Xa inhibitors. N Engl J Med. 2019;380(14):1326–35.
12. Li X, Sun Z, Zhao W, Chen J, Li Y, et al. Effect of acetylsalicylic acid usage and platelet transfusion on postoperative hemorrhage and activities of daily living in patients with acute intracerebral hemorrhage. J Neurosurg. 2013;118:94–103.
13. Baharoglu MI, Cordonnier C, Al-Shahi Salman R, de Gans K, Koopman MM, et al. Platelet transfusion versus standard care after acute stroke due to spontaneous cerebral hemorrhage associated with antiplatelet therapy (PATCH): a randomised, open-label, phase 3 trial. Lancet. 2016;387:2605–13.
14. Hemphill JC III, Greenberg SM, Anderson CS, Becker K, Bendok BR, et al. Guidelines for the management of spontaneous intracerebral hemorrhage: a guideline for healthcare professional from the American Heart Association/American Stroke Association. Stroke. 2015;46:2032.
15. Mendelow AD, Gregson BA, Fernandes HM, et al. Early surgery versus initial conservative treatment in patients with spontaneous supratentorial intracerebral haematoma in the international surgical trial in intracerebral hemorrhage (STICH: a randomised trial). Lancet. 2005;365:387–97.
16. Mendelow AD, Gregson BA, Rowan EN, Murray GD, Gholkar A, et al. Early surgery versus initial conservative treatment in patients with spontaneous supratentorial lobar intracerebral haematoma (STICH II): a randomised trial. Lancet. 2013;382:397–408.
17. Burns JD, Fisher JL, Cervantes-Arslanian. Recent advances in the acute management of intracerebral hemorrhage. Neurol Clin. 2017;35:737–49.
18. Hanley DF, Thompson RE, Rosenblum M, Yenokyan G, Lane K, McBee N, et al. MISTIE III Investigators. Efficacy and safety of minimally invasive surgery with thrombolysis in intracerebral haemorrhage evacuation (MISTIE III): a randomised, controlled, open-label, blinded endpoint phase 3 trial. Lancet. 2019;393(10175):1021–32.
19. Hanley DF, Lane K, McBee N, Ziai W, Tuhrim S, Lees KR, et al. CLEAR III Investigators. Thrombolytic removal of intraventricular haemorrhage in treatment of severe stroke: results of the randomised, multicentre, multiregion, placebo-controlled CLEAR III trial. Lancet. 2017;389(10069):603–11.

20. Diringer MN, Edwards DF. Admission to a neurologic/neurosurgical intensive care unit is associated with reduced mortality rate after intracerebral hemorrhage. Crit Care Med. 2001;29:635–40.
21. Passero S, Ciacci G, Ulivelli M. The influence of diabetes and hyperglycemia on clinical course after intracerebral hemorrhage. Neurology. 2003;61:1351–6.
22. Greer DM, Funk SE, Reaven NL, Ouzounelli M, Uman GC. Impact of fever on outcome in patients with stroke and neurologic injury: a comprehensive meta-analysis. Stroke. 2008;39:3029–35.
23. CLOTS Trials Collaboration, Dennis M, Sandercock P, Reid J, Graham C, et al. Effectiveness of intermittent pneumatic compression in reduction of risk of deep vein thrombosis in patients who have had a stroke (CLOTS 3): a multicentre randomised controlled trial. Lancet. 2013;382:516–24.
24. Hemphill JC 3rd, Bonovich DC, Besmertis L, Manley GT, Johnston SC. The ICH score: a simple, reliable grading scale for intracerebral hemorrhage. Stroke. 2001;32:891–7.
25. Hemphill JC 3rd. Intracerebral hemorrhage (ICH) score. MDCalc Cited May 16, 2019. Available from: https://www.mdcalc.com/intracerebral-hemorrhage-ich-score.
26. Rost NS, Smith EE, Chang Y, Snider RW, Chanderraj R, et al. Prediction of functional outcome in patients with primary intracerebral hemorrhage: the FUNC score. Stroke. 2008;39:2304–9.
27. Rost NS. Functional outcome in patients with primary intracerebral hemorrahge (FUNC) score. MDCalc. Cited May 16, 2019. Available from: https://www.mdcalc.com/functional-outcome-patients-primary-intracerebral-hemorrhage-func-score.
28. Hwang DY, Dell CA, Sparks MJ, Watson TD, Langefeld CD, et al. Clinical judgment vs formal scales for predicting intracerebral hemorrhage outcomes. Neurology. 2016;86:126–33.

Chapter 12
Aneurysmal Subarachnoid Hemorrhage

Sudhir Datar

Diagnostic Key Points
- Thunderclap headache is a classic but nonspecific presenting symptom.
- CT scan of the brain has a very high sensitivity for detecting subarachnoid blood.
- Lumbar puncture may be indicated in patients with a high degree of suspicion and a negative CT scan.
- Catheter cerebral angiogram remains the gold standard test for the detection of aneurysm and analysis of its morphology.

Treatment Priorities
- Initial stabilization of circulation and airway, endotracheal intubation if needed
- Control of blood pressure and immediate correction of any coagulation abnormality
- Placement of external ventricular drain for early symptomatic hydrocephalus
- Neurosurgical clipping or endovascular coiling of aneurysm as soon as feasible
- Admission to a dedicated neurosciences intensive care unit for post interventional care

S. Datar (✉)
Department of Neurology, Wake Forest University Baptist Medical Center, Winston-Salem, NC, USA
e-mail: sdatar@wakehealth.edu

> **Prognosis at a Glance**
> - Failure to improve in neurological grade within 48 hours in poor-grade aSAH (IV-V) despite external ventricular drainage is associated with a poor outcome.
> - Delayed cerebral ischemia can worsen the outcome particularly if severe and resistant to treatment.
> - Significant recovery months later is not uncommon, and thus one must have a low threshold to continue aggressive care for patients "looking bad" during the acute hospitalization in the absence of compelling reasons not to do so.

Introduction

Subarachnoid hemorrhage due to a ruptured aneurysm (aSAH) is a complex disorder with a potential for causing devastating neurological injury if not recognized and treated in a timely fashion. The incidence of aSAH varies, but overall it is about 10 cases per 100,000 persons per year [1]. The aneurysms form usually at the branching points of vessels along the circle of Willis at the base of the brain. Some of the early complications are re-rupture of the aneurysm, neurogenic pulmonary edema, cardiac arrhythmias sometimes leading to cardiovascular collapse, and obstructive hydrocephalus. Following initial stabilization, there is a period of relative calm which may be followed by a second phase of deterioration due to vasospasm and delayed cerebral ischemia. The focus of management is early stabilization and aneurysm treatment with neurosurgical clipping or endovascular coiling. Patients then need close monitoring by a multidisciplinary team in a dedicated neurosciences intensive care unit for early detection of cerebral vasospasm and delayed cerebral ischemia. Fever, hyponatremia due to cerebral salt wasting or syndrome of inappropriate antidiuretic hormone, hospital- and ventilator-associated infections, and sometimes seizures complicate the hospital course.

Clinical Presentation

Common predisposing factors for aSAH are hypertension, smoking, heavy drinking, black race, and female gender. Patients with a family history of aSAH are at greater risk. Other risk factors include a history of polycystic kidney disease and connective tissue disorders such as Ehlers-Danlos syndrome or systemic lupus erythematosus. Patients often present with the "worst headache of my life" sometimes occurring during exertion, such as strenuous exercise or sexual intercourse. This headache is classically referred to as a "thunderclap headache" characterized by severe pain that reaches peak intensity almost instantaneously after the onset. The diagnosis can be challenging and may be missed in patients with severe chronic uncontrolled headaches with frequent emergency room visits. A history of a change in the character of the pain as well as intensity should alert the physician to the possibility of aSAH. In the absence of a previous history of chronic headache, patients may report a transient headache preceding the primary ictus by a few weeks. This is known as a "sentinel hemorrhage" caused by a brief and self-contained rupture of the aneurysm leading to leakage of a small amount of blood in the subarachnoid space.

Headache can be accompanied by severe vomiting and is sometimes misdiagnosed as a viral gastroenteritis if adequate attention is not paid to the rest of the history. Nuchal rigidity due to meningeal irritation is a common symptom. Loss of consciousness for a variable amount of time can occur, following aneurysm rupture. With arterial blood ejecting under systemic pressure, intracranial pressure (ICP) rises rapidly and can cause transient cessation of the intracranial circulation if the ICP becomes equal to or greater than the mean arterial pressure (MAP). Extensor posturing or a few myoclonic jerks occurring at the time of loss of consciousness can be confused for seizures by an inexperienced provider. A true focal or generalized seizure can occur at the onset and has been reported in about 10% of the patients. Status epilepticus is rare, but prolonged unconsciousness following a seizure in the absence of an alternative explanation such as re-bleeding or hydrocephalus should alert the physician to investigate this possibility. Focal neurological deficit in the form of hemiparesis, language impairment, and gaze preference or deviation can occur and may signal associated intracerebral hemorrhage. Third or sixth nerve palsies leading to a dysconjugate gaze and pupillary dilation from involvement of parasympathetic fibers are associated with basilar or posterior communicating artery aneurysms.

Diagnosis

A diagnosis of aSAH is suspected using clinical constellation of symptoms and is often confirmed with a non-contrast brain CT scan (Fig. 12.1) with a sensitivity exceeding 98% for detecting subarachnoid blood in the first 2–3 days after the onset of hemorrhage (in fact, a good quality CT scan, nearly conclusively excludes aSAH when performed within 6 hours of headache onset) [2]. The pattern of hemorrhage can provide a clue to the potential location of the aneurysm. For example, hemorrhage predominantly located in the interhemispheric fissure may be due to an aneurysm involving the anterior cerebral artery whereas concentration of blood in the perimesencephalic cistern and posterior fossa can suggest aneurysm arising in the basilar artery. In some cases, if the volume of blood is very small, hemorrhage may not be readily visible on the CT scan of the brain especially if not done early after the onset of symptoms. aSAH is not ruled out in this situation without a lumbar puncture. It is important however that at least 6, preferably 12 hours have

Fig. 12.1 Non-contrast brain CT scan showing characteristic hyperdense appearance of extravasated blood in the basal cisterns (green arrow)

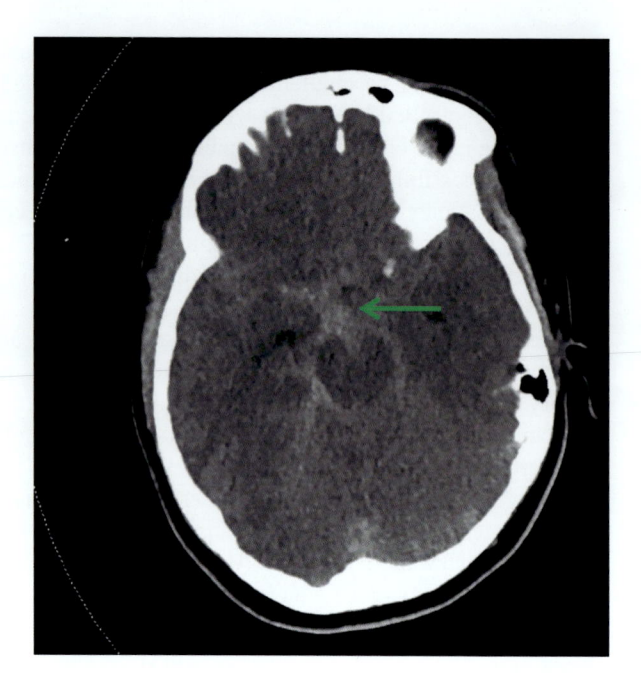

elapsed since the onset of the headache to allow sufficient time for xanthochromia to develop. Xanthochromia is far more reliable to differentiate traumatic tap from true aSAH than a drop in the red cell count between the first and the fourth tube.

CT angiogram of the brain (CTA) can be useful for a quick assessment of the location and morphology of the aneurysm especially if a catheter angiogram cannot be immediately obtained. One disadvantage of CTA is its potential to miss a small aneurysm or misdiagnose a bulge in the vessel as aneurysm. Catheter angiogram remains the gold standard test for detection of an intracranial aneurysm and for detailed examination of its morphology. Treatment of the aneurysm using platinum coils can be pursued during the same intervention. With an experienced operator, the risk of complications with catheter angiography is low, with one study reporting a neurological complication rate of 0.2% [3]. MRI with FLAIR (fluid-attenuated inversion recovery) is a reliable method of detecting SAH, but MRI is impractical as scanning takes longer, is not always readily available, and can be of poor quality in a restless patient. MRI can however identify the site of the hemorrhage in a patient with negative CT scan and positive lumbar puncture.

Initial Stabilization

In a patient with aSAH, ensuring adequate airway and circulation is a priority at the point of first contact. Acute respiratory failure can occur either due to aspiration injury from vomiting, failure to protect airway due to severe drowsiness, or neurogenic pulmonary edema [4]. When mechanical ventilation is needed, the mode that provides low tidal volume (6 ml/kg ideal body weight), low airway pressure, and maximum comfort should be selected. Pressure support ventilation (PSV) and synchronized intermittent mandatory ventilation (SIMV) may be better tolerated than controlled mechanical ventilation (CMV). Adequate analgesia is important, especially until the aneurysm is secured to prevent blood pressure and ICP swings that might increase the risk of re-rupture. However, ongoing sedation should consider the fine balance between keeping the patient at ease but also allowing neurological function to be adequately assessed to detect early complications such as re-rupture and obstructive hydrocephalus. As much as possible, patients should be liberated early from mechanical ventilation as that may not only lower the probability of ventilator-associated pneumonia but also eliminate the need for sedation thus allowing the clinician to accurately monitor neurological examination.

Vomiting and prolonged unresponsiveness can lead to dehydration and hypotension which are both delirious to the injured brain. Clinical assessment of fluid status is essential with adequate repletion of the lost volume with isotonic fluids (normal saline or Plasmalyte) to restore or maintain adequate cerebral perfusion. Precise blood pressure targets are not well established; however, it is reasonable to treat hypertension targeting for initial systolic blood pressure below 160 mmHg or mean arterial pressure below 110 mmHg [5]. Hydrocephalus after aSAH has been reported to occur in up to 67% of the cases [6]. It may be visible on the initial CT scan or may develop within the first few hours after the presentation. Hydrocephalus is clinically difficult to detect in poor-grade patients in whom a high index of suspicion and a low threshold for obtaining repeat CT scan are necessary. Placement of an EVD allows relief of intracranial hypertension by diverting the flow of CSF.

Seizures often occur at the onset of the hemorrhage; however, they need to be differentiated from extensor posturing or few brief myoclonic jerks sometimes seen at the moment of loss of consciousness. True seizures need to be treated with anti-seizure medication. Levetiracetam is often preferred due to its favorable side effect profile. Prophylactic anti-seizure medications are best avoided except in certain specific situations such as temporal lobe hemorrhage, previous history of seizures, or severe elevation of ICP with a risk of precipitous worsening with increased cerebral blood flow due to a seizure. When used prophylactically, a short course for 3–7 days is recommended. Phenytoin has been shown to worsen the outcome in patients with aSAH possibly due to increased metabolism of nimodipine from induction of cytochrome P450 system [7]. Status epilepticus is rare but should be considered in cases of persistent loss of consciousness following a seizure; these patients should be evaluated with electroencephalography.

Early Deterioration Following Aneurysm Rupture

Aneurysm re-rupture presents with a sudden clinical deterioration. Patients often become rapidly comatose, may have gasping or agonal breathing requiring immediate intubation, can have acute onset of supraventricular or ventricular arrhythmias, and are often hypertensive from acute sympathetic surge. Neurogenic pulmonary edema can lead to acute respiratory failure. New onset cranial nerve abnormalities can be seen, including pupillary dilation. If patients already have an external ventricular drain (EVD), fresh blood may be noted draining into the bag. As opposed to a sudden deterioration seen with aneurysm re-rupture, a more gradual deterioration over a matter of several hours to a day or two can signal development of obstructive hydrocephalus. This usually presents with worsening headache, confusion, and inattention followed by progressively worsening drowsiness. A prominent ocular finding is up-gaze palsy and/or downward gaze deviation which occurs due to compression of the dorsal midbrain by the third ventricle as the cerebrospinal fluid (CSF) pressure builds up. Untreated hydrocephalus will eventually lead to a comatose state and then to brain herniation.

Assessment of Severity and Prediction of Vasospasm

The World Federation of Neurological Surgeons scoring system (WFNS) utilizing Glasgow Coma Scale and motor deficits is a useful and simple clinical tool to assess the severity of aSAH and predict prognosis (Table 12.1) [8]. Grades I–III are considered good and grades IV and V are considered poor from a practical standpoint. The Fisher score predicts the risk of vasospasm based upon the thickness of blood in specific locations on brain CT scan [9]. The original scoring system has been modified incorporating the higher risk of vasospasm in patients with intraventricular hemorrhage (Table 12.2) [10].

Treatment of the Aneurysm

There are two primary modalities for treatment of cerebral aneurysms, endovascular coiling (Fig. 12.2) or open neurosurgical clipping. The pros and cons of each and detailed selection criteria are beyond the scope of this chapter; however, a few are outlined here. First and foremost factor driving the choice of the treatment modality is the aneurysm location. Aneurysms at locations that are difficult to access with

Table 12.1 Clinical grading scale for patients presenting with aneurysmal subarachnoid hemorrhage

Grade	WFNS grading system
I	GCS sum score 15 without motor deficit
II	GCS sum score 14–13 without motor deficit
III	GCS sum score 14–13 with motor deficit
IV	GCS sum score 12–7 with or without motor deficit
V	GCS sum score 6–3 with or without motor deficit

GCS Glasgow Coma Scale, *WFNS* World Federation of Neurological Surgeons

12 Aneurysmal Subarachnoid Hemorrhage

Table 12.2 Modified Fisher radiological grading scale

Scale	Modified Fisher scale
0	No SAH or IVH
1	Minimum or thin SAH, no IVH in either lateral ventricle
2	Minimum or thin SAH with IVH in both lateral ventricles
3	Thick SAH[a], no IVH in either lateral ventricle
4	Thick SAH[a] with IVH in both lateral ventricles

SAH subarachnoid hemorrhage, *IVH* intraventricular hemorrhage
[a]Completely filling ≥1 cistern or fissure

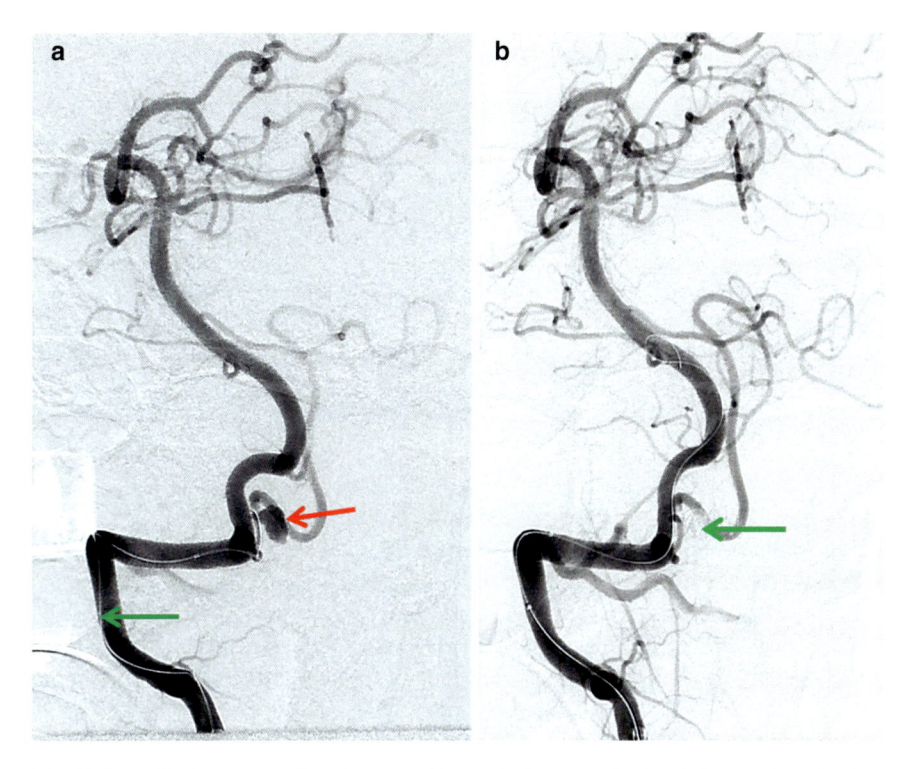

Fig. 12.2 (**a**) Catheter cerebral angiogram with vertebral artery injection in lateral view showing the aneurysm originating from the posterior inferior cerebellar artery (red arrow) and the microcatheter in the vessel positioned for coiling the aneurysm (green arrow). (**b**) Catheter cerebral angiogram with vertebral artery injection in lateral view showing a coiled aneurysm originating from the posterior inferior cerebellar artery (green arrow) and now excluded from the circulation

open surgery, such as the top of the basilar artery, are best treated with endovascular coiling. On the other hand, middle cerebral artery (MCA) aneurysms are often easier to access and can be treated with neurosurgical clipping. The second factor which determines the mode of treatment is the morphology. Aneurysms with a narrow neck can be coiled as the coil mass will be retained by the narrow neck as opposed to a wide-neck aneurysm which may not hold the coils. Typically a dome to neck ratio of greater than 2 is favorable for coiling. MCA aneurysms can have a vessel originating from the sac, and coiling the aneurysm would sacrifice that vessel leading to a stroke in the corresponding part of the brain. Clipping can get around this issue by carefully avoiding the branching arteries. All that said, when both coiling and clipping are technically feasible, randomized controlled trial data favors coiling over clipping in patients with good clinical grade [11].

Prevention and treatment of hyperglycemia in patients with aSAH is recommended. A reasonable blood sugar target is between 100 and 180 mg/dL. Neurocritical Care Society guidelines recommend maintaining serum glucose below 200 mg/dL [12].

Cardiovascular Support and Fluid Management

Blood pressure goal is typically relaxed after the aneurysm is secured as long as there are no compelling reasons for continued tight blood pressure control, such as concomitant myocardial infarction, severe heart failure, or aortic dissection. This so-called permissive hypertension is used to maintain cerebral perfusion, especially in patients at high risk of vasospasm. It is common practice to allow patients to autoregulate their systolic blood pressure to levels up to 180–200 mmHg once the aneurysm is secured. In addition, maintenance of optimal intravascular volume is crucial. Monitoring fluid intake and output and following daily weight allow for adequate replacement of lost fluid in the urine and through insensible losses. Swan Ganz catheters have fallen out of favor and are now seldom used solely for the purpose of managing fluid status. Central venous pressure monitoring can be used as an adjunct tool with a recommended pressure range between 6 and 8 mmHg, but correlation between intravascular volume and central venous pressure is fairly poor. Hypotonic fluids such as free water, dextrose water, half-normal saline, or Ringer lactate are best avoided as these fluids can worsen cerebral edema and hyponatremia. Normal saline and Plasmalyte are the two isotonic fluids of choice for maintaining euvolemia. In some cases, hypertonic fluids (1.5%, 2%, or 3% saline) may be needed for simultaneous correction of hyponatremia.

Management of Vasospasm and Delayed Cerebral Ischemia (DCI)

Oral nimodipine has been shown to reduce the frequency of DCI and improve outcome after aSAH, although the exact mechanism of action remains incompletely understood [13, 14]. The trials supporting the value of oral nimodipine did not show a significant impact on angiographically proven large vessel spasm, and consequently its benefit has been attributed to neuroprotection, though it is possible that the benefit of the drug may result from improvement of spasm in smaller arteries. The usual dose is 60 mg every 4 hours administered for 21 days. Dose adjustment to 30 mg every 2 hours may be necessary to mitigate hypotensive effect.

Vasospasm typically manifests between days 4 and 14 following the initial ictus. From a practical standpoint, if vasospasm does not appear by day 10, it is quite unlikely that it will start later. Monitoring for vasospasm and DCI is one of the cornerstones of neurocritical care. Clinical examination is the key component of daily assessment for DCI. However, clinical examination alone may not be sufficient, especially in patients with poor-grade hemorrhage (i.e., stuporous or comatose), or not reliable (because of confounding effects of sedation) and requires the clinician to monitor patients with other tools. A simple bedside noninvasive tool is transcranial Doppler ultrasonography (TCD) which measures the velocity of blood flow in the proximal large arteries at the base of the brain through transcranial windows. The velocity of blood flow increases as the diameter of the vessel is reduced by spasm. The Lindegaard ratio (the ratio of MCA velocity to extracranial carotid artery velocity) is also useful for vasospasm monitoring. Certain hyperdynamic circulatory states such as hemodynamic augmentation therapy, fever, anemia, or increased cardiac output can increase the intracranial flow velocities detected using TCD. The Lindegaard ratio helps to differentiate true vasospasm from a diffuse increase in flow from a hyperdynamic state. An absolute velocity greater than 120 cm/sec with a Lindegaard ratio > 3 has been most validated for the MCA and is considered the threshold for sonographic vasospasm [15]. One major limitation of TCD is the need for the study to be performed by trained operators in order to obtain reliable measurements. In reliable hands, TCD has a high sensitivity (90%) and negative predictive value (92%) for predicting DCI. As TCD looks only at the large arteries at the base of the brain, the study can miss vasospasm in the smaller distal vessels. Brain CT perfusion scan with CT angiogram generates a map of perfusion mismatch of brain tissue at risk of infarction thus providing data on small arterial spasm and, in some cases, can directly demonstrate spasm of large arteries [16].

Vasospasm occurs in approximately two-thirds of patients with aSAH and one-third become symptomatic. Traditional triple-H therapy involving hypervolemia, hemodilution, and hypertension has fallen out of favor as the hypervolemia leads to cardiopulmonary complications from volume overload and is not sufficient to cause a sustained increase in cerebral perfusion. By causing hemodilution, the O2-carrying capacity of the blood is lowered as well. Augmenting the blood pressure while maintaining normal intravascular volume is currently considered the mainstay of medical management for DCI. Choice of vasopressors depends on the general medical condition. In patients with impaired cardiac contractility, norepinephrine is preferred due to its beta agonistic effect which augments cardiac output, and pure alpha agonists such as phenylephrine are best avoided in these cases. Phenylephrine, which causes reflex bradycardia, is a good choice in patients with baseline tachycardia or those at risk of cardiac tachyarrhythmias. Pure cardiac ionotropic agents such as dobutamine or milrinone can be added to augment cardiac contractility, and there are reports of improvement in cerebral blood flow independent of the blood pressure with these agents. Blood pressure targets are variable throughout the literature.

Increasing the MAP by 20–25% above baseline is a reasonable starting point. If the patient has elevated ICP, a target cerebral perfusion pressure (CPP) can be used instead of the MAP to guide management. Hemodynamic augmentation is generally safe in patients with concomitant small, unruptured, unsecured aneurysms.

If there is no clinical improvement after hemodynamic augmentation, catheter angiogram should be considered within at most a few hours to prevent cerebral infarction. Balloon angioplasty of the proximal major intracranial vessels is effective in the treatment of focal large artery vasospasm with angiographic success rates of greater than 90% [17]. Balloon angioplasty is not practical for treating distal smaller vessels due to a greater risk of perforation. Intra-arterial injection of vasodilators such as verapamil or nicardipine is an option, albeit much less durable. Complications of angioplasty include rupture of the cerebral vessel, dissection, thrombosis, and cerebral embolism. Groin puncture hematomas and rarely thrombosis of the femoral artery can occur. It is to be noted that vasospasm is just one of the causes and that DCI can occur from other mechanisms [18].

Hyponatremia

The incidence of hyponatremia in patients with SAH is up to 40% and is usually asymptomatic. It can be either due to cerebral salt wasting (CSW) or the syndrome of inappropriate antidiuretic hormone (SIADH). Polyuria may signal CSW over SIADH although this is not pathognomonic. A battery of tests to differentiate SIADH from CSW is usually not necessary as salt replacement is the common treatment for both in this situation and both disorders are usually self-limited. Fluid restriction as would be otherwise indicated for SIADH is contraindicated in patients with aSAH as the dehydration can worsen DCI. Mild hyponatremia (up to 130 mEq/L) is generally asymptomatic. Seizures, alteration of consciousness, or worsening of cerebral edema can occur with severe hyponatremia (<120 mEq/L). It is reasonable to start infusion of intravenous hypertonic salt solutions (1.5%, 2%, or 3% saline) when the serum sodium drops below 130 mEq/L. In patients with high urine output, oral fludrocortisone acetate (0.2 mg two times per day) is a useful adjunctive treatment option, although it only confers a modest benefit.

Fever

Fever is common in the course of aSAH and worsens neurological outcome [19]. Common causes include pulmonary or urinary infection, drug fever, and central fever due to injury to the nervous system. Examination of a urine sample, sputum analysis and culture, blood culture, and chest radiographs are indicated to exclude infection. CSF examination obtained via EVD is confounded by the subarachnoid blood and the only reliable signs of ventriculitis are a positive Gram stain and/or culture. Fever control can be achieved with pharmacologic measures such as acetaminophen or ibuprofen (after securing the aneurysm as ibuprofen has antiplatelet effect) and, in refractory cases, using surface or endovascular cooling devices.

Hydrocephalus

Hydrocephalus often manifests early after aSAH and needs CSF diversion. The cause of hydrocephalus can be either from obstruction to the flow of CSF from intraventricular blood (obstructive) or impaired reabsorption of CSF (communicating) or both. EVD is necessary when the hydrocephalus is obstructive (the obstruction typically occurs at the level of the aqueduct and manifests with dilatation of the third but not the fourth ventricle). Lumbar drainage is a valid alternative in patients with nonobstructive (communicating) hydrocephalus. Once an EVD is placed, it is not uncommon for the drain to remain in place for up to 7–10 days. Once most of the ventricular blood is cleared and severe vasospasm is ruled out, a "weaning process" begins by raising the level of the drain gradually. If the weaning process is tolerated, EVD is removed. Patients who fail EVD weaning trials need internalization of the EVD usually in the form of ventriculoperitoneal shunt. The reported incidence of shunt dependency varies widely across series (10–40%).

Monitoring and Treatment of Intracranial Hypertension

The frequency of increased ICP can be as high as 80% according to some estimates particularly in patients with poor-grade subarachnoid hemorrhage, though ICP elevations are generally not sustained. EVD serves dual purpose in patients with aSAH, namely, ICP monitoring and drainage of CSF to treat intracranial hypertension. Sustained high ICP is associated with deranged cerebral metabolism and poor outcome. Aggressive control of fever and treatment of seizures can improve ICP by reducing brain metabolism. Usual ICP target is <20 mmHg. If ICP cannot be controlled by conservative measures and CSF drainage, osmolar therapy is indicated. In patients with aSAH, hypertonic saline is often preferred over mannitol because it leads to intravascular volume expansion and augmentation of cardiac output as compared to mannitol which can cause volume depletion from osmotic diuresis. In severe cases, sedation may be necessary, but with the clear disadvantage of confounding neurological examination. Short-acting agents such as propofol are preferred as they can be quickly held for neuro checks; in addition, propofol has an independent ICP-lowering effect. In recalcitrant cases, decompressive hemicraniectomy can be considered. Due to lack of evidence suggesting a benefit, barbiturate infusion and hypothermia are only used as a last resort when all other methods fail.

Continuous EEG Monitoring

Continuous EEG monitoring can be utilized for early detection of cortical hypoperfusion which may precede the onset of ischemic symptoms. Reductions in the alpha/delta ratio (ADR) or in alpha variability are most sensitive and specific for predicting DCI [20]. EEG can also potentially serve as a therapeutic target with hemodynamic therapy titrated to normalize ADR. However, due to limited resources and its labor-intensive nature, continuous EEG monitoring is rarely utilized for this purpose.

Subclinical status epilepticus in aSAH has been reported in 3% to 10% of the cases [21]. In patients with unexplained depression of consciousness or marked fluctuations, EEG monitoring is useful to detect subclinical seizures. Seizures should be treated with anti-seizure medications. Phenytoin has been associated with functional and cognitive disability and is therefore best avoided in patients with aSAH [7]. There is no data for prophylactic use of anti-seizure medications; however, if used, a short course (3–7 days) is recommended [12].

Prognosis

One in six patients with aSAH expires upon aneurysm rupture. However, among those who survive the ictus, mortality has declined considerably over the last three decades [22]. This favorable trend may be explained by the advent of coiling (providing an option for patients who cannot be clipped safely) and improvements in neurocritical care. With optimal care, patients with aSAH can regain excellent function, and, in fact, such outcome can be expected in patients who have no initial parenchymal damage unless delayed ischemic infarctions occur [23]. Cognitive difficulties are the most frequent sequelae, and optimal treatment of hydrocephalus may be particularly important to minimize these problems.

> **Cardinal Messages**
> - aSAH is a complex disorder with a high risk of mortality and morbidity, but often with good prognosis if optimal neurocritical care is delivered.
> - Hydrocephalus and aneurysm re-bleeding are two major causes of early decline.
> - Treatment of the aneurysm at the earliest possible opportunity minimizes the chances of re-bleeding.
> - Catheter cerebral angiogram remains the gold standard test for the detection of intracranial aneurysms and offers the possibility of treatment of the aneurysm with platinum coils.

- Cerebral vasospasm and delayed cerebral ischemia lead to secondary brain insults that worsen the outcome.
- Careful clinical examination, transcranial Doppler ultrasonography, CT perfusion imaging, and catheter angiography are used for monitoring delayed cerebral ischemia.
- Hemodynamic augmentation and maintenance of normal intravascular volume are the key elements in the treatment of delayed cerebral ischemia.
- A pessimistic prognosis is not warranted in aSAH unless major parenchymal injury is documented.

References

1. Linn FH, Rinkel GJ, Algra A, van Gijn J. Incidence of subarachnoid hemorrhage: role of region, year, and rate of computed tomography: a meta-analysis. Stroke. 1996;27(4):625–9.
2. Dubosh NM, Bellolio MF, Rabinstein AA, Edlow JA. Sensitivity of early brain computed tomography to exclude aneurysmal subarachnoid hemorrhage: a systematic review and meta-analysis. Stroke. 2016;47(3):750–5. Epub 2016 Jan 21
3. Report of World Federation of Neurological Surgeons Committee on a Universal Subarachnoid Hemorrhage Grading Scale. J Neurosurg. 1988;68(6):985–6.
4. Fisher CM, Kistler JP, Davis JM. Relation of cerebral vasospasm to subarachnoid hemorrhage visualized by computerized tomographic scanning. Neurosurgery. 1980;6(1):1–9.
5. Connolly ES Jr, Rabinstein AA, Carhuapoma JR, Derdeyn CP, Dion J, Higashida RT, Hoh BL, Kirkness CJ, Naidech AM, Ogilvy CS, Patel AB, Thompson BG, Vespa P. American Heart Association stroke council; council on cardiovascular radiology and intervention; council on cardiovascular nursing; council on cardiovascular surgery and anesthesia; council on clinical cardiology. Guidelines for the management of aneurysmal subarachnoid hemorrhage: a guideline for healthcare professionals from the American Heart Association/american Stroke Association. Stroke. 2012;43(6):1711–37. Epub 2012 May 3
6. Claassen J, Bernardini GL, Kreiter K, et al. Effect of cisternal and ventricular blood on risk of delayed cerebral ischemia after subarachnoid hemorrhage: the Fisher scale revisited. Stroke. 2001;32(9):2012–20.
7. Kaufmann TJ, Huston J 3rd, Mandrekar JN, Schleck CD, Thielen KR, Kallmes DF. Complications of diagnostic cerebral angiography: evaluation of 19,826 consecutive patients. Radiology. 2007;243(3):812–9.
8. Busl KM, Bleck TP. Neurogenic pulmonary edema. Crit Care Med. 2015;43(8):1710–5.
9. Adams H, Ban VS, Leinonen V, et al. Risk of shunting after aneurysmal subarachnoid hemorrhage: a collaborative study and initiation of a consortium. Stroke. 2016;47(10):2488–96.
10. Naidech AM, Kreiter KT, Janjua N, et al. Phenytoin exposure is associated with functional and cognitive disability after subarachnoid hemorrhage. Stroke. 2005;36(3):583–7.
11. Lindgren A, Vergouwen MD, van der Schaaf I, Algra A, Wermer M, Clarke MJ, Rinkel GJ. Endovascular coiling versus neurosurgical clipping for people with aneurysmal subarachnoid haemorrhage. Cochrane Database Syst Rev. 2018;(8):CD003085.
12. Diringer MN, Bleck TP, Claude Hemphill J 3rd, et al. Critical care management of patients following aneurysmal subarachnoid hemorrhage: recommendations from the Neurocritical Care Society's Multidisciplinary Consensus Conference. Neurocrit Care. 2011;15(2):211–40.

13. Allen GS, Ahn HS, Preziosi TJ, et al. Cerebral arterial spasm—a controlled trial of nimodipine in patients with subarachnoid hemorrhage. New Engl J Med. 1983;308(11):619–24.
14. Dorhout Mees SM, Rinkel GJ, Feigin VL, et al. Calcium antagonists for aneurysmal subarachnoid haemorrhage. Cochrane Database Syst Rev. 2007;(3):CD000277.
15. Kumar G, Alexandrov AV. Vasospasm surveillance with transcranial Doppler sonography in subarachnoid hemorrhage. J Ultrasound Med. 2015;34(8):1345–50.
16. Rabinstein AA, Lanzino G, Wijdicks EF. Multidisciplinary management and emerging therapeutic strategies in aneurysmal subarachnoid haemorrhage. Lancet Neurol. 2010;9(5):504–19.
17. Chalouhi N, Tjoumakaris S, Thakkar V, et al. Endovascular management of cerebral vasospasm following aneurysm rupture: outcomes and predictors in 116 patients. Clin Neurol Neurosurg. 2014;118:26–31.
18. Rabinstein AA. Secondary brain injury after aneurysmal subarachnoid haemorrhage: more than vasospasm. Lancet Neurol. 2011;10(7):593–5.
19. Rabinstein AA, Sandhu K. Non-infectious fever in the neurological intensive care unit: incidence, causes and predictors. J Neurol Neurosurg Psychiatry. 2007;78(11):1278–80.
20. Claassen J, Hirsch LJ, Kreiter KT, et al. Quantitative continuous EEG for detecting delayed cerebral ischemia in patients with poor-grade subarachnoid hemorrhage. Clin Neurophysiol: Off J Int Fed Clin Neurophysiol. 2004;115(12):2699–710.
21. Claassen J, Hirsch LJ, Frontera JA, et al. Prognostic significance of continuous EEG monitoring in patients with poor-grade subarachnoid hemorrhage. Neurocrit Care. 2006;4(2):103–12.
22. La Pira B, Singh TD, Rabinstein AA, Lanzino G. Time trends in outcomes after aneurysmal subarachnoid hemorrhage over the past 30 years. Mayo Clin Proc. 2018;93(12):1786–93.
23. Pegoli M, Mandrekar J, Rabinstein AA, Lanzino G. Predictors of excellent functional outcome in aneurysmal subarachnoid hemorrhage. J Neurosurg. 2015;122(2):414–8. Epub 2014 Dec 12

Chapter 13
Management of Severe Traumatic Brain Injury: A Practical Approach

Daniel Agustin Godoy, Ahsan Ali Khan, and Andres M. Rubiano

> **Diagnostic Keys**
> - Physical examination remains a fundamental pillar in the management of TBI.
> - Detailed evaluation of the head CT scans is indispensable to guide patient care.
> - Monitoring of intracranial pressure is an extremely useful diagnostic addition, which also allows for evaluation of cerebral perfusion pressure.

D. A. Godoy (✉)
Department of Critical Care, Hospital San Juan Bautista, Sanatorio Pasteur, Catamarca, Catamarca, Argentina

Neurointensive Care Unit, Sanatorio Pasteur, Catamarca, Catamarca, Argentina

Intensive Care Unit, Hospital San Juan Bautista, Catamarca, Catamarca, Argentina

A. A. Khan
Departments of Clinical Research and Neurotrauma, Meditech Foundation/Barrow Neurological Institute at PCH/University of Cambridge, Cali, Valle del Cauca, Colombia

A. M. Rubiano
Department of Clinical Research/Neurosciences Institute, El Bosque University/Meditech Foundation, Bogotá, Cundinamarca, Colombia

© Springer Nature Switzerland AG 2020
A. A. Rabinstein (ed.), *Neurological Emergencies*,
https://doi.org/10.1007/978-3-030-28072-7_13

> **Treatment Priorities**
> - Achieve physiological homeostasis.
> - Avoid secondary and tertiary insults.
> - Control intracranial hypertension.
> - Ensure adequate cerebral perfusion and oxygenation.
> - Avoid metabolic crises and energy dysfunction.

> **Prognosis at Glance**
> - Prognostic scales have been developed and validated to estimate the risk of mortality in large cohorts, but their value for individual patients is questionable.
> - Evidence of diffuse axonal damage involving the brainstem in patients with prolonged post-traumatic coma is associated with worse prognosis.
> - It is imperative to avoid therapeutic nihilism. Patients with severe TBI may regain meaningful function even after prolonged coma, especially if young.

Introduction

Severe traumatic brain injury (TBI) remains one of the leading causes of untimely death, severe cognitive and physical disability, and tremendous healthcare costs throughout the world [1, 2]. Its prevalence is particularly high in developing countries, affecting young individuals at their peak productive age as a result of road accidents and violence. In developed countries it affects older individuals with multiple comorbidities, many of them taking antithrombotic medications, with falling being the most frequent mechanism. The last decades have been marked by increased understanding of the complex pathophysiology of severe TBI together with technological advances, especially in neuromonitoring [3, 4]. Yet, the evidence supporting most medical and surgical treatment decisions in TBI remains limited [5, 6].

Definition

Severe TBI is defined by a sum score of 8 points or less in the Glasgow Coma Scale (GCS) after cardiopulmonary stabilization [3, 5]. This clinical definition takes into account ocular, verbal, and motor response, but not provides information about the pathophysiology or the type of injury.

Pathophysiology

Severe TBI is a heterogeneous disease with a complex pathophysiology [3–5]. The damage occurs as a result of the external energy applied to and absorbed by the different cranial structures (scalp, skull, brain parenchyma, cerebrospinal fluid (CSF), blood vessels). The injury type will depend on the location and severity of the applied mechanical load [7]. There are different types of mechanical load: coup or direct impact, kickback, acceleration-deceleration inertial phenomena, rotation, translation, angulation, and penetrating injuries with or without expansive waves [7]. These mechanisms can transmit energy over the static or moving (dynamic) skull [7]. The nature, intensity, and duration of the aforementioned forces determine the pattern and extent of the damage. The primary injury is then followed by secondary insults [3, 4, 7].

Primary Injuries

They occur immediately after the impact [3, 4, 7]. Their development continues during the first hours and days after the trauma. The consequence will be functional or structural, and lesions may be focal or diffuse [3, 4, 7]. Primary lesions are irreversible and do not have treatment.

Macroscopically, the primary damage may include cerebral contusions, extra-axial (subdural, extradural) or intraparenchymal hematomas, subarachnoid hemorrhage, or cerebral edema [3, 4, 7]. At the microscopic level, cell injury, lacerations, tearing and retraction of the axons, rupture, vascular torsion, and microbleeds may be evident. Diffuse axonal injury (DAI) is the classic form of diffuse brain damage; it is produced by rotation of the gray matter on the white matter due to forces acting on the axons in a linear or angular direction [3, 4, 7]. Macroscopically, it is characterized by multiple and small lesions in specific brain areas, such as the centrum semiovale, corpus callosum, pontomesencephalic tegmentum, cerebellar peduncles, and medulla [3, 4, 7].

Ischemic brain damage usually accompanies these primary lesions. Immediately after the trauma, a series of excitotoxic and inflammatory cascades are triggered, which eventually may result in energy failure and ischemia [3, 4, 7].

Secondary Insults

Secondary insults appear minutes, hours, or days after trauma and contribute to worsening the primary injury [3, 6, 8].

The toxic cascades initiated by the primary injury have different components: release of oxygen free radicals, lipid peroxidation, release of excitatory amino acids, calcium-mediated cell damage, microcirculation thrombosis, inflammation, mitochondrial dysfunction, activation of genes that trigger apoptosis, and increase in permeability of the blood-brain barrier. These phenomena result in loss of autoregu-

Table 13.1 Secondary insults

Systemic	Hypotension
	Hypoxemia
	Acidosis
	Hyper- and hypocapnia
	Agitation
	Pain
	Fever
	Hypo- and hypernatremia
	Hypo- and hyperglycemia
	Severe anemia
	Disseminated intravascular coagulation
	Inflammatory systemic response
Intracranial	Late brain hematomas
	Cerebral edema
	Hyperemia
	Vasospasm
	Sympathetic hyperactivity
	Seizures
	Spreading depolarizations
	Metabolic crises
	Cerebral vascular reactivity disorders
	Cerebral hyperthermia
	CSF disorders (hydrocephalus and intracranial hypotension)

CSF Cerebrospinal fluid

lation, decrease in cerebral blood flow (CBF), intracranial hypertension (IHT), tissue hypoxia, and energy failure [3, 6, 8].

Secondary insults may have an intracranial or systemic origin (Table 13.1). Among the systemic causes, the most detrimental are arterial hypotension and hypoxemia [3, 6, 8]. Among the intracranial mechanisms of secondary injury, IHT is particularly important because it may be life-threatening but also represents a major treatable target [3, 6, 8, 9]. IHT exerts its deleterious effect by cerebral ischemia by decreasing cerebral perfusion pressure (CPP) or by causing herniation of the parenchyma with compression and displacement of vital structures, particularly the brainstem [3, 6, 9]. Although most cases of IHT are explained by intracranial processes (mass lesions or severe edema), in some instances it can be generated by extracranial disease (increased pressure in the thoracic or abdominal compartments) [9].

Tertiary Injuries

We categorize as tertiary insults those that occur as consequence of patient care [4, 9]. In this group we include sepsis (related to urinary catheters, indwelling venous catheters, or ventricular drainage catheters; ventilator-associated pneumonia);

injury to the lung from mechanical ventilation; and toxicity from medications such as renal dysfunction (e.g., osmotherapy), intestinal ischemia (from vasopressors), myocardial depression (e.g., barbiturates), reactions to transfusion of blood products, etc. [4, 9].

Initial Assessment: Role of Neuroimaging

Clinically, it is important to follow ATLS standards (first and second exam) in an orderly and systematic manner [10]. Rapid neurological examination can be guided by the GCS or FOUR scores; the latter provides more information on brainstem responses and is not limited by orotracheal intubation (refer to Chap. 1 for a more detailed discussion on the evaluation of comatose patients) [11, 12]. Spine immobilization is indicated until obtaining adequate diagnostic images to rule out spinal cord injury [13].

Once clinically stabilized, the neurological evaluation is completed with non-contrasted computed tomography (CT), the technique of choice in the acute phase of severe TBI for several reasons:

- Widely available
- Provides diagnostic information with therapeutic and prognostic implications
- Fast full-body scanning
- Allows simultaneous resuscitation
- Can be safely performed in patients on mechanical ventilation

The classification system developed by Marshall et al. combines practicality and validated therapeutic and prognostic guidance (Fig. 13.1) [14].

Pathophysiology

Brain trauma initiates a cascade of complex pathophysiological mechanisms that compromise cellular function. Disturbances occur at different levels:

A. *Cerebral Blood Flow (CBF)*. It depends mainly on the metabolic activity in different parts of the brain [3, 9, 13, 14]. Its main determinants are the CPP and the diameter of the resistance vessels, which will depend on the state of autoregulation, that aims to maintain the CBF constant despite fluctuations in the CPP [3, 9, 13, 15]. Cerebral autoregulation in the early phase of the severe TBI may be compromised, thus rendering the CBF passively dependent on systemic blood pressure and the brain more susceptible to ischemia if systemic hypotension occurs [3, 9, 13, 15]. Additionally, CBF follows a temporal profile of three phases: an initial decrease, especially in the first 24 hours, followed by a phase of relative hyperemia from the second to fifth day and then possible CBF compromise because of vasospasm until about day 10 [3, 9, 13, 15].

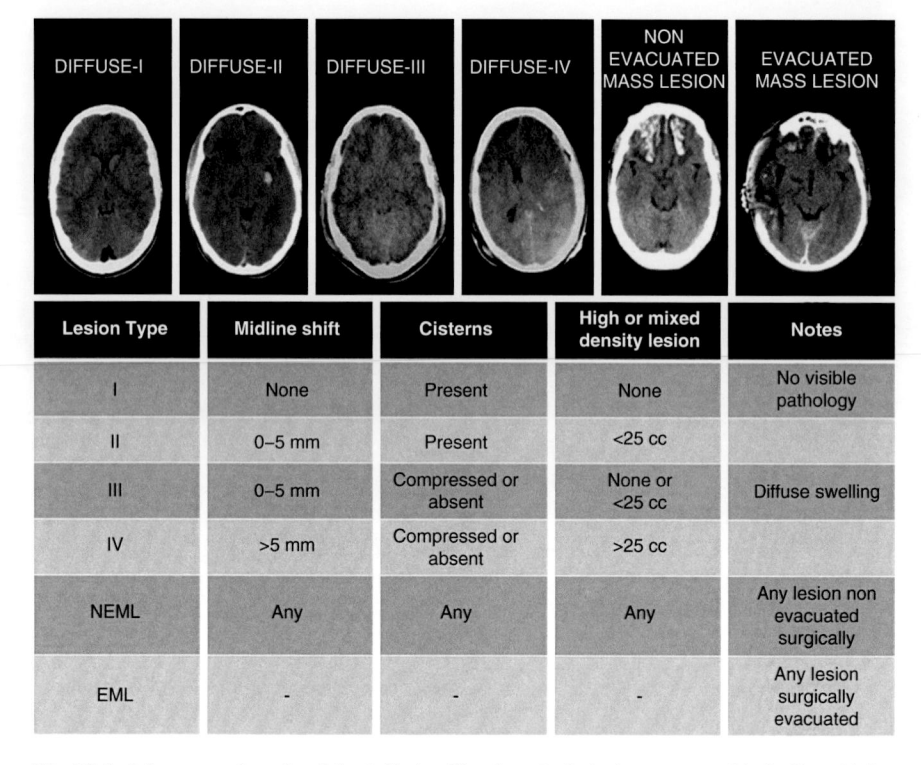

Lesion Type	Midline shift	Cisterns	High or mixed density lesion	Notes
I	None	Present	None	No visible pathology
II	0–5 mm	Present	<25 cc	
III	0–5 mm	Compressed or absent	None or <25 cc	Diffuse swelling
IV	>5 mm	Compressed or absent	>25 cc	
NEML	Any	Any	Any	Any lesion non evacuated surgically
EML	-	-	-	Any lesion surgically evacuated

Fig. 13.1 Injury types based on Marshall classification of admission tomographic findings [14]

B. *Intracranial Pressure (ICP)*. IHT is prevalent in severe TBI, but it is not always present [3, 9, 13, 15]. Its etiology is multifactorial. Following the doctrine of Monro-Kellie, the brain is inside an inextensible cavity; therefore, the ICP is the result of the sum of the pressures exerted by each of the intracranial components. The increase of ICP occurs after compensatory mechanisms become exhausted (as illustrated by the volume pressure or compliance curve), and it can be triggered as a result of a new space-occupying lesion (contusions, hematomas), increased volume of the brain parenchyma (edema), alterations in the CSF dynamics (hydrocephalus), or increase in cerebral blood volume (arterial vasodilatation, venous congestion) [3, 9, 13, 15]. Additionally, in the context of polytrauma, different situations outside the skull can cause IHT, mainly associated with elevations in intrathoracic pressure (pneumothorax, asynchrony with mechanical ventilation, inadequate PEEP) or intra-abdominal pressure (pneumoperitoneum, intra-abdominal hemorrhages, positive fluid balance, ileus) [3, 9, 13, 15].

C. *Brain Oxygenation*. The brain is metabolically very active and utilizes 20% of the oxygen consumed by the entire body [3, 13, 15]. Cerebral tissue hypoxia can originate from disorders affecting any of the components of the oxygen transport system: CBF, arterial oxygen content (which includes dissolved oxygen and oxygen bound to hemoglobin), oxygen delivery (which depends in part on the state of the dissociation curve of O2 from hemoglobin that may be influenced by temperature, acidity, or alkalinity of the blood and the 2,3-diphosphoglycerate concentration), and oxygen utilization by the cells. Alterations of the microcirculation (shunts), mitochondrial dysfunction or increased metabolic activity (seizures, sepsis, sympathetic hyperactivity), or the distance that the oxygen must cross between the capillary and the cell (edema) may cause cerebral hypoxia at the tissue level [3, 13, 15].

D. *Cerebral Metabolism.* The traumatized brain is highly vulnerable to the deficit of its energy substrates: oxygen and glucose [15, 16]. After severe TBI, the metabolic rate of oxygen usually decreases, but the metabolic rate of glucose increases, a condition called hyperglycolysis [16]. The brain utilizes 25% of the glucose consumed by the body and it lacks glucose reserves; therefore it depends on constant glucose supply. When fuel supply is insufficient, the brain suffers a "metabolic crisis." Two types of metabolic crises have been recognized: type I or ischemic, associated with oxygen deficiency, and type II or nonischemic, closely linked to glucose metabolism [15].

E. *Systemic Derangements.* Severe TBI is generally associated with a hyperadrenergic state [17]. Inflammatory and coagulation cascades are activated predisposing patients to organ dysfunction, thrombosis, and sepsis [16].

Multimodal Neuromonitoring

Technological advances now allow us to monitor multiple physiological variables that can be integrated to better understand dynamic changes in brain function in real time. Multimodality monitoring can thus be used to individualized therapeutic decisions [3, 15–18] (Fig. 13.2).

Both ICP and CPP are the parameters most commonly monitored, but they may be insufficient to detect secondary insults [3, 13, 14, 16, 17]. Brain oxygenation and energy metabolism may be impaired despite relatively normal ICP and CPP. Consequently, monitoring of local-regional brain oxygenation (ptiO2) through intracerebral probes, hemispheric-global oxygenation (SvJO2) through jugular bulb catheters, electrical function (as a surrogate of metabolic function) through continuous electroencephalography (EEG), and local cerebral metabolism through microdialysis can be useful adjuncts [3, 13, 15–17].

Transcranial Doppler provides information about flow resistance (pulsatility index) and high flow states (vasospasm, hyperemia), and it may allow testing of autoregulation (and calculation of the pressure reactivity index or PRx) and response to therapy (hyperventilation, vasopressors). Meanwhile, in addition to provide oxygenation data, ptiO2 allows us to optimize CPP through calculation of the "oxygen reactivity index" (ORx) [3, 13, 15–17].

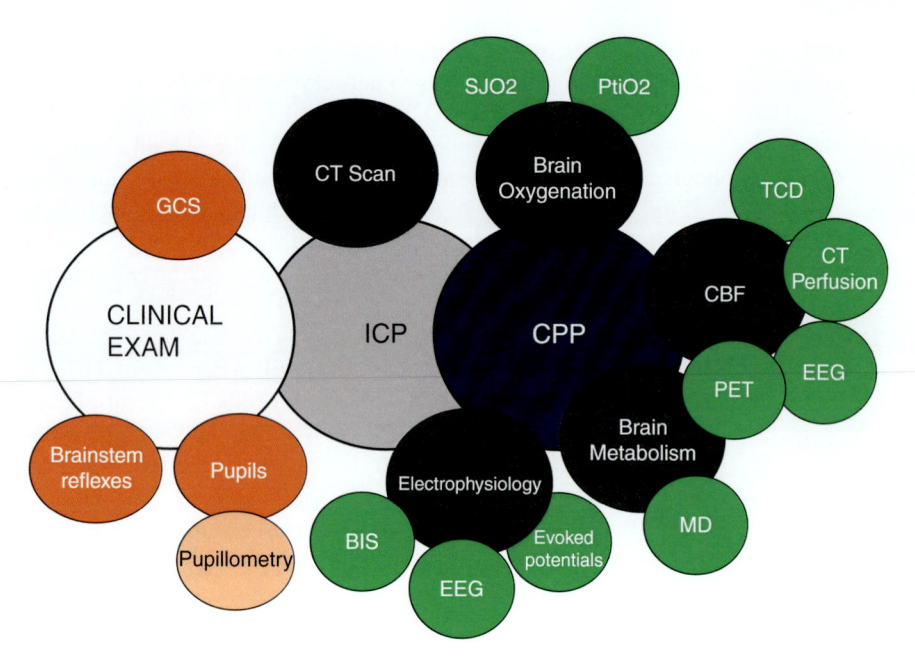

Fig. 13.2 Multimodal neuromonitoring. GCS Glasgow Coma Scale, CT computed tomography, ICP intracranial pressure, CPP cerebral perfusion pressure, SJO2 jugular vein oxygen saturation, PtiO2 brain oxygen parenchymal pressure, TCD transcranial Doppler, CBF cerebral blood flow, PET positron emission tomography, EEG electroencephalography, MD microdialysis, BIS bispectral index

Energy failure can be monitored with microdialysis, which provides data on lactate, pyruvate, and their ratio (*L*/*P*). A high *L*/*P* ratio is indicative of anaerobic metabolism. Lack of spatial resolution (i.e., it only measures concentrations within a very small area of the brain surrounding the microdialysis catheter) is a major limitation of this technique, as it is also the case for ptiO2. Positron emission tomography (PET) provides high-quality information about metabolic rates for glucose and oxygen (CMRO2, CMRgl) throughout the brain, but this technique is generally unavailable and can only offer snapshots of the situation at certain times [3, 13–17].

In summary, multimodality monitoring may facilitate individualization of therapies for specific pathophysiological processes [3, 13–18]. Examples are the use of hyperventilation in presence of hyperemia, osmotherapy for cerebral edema when autoregulation is preserved, or the use of blood pressure augmentation in the presence of mildly increased ICP with nonoptimal CPP. While this approach is intellectually appealing, it is hindered by the fact that pathophysiology is usually complex and mixed, and global monitors of brain physiology may miss focal abnormalities, while focal monitors may miss areas of ongoing damage [3, 13–17].

The Cornerstones of Medical Therapy

Physiological Neuroprotection to Avoid Secondary Insults

It is key to avoid, recognize, and correct secondary insults of systemic origin. The aim is to create a microenvironment that favors the survival and functional recovery of damaged cells [3, 9, 13, 15–17]. Physiological neuroprotection is the set of usual measures in the ICU aimed at maintaining the homeostasis of basic physiological variables, which, if altered, negatively affect brain function as well as being closely associated independently with poor outcome [3, 9, 13, 15–17] (Fig. 13.3).

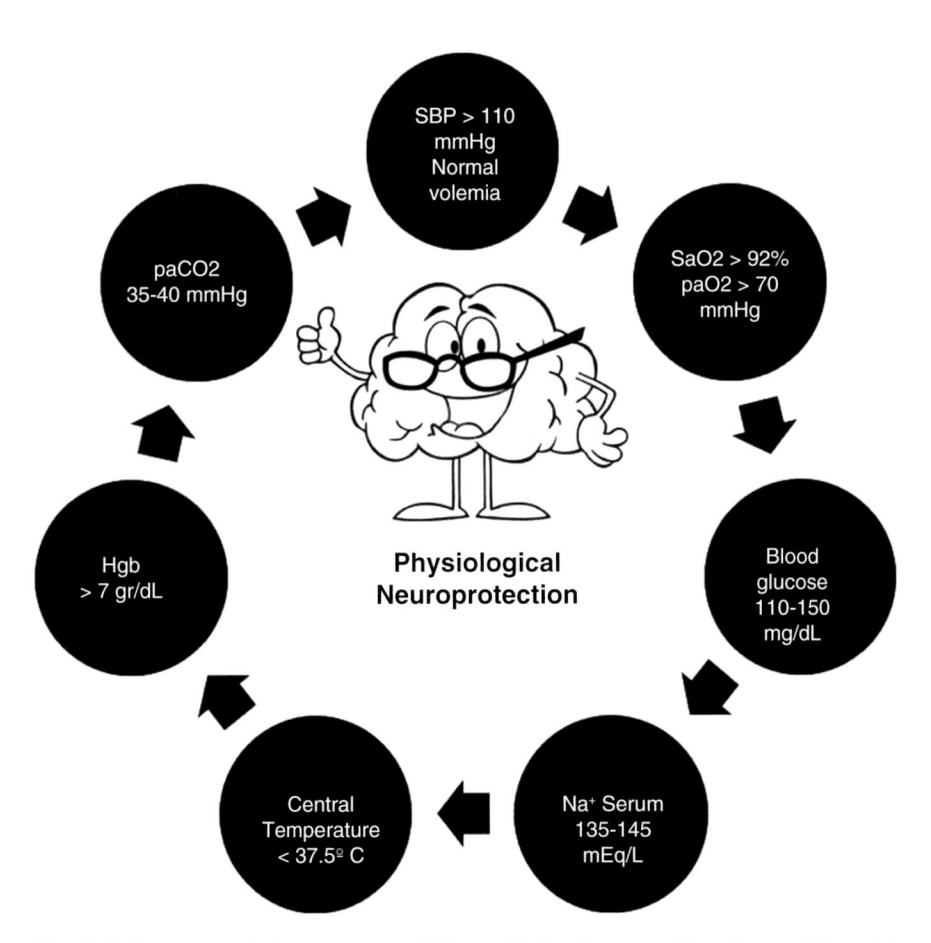

Fig. 13.3 Target physiological parameters. SBP systolic blood pressure, Na sodium, paO2 arterial oxygen pressure, SaO2 arterial oxygen saturation, paCO2 arterial carbon dioxide pressure

Patients with severe TBI often have respiratory failure. As general rule, orotracheal intubation is mandatory in patients with TBI and coma. When getting ready to intubate trauma patients, it is crucial to consider the possibilities of cervical spinal cord injury and intracranial hypertension. Thus, rapid sequence intubation with in-line spine stabilization is mandatory.

Mechanical ventilation should then be adjusted to maintain adequate ventilation and oxygenation. The therapeutic goals to achieve are:

- Normal arterial oxygenation: this is SaO2 > 92% in healthy young individuals or > 95% in patients with reduced cardiopulmonary reserve, paO2 > at 90 mmHg, always with the lowest inspired oxygen fraction to avoid oxygen toxicity. Hyperoxia does not provide additional value [17].
- Normocapnia: PaCO2 between 35 and 40 mmHg [17]. Hyperventilation targeted to induce moderate hypocapnia (PaCO2 28–32 mmHg) can be used to treat acute ICP elevations or signs of herniation, but prolonged hyperventilation and pronounced hypocapnia should be avoided because they can result in ischemia from excessive cerebral vasoconstriction [19].

The hemodynamic management should focus on maintaining adequate cerebral perfusion. Arterial hypotension should be strictly avoided. The current recommendation is to maintain systolic blood pressure greater than 110 mmHg, if possible [6]. Once ICP and CPP are available, blood pressure should be adjusted to maintain CPP values between 60 and 70 mmHg [6].

Hypotension is common shortly after severe trauma. Immediate fluid resuscitation is generally provided with crystalloids (balanced solutions may be preferable) [20]. Blood and plasma should be administered in cases of hemorrhagic shock. Two situations should be avoided:

- Fluid restriction, unless it is necessary because of decompensated cardiac failure.
- Use of hypotonic solutions (5% dextrose, lactate Ringer, 0.45% sodium chloride), because they may worsen brain edema. Glucose solutions may also provoke local acidosis, vasodilation, increased cerebral blood volume, and IHT, while providing substrate for the formation of neurotoxic substances such as glutamate [15, 17, 20].

If blood pressure goals are not rapidly achieved after fluid resuscitation, vasopressors and/or inotropic drugs must be used, and hemodynamic investigations must proceed to identify the cause of the persistent hypotension.

Hyperthermia is another highly prevalent neurotoxic secondary insult of multifactorial origin. During the acute phase of the trauma, it is generally attributed to the systemic inflammatory response and the central increase in sympathetic activity. Fever increases ICP and cerebral metabolism, which can cause tissue hypoxia, and it also decreases the seizure threshold. Normothermia can be achieved with the use of external (ice, thermal blankets, surface cooling device), pharmacological (acetaminophen, ibuprofen), or intravascular strategies [21]. Shivering should be recognized and treated promptly as it can increase metabolic demands.

The brain cells are vulnerable to alterations in the internal environment. Disorders of sodium and water metabolism are common and are associated with osmolarity alterations and changes in brain volume. Hyponatremia (serum sodium <135 mEq/L) is relatively common. Correction of hyponatremia is necessary because it can exacerbate brain edema. Hypernatremia (serum sodium >145 mEq /L) is often an iatrogenic occurrence related to the administration of osmotic agents. Yet, diabetes insipidus should be ruled out when the hypernatremia is severe and accompanied by polyuria. In general, there is no need to correct hypernatremia unless it exceeds 155–160 mEq/L.

As previously mentioned, the acutely injured brain is highly dependent on the constant supply of glucose to maintain its increased metabolic demands. Thus, maintaining normoglycemia is essential [16]. In fact, increased L/P ratio has been documented with serum glucose levels within the usual normal range (60–90 mg/dl) and no evidence of ischemia, underscoring the increased susceptibility to neuroglycopenia in patients with TBI [16].

Conversely, severe hyperglycemia can contribute to exacerbate brain damage by various local and systemic mechanisms: increased permeability of the blood-brain barrier, inflammation and thrombosis of the microcirculation, osmotic diuresis, hypovolemia, and increased susceptibility to infections [16]. Regular insulin is the treatment of choice of hyperglycemia due to its neuroprotective effects. Routine and periodic blood glucose monitoring is mandatory. We recommend starting treatment when serum glucose exceeds 180 mg/dl [15].

Anemia is frequent, multifactorial, and associated with worse prognosis. However, transfusions can cause various serious complications [22–25]. In a randomized controlled trial, neither the administration of erythropoietin nor maintaining hemoglobin concentration > 10 g/dL (as opposed to 7 g/dL) resulted in improved neurological outcome at 6 months [24]. Therefore, a restrictive transfusion strategy targeting a hemoglobin >7 g/dL is generally advisable. Although there are certain circumstances that may justify a more aggressive transfusion strategy (e.g., ptiO2 < 15 mmHg or an L/P ratio > 25), maintaining a hemoglobin concentration > 10 g/dL has been associated with increased risk of progressive hemorrhagic lesions, especially in the first 48 hours, and worse functional outcomes [23].

Clinical practice guidelines suggested in trauma patients [24]:

- Do not transfuse if hemoglobin ≥10 g/dL.
- Transfuse if hemoglobin <7 g/dL.
- Consider the clinical context (age, ischemic heart disease, hemorrhagic shock).
- Avoid transfusion of blood stored for more than 3 weeks.

Management of Intracranial Hypertension

Optimal management of IHT requires a systematic approach. The first step is to establish the cause or causes, whether inside or outside the cranium. Therapeutic measures should be adopted in a sequential and stepwise manner, from the least to the most aggressive in terms of their potential to generate undesirable effects. These treatment measures must be additive, meaning that when we decide to implement the next one, we do not abandon the previous one. It is important to take a time to evaluate the effectiveness of each measure taken before moving to the next step of the algorithm [17, 18] (Fig. 13.4).

As a general principle, space-occupying lesions (extra-axial hematomas, large hemorrhagic contusions) should be evacuated when possible. Ventricular drainage

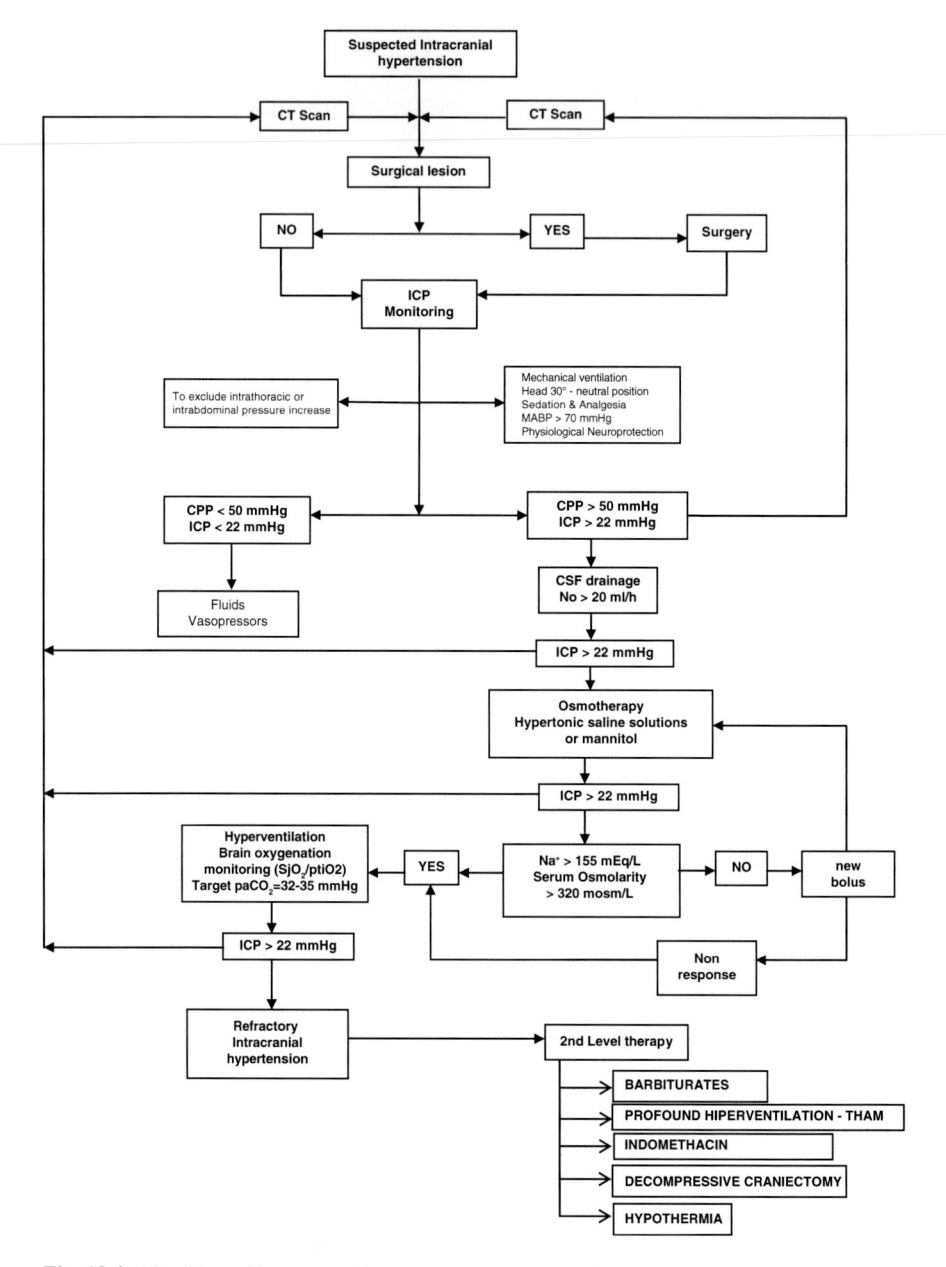

Fig. 13.4 Algorithm of intracranial hypertension management

is indicated when there is hydrocephalus and may be a useful therapeutic intervention even in patients without ventricular dilatation.

First-level measures start by placing the head in neutral position (not flexed nor extended), aligned with the rest of the body and raised to 30 degrees from the horizontal. It is important to ensure that the jugular veins are not compressed to facilitate the venous drainage from the brain. Agitation, anxiety, and pain significantly increase blood pressure and ICP; therefore, analgesia and sedation are essential for the control of IHT. We prefer using short-acting agents (remifentanil/propofol) to allow brief interruptions for neurological examination. The determination of the adequacy of analgesia and sedation for these patients still relies on the observation of indirect clinical signs (tachycardia, systemic hypertension, ICP increase) and should be monitored with a formal scale (such as the Richmond Agitation Scoring System or RASS). Some centers favor the use of the bispectral index.

Osmotherapy is the cornerstone of pharmacological treatment for the control of IHT [3, 5, 9, 13, 17]. Osmotic agents work by creating gradients causing fluid shift from the interstitial space to the intravascular space, and they improve the rheological properties of the blood, thus increasing CBF and in turn causing a compensatory vasoconstriction that lowers the ICP. The most common agents are mannitol and hypertonic saline solutions (HSS). Both share pharmacological properties: low molecular weight, similar distribution in the extracellular space, and similar half-life.

Mannitol is administered as a 20% solution in bolus doses usually ranging from 0.25 to 1 g/kg. It can be safely administered through a peripheral vein. The maximal effects of mannitol are observed after 30–40 minutes, but ICP may start to decline within minutes and the effect can last for several hours. Mannitol requires monitoring of serum osmolality (or ideally the osmolar gap) and intravascular volume status. A serum osmolality >320 mOsm/L is associated with higher risk of acute renal injury; this risk can be reduced by strictly avoiding intravascular volume contraction.

HSS rapidly expands the intravascular space and can improve cardiac output. It may have a greater and longer effect (18–24 hours) on ICP than mannitol and may also have a better effect on CPP [26]. Administration practices vary across centers, but any concentration $\geq 3\%$ should be infused into a central vein. Concentrations used go from 3% to 23.4% and the volumes of the bolus depend on the concentration chosen. Monitoring of serum sodium is necessary, and HSS administration is generally stopped when hypernatremia exceeds 155–160 mEq/L. Congestive heart failure and hyperchloremic acidosis are the major side effects.

Hypertonic lactate (0.5 molar) has emerged as an alternative osmotic agent [13]. It avoids the risk of hyperchloremia and can help to mitigate the increase in energetic demands because lactate can be used as fuel by astrocytes and neurons [14].

Hyperventilation decreases PaCO2, thus inducing vasoconstriction by alkalinizing CSF, which in turn reduces CBV and lowers ICP. However, effects are transient because of re-equilibration of the pH on the CSF, and, most notably, cerebral vasoconstriction may result in ischemia if excessive. Consequently, hyperventilation should not be used prophylactically, and it should be limited to the emergency management of life-threatening IHT only until other treatments can be initiated. While inducing hyperventilation, it is recommended to continuously monitor expired (end-tidal) CO2, regional cerebral oxygenation, or both [19].

Refractory ICH is defined by the failure of first-level measures and osmotherapy to control ICP, a situation that occurs in approximately 10–15% of cases [3, 5, 13]. Refractoriness denotes a poor prognosis with mortality rates that may exceed 80%. In this situation, rescue therapeutic measures become necessary, though they carry high risks of serious adverse effects.

Barbiturates at high doses are an option [3, 5, 13]. Barbiturates decrease cerebral metabolism, causing a consequent reduction in CBF. Thiopental has a half-life of 9–27 hours; it is administered in a loading dose of 300–500 mg, which can be repeated every 30 minutes, followed by continuous infusion at the rate of 1–6 mg/kg/h. Pentobarbital is generally given as a bolus of 5–10 mg/kg, which can be repeated every 15–20 minutes, followed by continuous infusion between 1 and 5 mg/kg/h. These agents can cause arterial hypotension, myocardial depression, and potentially severe reductions of CPP. Additionally, barbiturates have immunosuppressant properties and therefore increase the susceptibility to infections, particularly pneumonia. Adynamic ileus, hepatotoxicity, and very prolonged sedation are additional untoward effects.

Indomethacin is a nonsteroidal anti-inflammatory drug, unique for its vasoactive properties at the level of resistance vessels, causing vasoconstriction with CVB and ICP decrease [13]. After indomethacin bolus, CBF decreases on average by around 30%. In theory, this effect could induce cerebral ischemia, but such complication has never been demonstrated which may be explained by the coupled reduction in cerebral metabolic rate of oxygen [13]. Other side effects of indomethacin include renal failure, bleeding from platelet anti-aggregation, and peptic ulcers. Abrupt discontinuation is not recommended because ICP can increase suddenly as a rebound effect [13].

Induced hypothermia can reduce ICP, but a randomized controlled trial showed that therapeutic cooling (32–35 °C) was associated with worse functional outcomes (including a higher mortality rate) as compared with standard care in patients with IHT [27].

To Maintaining Adequate Brain Oxygenation

Brain tissue hypoxia is defined as the inability of the body to provide enough oxygen to meet the cellular metabolic demands in the brain or the inability of the brain cells to use the oxygen that is provided. Brain oxygenation can be estimated by measuring the oxygen saturation in the jugular bulb (SvjO2), a hemispheric-global measure, or within the cerebral parenchyma (ptiO2), a local measure [3, 13, 14, 28]. Both parameters reflect the balance between supply and demand of oxygen, but both have limitations; consequently, it is ideal to have both measures simultaneously available. SvjO2 < 50% and ptiO2 < 20 mmHg indicate cerebral tissue hypoxia.

We recommend the analysis of the possible causes of hypoxia following the "oxygen route" from the ambient air to its final destination, the mitochondria (Fig. 13.5).

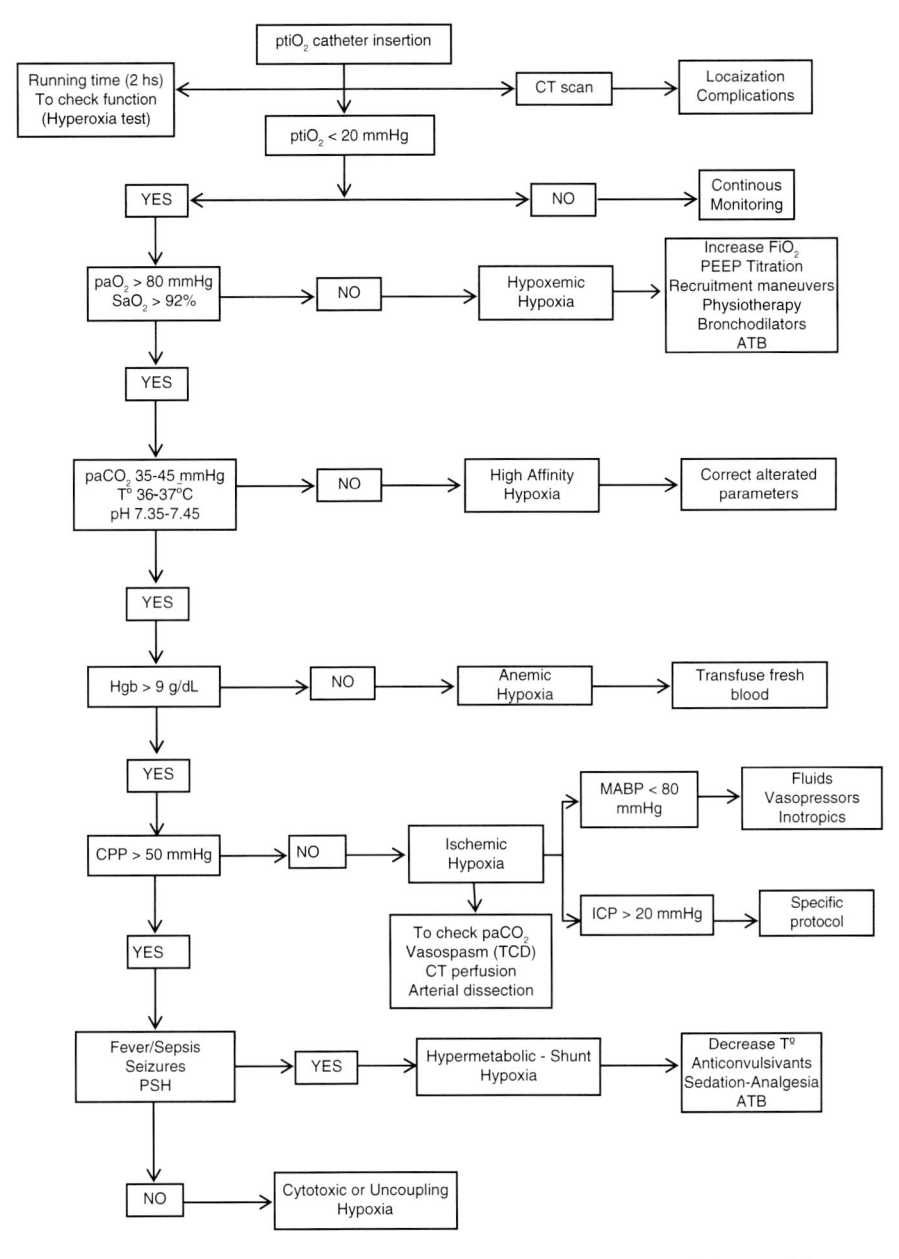

Fig. 13.5 Stepwise approach to brain hypoxia. PSH, paroxysmal sympathetic hyperactivity

Causes of tissue hypoxia:

A. Ischemic: from inadequate CBF.
B. Hypoxemic: from a gas exchange problem.
C. Anemic: from insufficient hemoglobin.

D. High hemoglobin affinity for oxygen: conditions that shift the oxygen-hemoglobin dissociation curve to the left, such as hyperventilation, metabolic alkalosis, hypothermia.
E. Diffusion: when the distance that the oxygen must travel to reach the cell increases as it happens with cerebral edema.
F. Hypermetabolic: from increased oxygen demand, as seen with seizures, sepsis, inflammation, sympathetic hyperactivity.
G. Hypoxia due to shunt, O2/ATP decoupling (mitochondrial failure), cytotoxic edema: they are diagnosed after discarding the previous causes.

General Care

It is important to highlight here that severe TBI is an entity with many systemic repercussions; therefore general measures inherent to any critically ill patients must be taken. They include:

A. Eye care
B. Frequent and periodic oral hygiene
C. Pulmonary toileting
D. Early initiation of nutrition, preferably through the enteral route
E. Prophylaxis of gastrointestinal bleeding, gastroparesis, ileus, and constipation
F. Deep vein thrombosis prophylaxis
G. Early physical therapy and mobilization

Pharmacological prophylaxis can reduce the risk of early seizures but does not lower the incidence of late epilepsy; thus, a short course (7–10 days) of an antiseizure medication is recommended [6]. Patients at higher risk for early seizures are those with depressed skull fractures, penetrating injuries, brain contusions, epidural or subdural hematomas, or previous seizures [3, 6]. It is not established which antiseizure drug is better. We favor levetiracetam because of its favorable side effect profile and lack of interaction with other drugs (see Chap. 2 for a detailed discussion on antiseizure medications).

Paroxysmal sympathetic hyperactivity is a common complication of severe TBI. It is manifested by episodes of fever, hypertension, tachycardia, tachypnea, diaphoresis, and sometimes tonic posturing. If left uncontrolled, they can substantially increase metabolic demands. Intravenous morphine sulfate is useful in aborting the episodes, and gabapentin, propranolol, and clonidine or dexmedetomidine are helpful in preventing their occurrence [29].

Surgical Management of TBI

The surgical treatment of patients with severe TBI primarily consists of interventions to relieve mass effect [30, 31]. Surgical indication depends on the clinical picture, image findings, and monitoring variables.

We favor the use of a mnemonic (ABCDE) to facilitate a methodical interpretation of the brain scan (Fig. 13.6):

A. Asymmetry and abnormality: Check for asymmetries or presence of abnormal hyperdensities (blood collections) or hypodensities (air, brain edema, infarcts).
B. Blood volume: Measure the volumes of the post-traumatic blood collections (Fig. 13.7).
    Epidural and intracerebral hematomas: (AxBxC)/2.
    Subdural hematoma: Measure the thickness of the hematoma.
C. Cisterns: Check for presence, partial absence, or full absence of the basal cisterns.
D. Deviation of the midline: Apply (A/2)—B method for evaluation of midline shift. A will be measured at the level of the foramen of Monro, from temporal to temporal bone. B will be measured on the side of the shift from the septum pellucidum to the temporal bone immediately behind line A.
E. External elements: Describe any other abnormal elements like foreign bodies, metal fragments, subarachnoid hemorrhage, infarcts, or pneumocephalus.

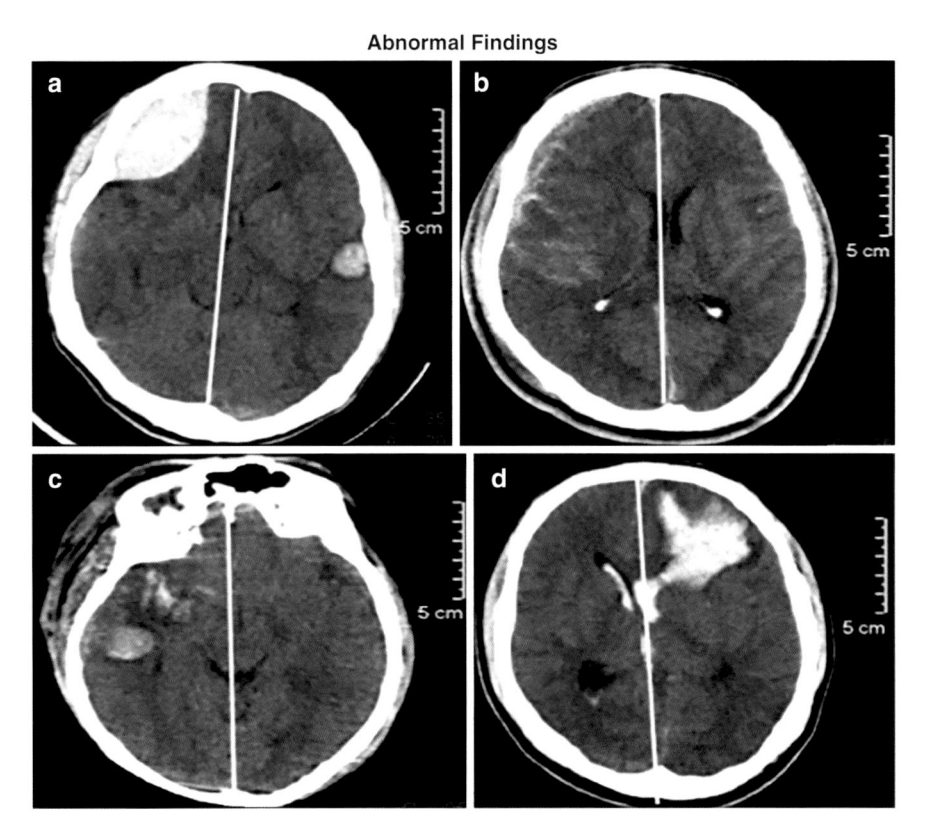

Fig. 13.6 The (**a–e**) proposed method for emergency interpretation of the head CT in traumatic brain injury. The sequence of reading includes asymmetry or abnormal findings, blood volume, cisternal compression, deviation of the midline, and external elements

Blood volume: Subdural

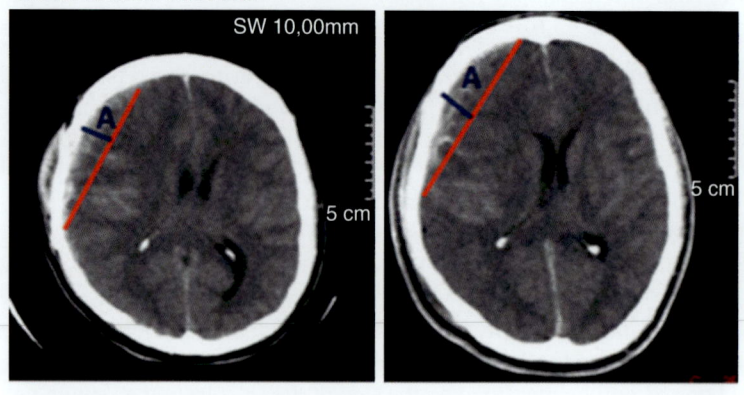

Blood volume: Epidural/intracerebral

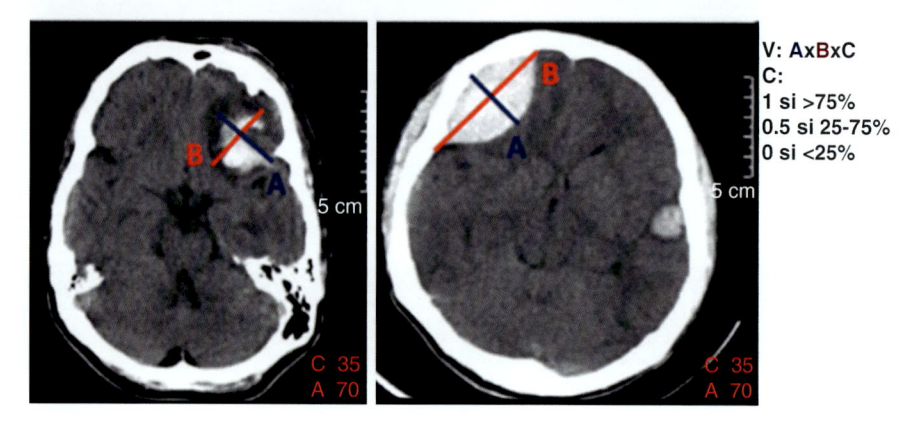

V: AxBxC
C:
1 si >75%
0.5 si 25-75%
0 si <25%

Cisternal Compression

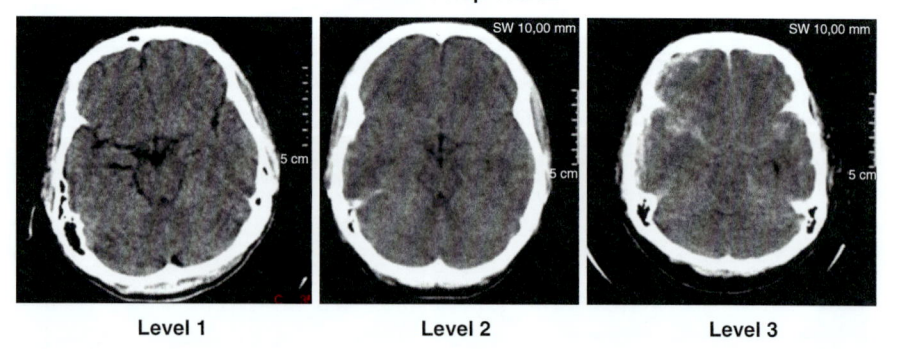

Level 1 Level 2 Level 3

Fig. 13.6 (continued)

Deviation of midline

DML: (A/2)-B
DML: (14/2)-4.5 = 2.5cm

External Elements

Fig. 13.6 (continued)

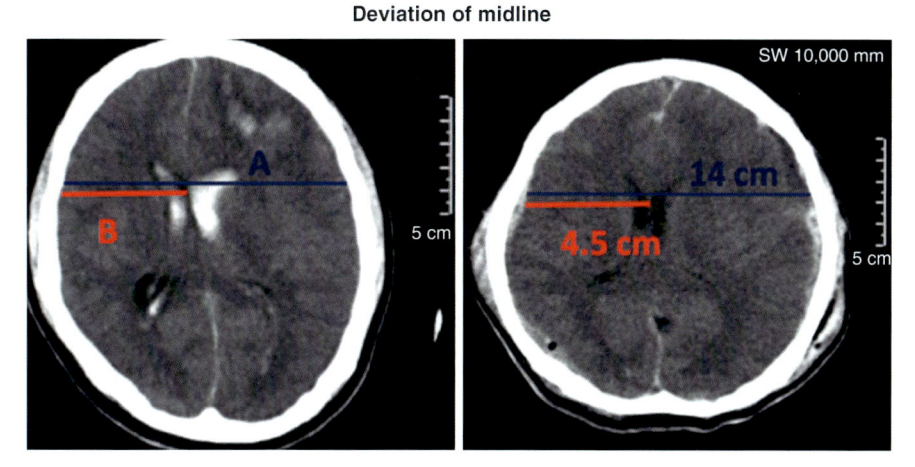

The Guidelines for Surgical Management of severe TBI [30] recommended surgery in the following cases:

- Epidural lesion of more than 30 cc independent of the GCS
- Subdural mass of more than 10 mm thickness independent of the GCS
- Subdural mass lesion with midline deviation of more than 5 mm
- Intracerebral mass lesion of more than 50 cc

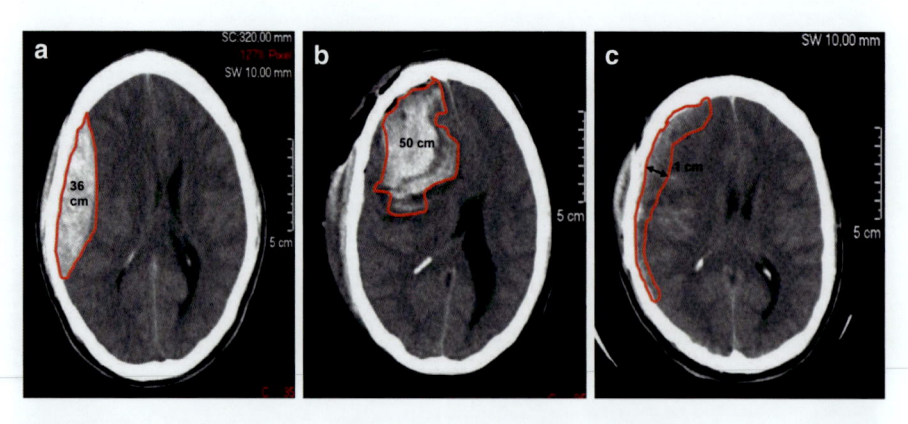

Fig. 13.7 (**a**) Epidural hematoma with a convex shape toward the midline with volume of 36 cc, which is a surgical indication independent of the patient's GCS. (**b**) Intraparenchymal hematoma of 50 cc of volume with midline deviation and compression of basal cisterns. In this case, there is surgical indication. (**c**) Acute subdural hematoma, with thickness greater than 1 cm. It is an emergency that requires surgery regardless of the patient's GCS

- Diffuse lesion with midline shift >5 mm or with obliteration of the basal cisterns compatible with a Grade II or III edema on the Marshall CT classification. Suggested management: unilateral or bilateral decompressive craniectomy

Surgical management of mass lesions can be restricted to evacuation only or combined with decompressive craniectomy. Open or markedly depressed skull fractures require surgical intervention. Closed fractures with depression less than 1 cm and without evidence of dural penetration or cerebrospinal fluid leak can be observed and managed conservatively.

In cases of refractory intracranial hypertension from diffuse brain injury, decompressive craniectomy may be indicated to reduce ICP and improve brain perfusion and oxygenation. Randomized controlled trials of decompressive craniectomy for severe TBI have shown conflicting results that can be at least partially explained by differences in patient selection [32, 33]. Decompressive craniectomy can be either unilateral or bilateral. Performing a wide craniectomy (at least 12 × 15 cm) is recommended to avoid complications, such as brain tissue herniation or tissue ischemia under the bony edge. In some cases, if there is no ICP control or there is an ipsilateral midline shift toward the site of the previous decompression, it is necessary to perform a bilateral procedure (Figs. 13.8 and 13.9).

Surgical approaches are applied also for the management of penetrating cranial injuries. Recently, the experience of military neurotrauma surgery in the Middle East has shown benefits of surgery for damage control in penetrating and blasting injuries. The benefits of surgery in penetrating injuries in civilian environments have also been reported. Factors associated with a poor neurological outcome in patients with penetrating injuries include involvement of two or more lobes, wound that crosses the midline, brainstem injury, transventricular wound, and presence of subarachnoid hemorrhage in basal cisterns (Fig. 13.10).

Prognosis

Although severe TBI, particularly when complicated with IHT, carries a high mortality and a high risk of cognitive and physical sequelae among survivors, gradual recovery is possible even after prolonged coma. Thus, it is imperative to avoid a nihilistic attitude.

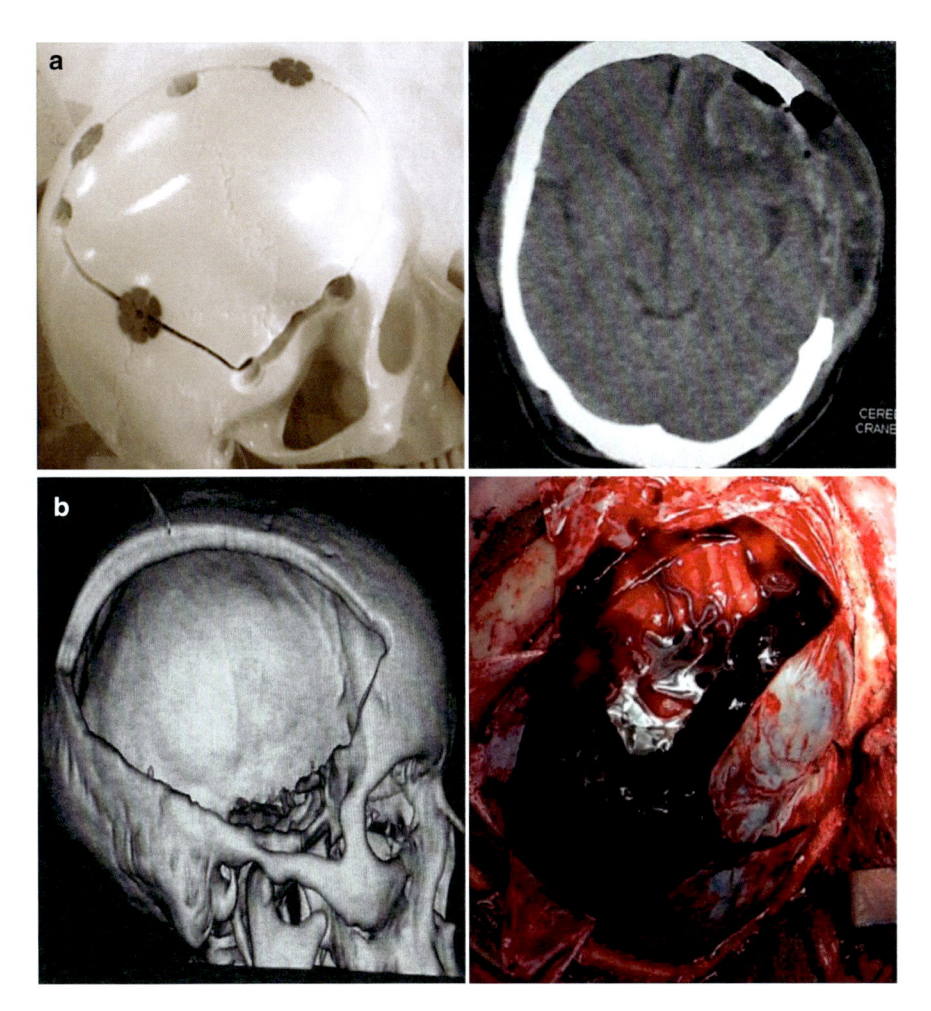

Fig. 13.8 The procedure of decompressive hemicraniectomy can effectively lower the intracranial pressure. Craniectomy should be wide. (**a**) Conventional technique in which a standard trauma flap incision is made, which resulted in restricted exposure in the low temporal region. (**b**) Limited decompression is evident. (**c**) The modified Kempe incision allows a larger craniectomy, including removal of the posterior and basal bone. (**d**) A wider decompression is evident after Kempe's incision

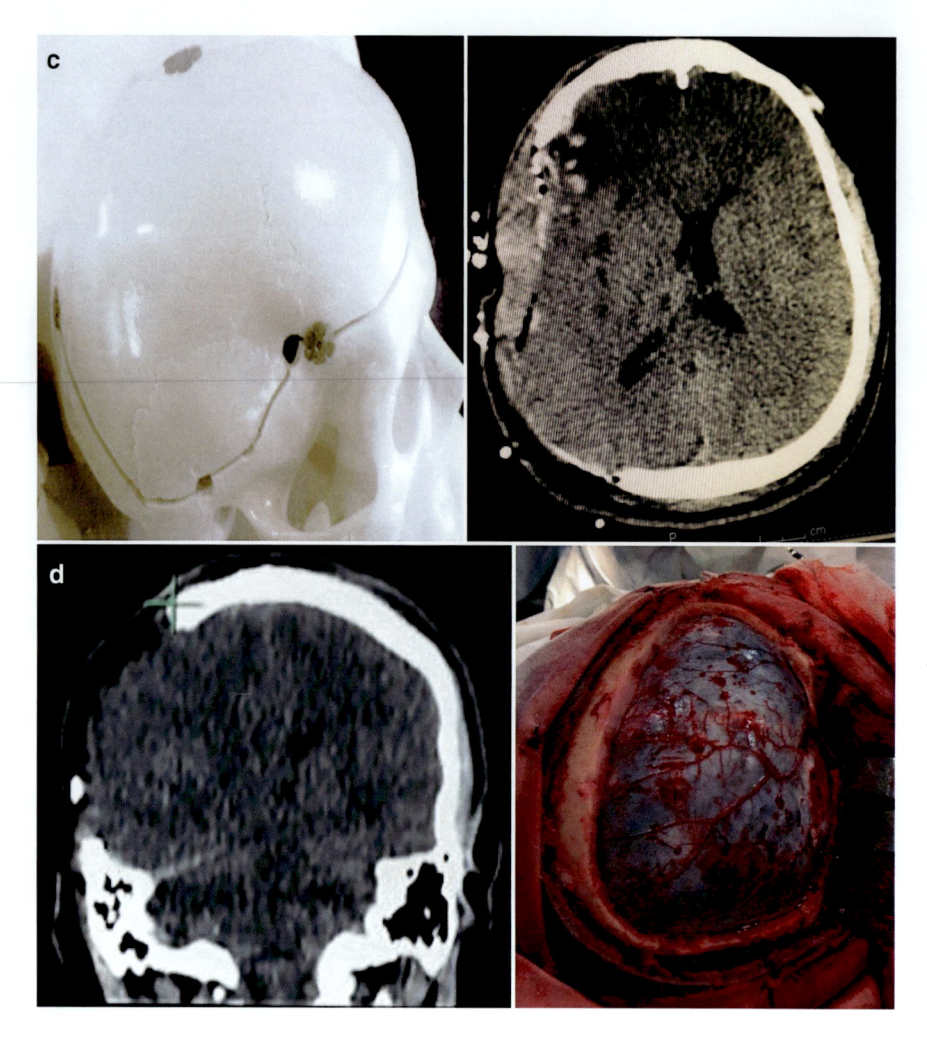

Fig. 13.8 (continued)

Older age, refractory IHT, and evidence of diffuse axonal injury affecting the brainstem on brain MRI are factors strongly associated with worse prognosis [17].

Prognostic scores derived from large cohorts (CRASH, IMPACT) are useful epidemiologically but should not be used for prognostication in individual cases. In addition, these scores were developed to predict mortality but not functional outcome in survivors.

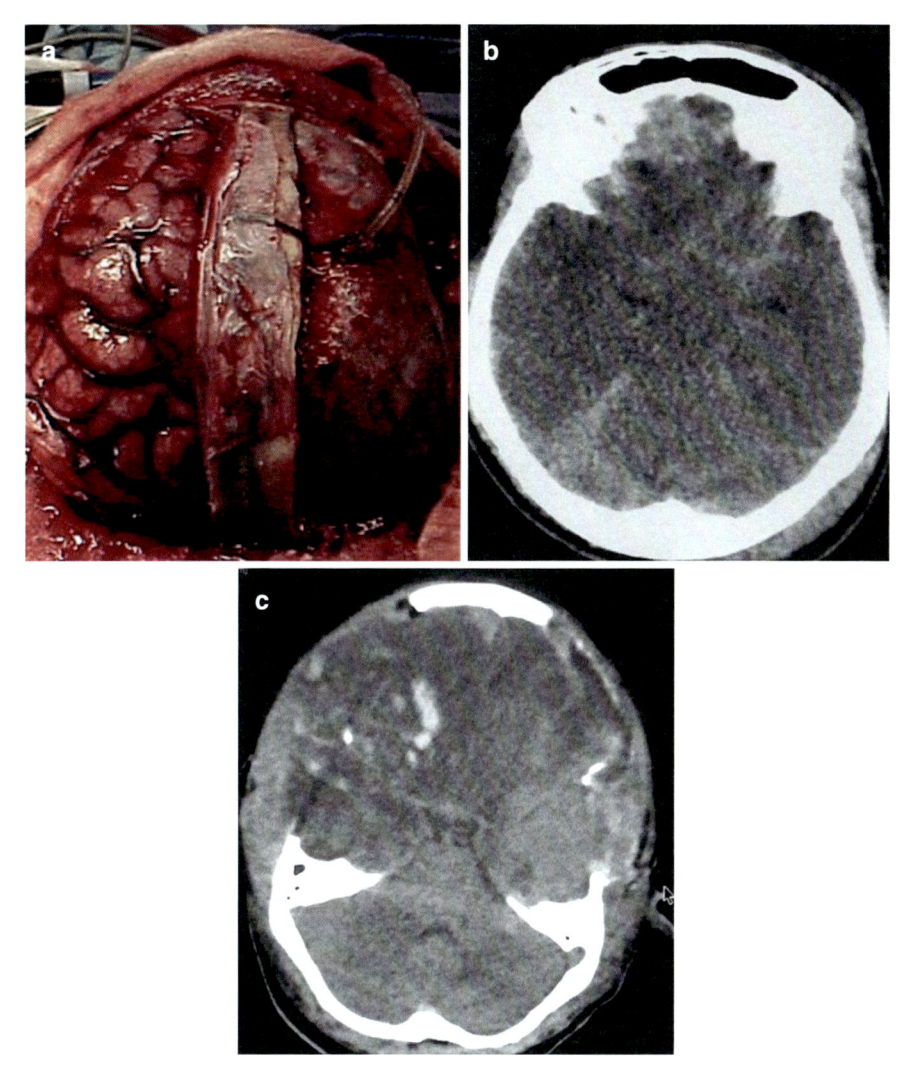

Fig. 13.9 (**a–c**) Bilateral bifrontal decompression in a patient with severe TBI and severe brain edema (Marshall grade III). From left to right: intraoperative photograph, preoperative CT scan, and postoperative CT scan

Fig. 13.10 Cranial wound due to low velocity projectile in right frontal region, single hemisphere compromise. This kind of injury can be managed with an early surgical decompression

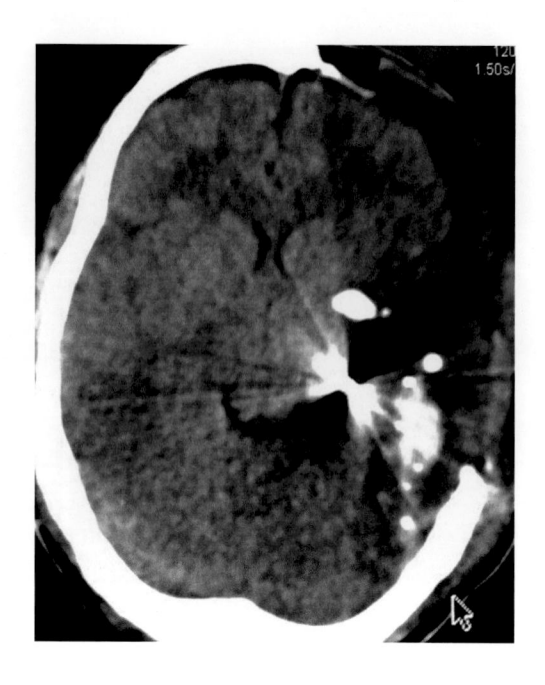

Cardinal Messages
- Severe traumatic brain injury (TBI) remains a major global health problem, with an epidemiological profile that changes according to the age group.
- The pathophysiology of severe TBI is complex and heterogeneous.
- Treatment priorities include surgical treatment of lesions causing mass effect and optimization of intracranial pressure and cerebral perfusion pressure.
- Modern management should be based on information obtained from multimodal monitoring.
- Optimal care of patients with severe TBI demands a multidisciplinary approach.
- Prolonged coma is not inconsistent with meaningful recovery, especially in young patients.

References

1. Rubiano AM, Carney N, Chesnut R, Puyana JC. Global neurotrauma research challenges and opportunities. Nature. 2015;527:S193–7.
2. Roozenbeek B, Maas AI, Menon DK. Changing patterns in the epidemiology of traumatic brain injury. Nat Rev Neurol. 2013;9:231–6.
3. Stochetti N, Carbonara M, Citerio G, Ercole A, Skrifvars MB, Smielewski P, et al. Severe traumatic brain Injury: targeted management in the intensive care unit. Lancet Neurol. 2017;16:452–64.

4. Chesnut RM. A conceptual approach to managing severe traumatic brain injury in a time of uncertainly. Ann N Y Acad Sci. 2015;1345:99–107.
5. Brain Trauma Foundation; American Association of Neurological Surgeons; Congress of Neurological Surgeons. Guidelines for the management of severe traumatic brain injury. J Neurotrauma. 2007;24(Suppl 1):S1–106.
6. Carney N, Totten AM, O'Reilly C, Ullman JS, Hawryluk GW, Bell MJ, Bratton SL, Chesnut R, Harris OA, Kissoon N, Rubiano AM, Shutter L, Tasker RC, Vavilala MS, Wilberger J, Wright DW, Ghajar J. Guidelines for the management of severe traumatic brain injury, Fourth Edition. Neurosurgery. 2017;80:6–15.
7. Gennarelli TA. Mechanisms of brain injury. J Emerg Med. 1993;11(Suppl 1):5–11.
8. Chesnut RM, Marshall LF, Klauber MR, et al. The role of secondary brain injury in determining outcome from severe head injury. J Trauma. 1993;34:216.
9. Godoy DA, Videtta W, Di Napoli M. Practical approach to posttraumatic intracranial hypertension according to pathophysiologic reasoning. Neurol Clin. 2017;35:613–40.
10. ATLS. Advanced trauma life support. 8th ed. Chicago, USA: American College of Surgeons; 2008.
11. Teasdale G, Maas A, Lecky F, Manley G, Stocchetti N, Murray G. The Glasgow Coma Scale at 40 years: standing the test of time. Lancet Neurol. 2014;13:844–54.
12. Wijdicks EF, Bamlet WR, Maramattom BV, Manno EM, McClelland RL. Validation of a new coma scale: The FOUR score. Ann Neurol. 2005;58:585–93.
13. Bouzat P, Sala N, Payen J-F, Oddo M. Beyond intracranial pressure: optimization of cerebral blood flow, oxygen, and substrate delivery after traumatic brain injury. Ann Intensive Care. 2013;3:23.
14. Marshall LF, Marshall SB, Klauber MR, van Berkum Clark M. A new classification of head injury based on computerized tomography. J Neurosurg. 1991;75(Suppl):S14–20.
15. Godoy DA, Lubillo S, Rabinstein AA. Pathophysiology and management of intracranial hypertension and tissular brain hypoxia after severe traumatic brain injury: an integrative approach. Neurosurg Clin N Am. 2018;29:195–212.
16. Godoy DA, Behrouz R, Di Napoli M. Glucose control in acute brain Injury: does it matter? Curr Opin Crit Care. 2016;22:120–7.
17. Menon DK, Ercole A. Critical care management of traumatic brain injury. Handb Clin Neurol. 2017;140:239–74.
18. Godoy DA, Murillo-Cabezas F, Egea-Guerrero JJ, Carmona-Suazo JA, Muñoz-Sánchez MA. Diagrams to interpret and solve physiopathological events triggered after severe traumatic brain injury. Med Intensiva. 2015;39:445–7.
19. Godoy DA, Seifi A, Garza D, Lubillo-Montenegro S, Murillo-Cabezas F. Hyperventilation therapy for control of posttraumatic intracranial hypertension. Front Neurol. 2017;8:250. eCollection 2017.
20. Oddo M, Poole D, Helbok R, Meyfroidt G, Stocchetti N, Bouzat P, Cecconi M, Geeraerts T, Martin-Loeches I, Quintard H, Taccone FS, Geocadin RG, Hemphill C, Ichai C, Menon D, Payen JF, Perner A, Smith M, Suarez J, Videtta W, Zanier ER, Citerio G. Fluid therapy in neurointensive care patients: ESICM consensus and clinical practice recommendations. Intensive Care Med. 2018;44:449–63.
21. Madden LK, Hill M, May TL, Human T, Guanci MM, Jacobi J, Moreda MV, Badjatia N. The implementation of targeted temperature management: an evidence-based guideline from the Neurocritical Care Society. Neurocrit Care. 2017;27:468–87.
22. Lelubre C, Taccone F. Transfusion strategies in patients with traumatic brain injury: which is the optimal hemoglobin target? Minerva Anestesiol. 2016;82(1):112–6.
23. Vedantam A, Robertson C, Gopinath S, et al. Progressive hemorrhagic injury after severe traumatic brain injury: effect of hemoglobin transfusion thresholds. J Neurosurg. 2016;125:1229–34.
24. Robertson CS, Hannay HJ, Yamal JM, Gopinath S, Goodman JC, Tilley BC, Investigators ESTBIT. Effect of erythropoietin and transfusion threshold on neurological recovery after traumatic brain injury: a randomized clinical trial. JAMA. 2014;312:36–47.

25. Napolitano LM, Kurek S, Luchette FA, Anderson GL, Bard MR, Bromberg W, Chiu WC, Cipolle MD, Clancy KD, Diebel L, Hoff WS, Hughes KM, Munshi I, Nayduch D, Sandhu R, Yelon JA, Corwin HL, Barie PS, Tisherman SA, Hebert PC, EAST Practice Management Workgroup; American College of Critical Care Medicine (ACCM) Taskforce of the Society of Critical Care Medicine (SCCM). Clinical practice guideline: red blood cell transfusion in adult trauma and critical care. J Trauma. 2009;67:1439–42.
26. Mangat HS, Wu X, Gerber LM, Schwarz JT, Fakhar M, Murthy SB, et al. Hypertonic saline is superior to mannitol for the combined effect on intracranial pressure and cerebral perfusion pressure burdens in patients with severe traumatic brain injury. Neurosurgery. 2019. pii: nyz046.
27. Andrews PJ, Sinclair HL, Rodriguez A, Harris BA, Battison CG, Rhodes JK, Murray GD, Eurotherm3235 Trial Collaborators. Hypothermia for intracranial hypertension after traumatic brain injury. N Engl J Med. 2015;373:2403–12.
28. Okonkwo DO, Shutter LA, Moore C, Temkin NR, Puccio AM, Madden CJ, et al. Brain Oxygen Optimization in Severe Traumatic Brain injury (BOOST) phase II: a phase II randomized trial. Crit Care Med. 2017;45:1907–14.
29. Hughes JD, Rabinstein AA. Early diagnosis of paroxysmal sympathetic hyperactivity in the ICU. Neurocrit Care. 2014;20:454–9.
30. Bullock MR, Chesnut R, Ghajar J, et al. Surgical management of traumatic brain injury author group. Neurosurgery. 2006;58(3 Suppl):S1–S75.
31. Adams H, Kolias AG, Hutchinson PJ. The role of surgical intervention in traumatic brain injury. Neurosurg Clin N Am. 2016;27:519–28.
32. Cooper DJ, Rosenfeld JV, Murray L, et al. Decompressive craniectomy in diffuse traumatic brain injury. N Engl J Med. 2011;364:1493–502.
33. Hutchinson PJ, Kolias AG, Timofeev IS, Corteen EA, Czosnyka M, Timothy J, RESCUEicp Trial Collaborators. Trial of decompressive craniectomy for traumatic intracranial hypertension. N Engl J Med. 2016;375:1119–30.

Chapter 14
Traumatic Spinal Cord Injury

Alejandro A. Rabinstein

Diagnostic Keys
- Spinal cord injury should always be suspected in patients with possible or confirmed neck trauma.
- Detailed motor and sensory examination should be performed to determine the level of injury and its severity (using the ASIA scale for categorization).
- Emergency imaging with CT scanning is essential for early management. MRI can subsequently characterize the extent of cord injury.

Treatment Priorities
- Immediate spine immobilization in the field is crucial to avoid additional cord injury during transportation.
- Early definite surgical stabilization of the spine (within 24–36 hours) may improve recovery.
- Patients with severe spinal cord injury are at continuous risk of major systemic complications throughout the acute and subacute phases and beyond. Prevention and treatment of these complications is crucial to optimize long-term prognosis.

A. A. Rabinstein (✉)
Department of Neurology, Mayo Clinic, Neuroscience ICU, Rochester, MN, USA
e-mail: Rabinstein.Alejandro@mayo.edu

© Springer Nature Switzerland AG 2020
A. A. Rabinstein (ed.), *Neurological Emergencies*,
https://doi.org/10.1007/978-3-030-28072-7_14

> **Prognosis at a Glance**
> - The severity of deficits on acute examination, typically categorized using the ASIA score, is the main determinant of functional outcome after traumatic spinal cord injury.
> - Avoid prognostic statements early after the injury. Deficits can be initially exacerbated by spinal shock and ongoing swelling.

Introduction

Traumatic spinal cord injury can be devastatingly disabling, particularly when involving the cervical spinal cord. Paraplegia and quadriplegia are the most overt manifestations of the injury, but multiple neurological and systemic complications also occur and exacerbate the morbidity of the disease. It often affects young patients, and consequently the societal costs are enormous, both from the high costs of acute and long-term care and the cumulative loss of productivity [1].

Basic Pathophysiology

Motor vehicle accidents and various forms of violence are the most common mechanisms of injury among young individuals, while falls predominate in older patients. Cord injuries affecting the cervical levels are most common at all ages, but particularly so in the young.

The cord may be injured by compression (transient or persistent at the time of first evaluation) or by direct damage (laceration or transection) in cases of penetrating injury [2]. Cord compression may be associated with vertebral fractures, vertebral subluxation, facet dislocation, disk herniation, and major ligamentous disruption. Individuals with narrow spinal canal and those with cervical spondylosis are at increased risk of suffering spinal cord injury because they develop worse compression with comparatively less severe neck injury. Flexion injuries tend to affect predominantly the anterior portions of the cord, whereas extension injuries affect more the posterior aspects.

In addition to the initial impact, the cord injury can be greatly worsened by secondary insults, in particular early hypoxia and ischemia. Inflammation with edema, reperfusion, microthrombosis, and oxidative damage from mitochondrial failure also play substantial contributing roles in the evolution and exacerbation of the cord injury.

Diagnosis

Physical examination and radiological assessment of the spine are the two pillars in the diagnosis of acute traumatic spinal cord injury. However, early evaluation cannot be restricted to the spine; coexistent traumatic injuries to the head and to internal organs are common, and therefore the initial trauma survey should be comprehensive.

Physical Examination

Even before starting the neurological examination, it is essential to evaluate ventilation, oxygenation, breathing pattern, and circulation. Patients with high cervical cord injury (above C5) typically present with respiratory failure (both hypoxemic and hypercapnic) because of compromise of diaphragmatic innervation. These patients exhibit paradoxical breathing pattern (the chest moves out but the abdomen moves in with inspiration). Injury to lower levels of the cervical cord can also produce less severe degrees of respiratory failure from loss of function of accessory thoracic and abdominal breathing muscles [3]. In such cases, the breathing pattern is characterized by inward movement of the chest with outward movement of the abdomen with inspiration. In addition, poor cough strength results in increased risk of aspiration.

Neurogenic shock manifests with hypotension and bradycardia due to loss of sympathetic function. It is seen with cervical and upper thoracic lesions and can be severe for several days. Other signs of sympathetic failure and unopposed vagal tone can also be found. Acute urinary retention is especially common.

The neurological examination should accomplish two main goals:

- Defining the level of the injury
- Defining the severity of the injury

The American Spinal Injury Association (ASIA) tool is broadly preferred to document and categorize the findings on neurological examination (*asia-spinalinjury.org/wp-content/uploads/2016/02/International_Stds_Diagram_Worksheet.pdf*). The neurological level of the injury is determined by the lowest segment with antigravity strength and intact sensation to pinprick. It should be established in both sides of the body. The injury is considered complete when there is no motor or sensory function below the level of injury. Otherwise, it is deemed incomplete. Even small degrees of preservation of function below the level of injury should be noted, as these findings can have prognostic importance. The examination should always include specific assessment of sacral function (anal contraction and anal sensation). Depending on the completeness of motor and sensory involvement, patients are classified into four grades (Table 14.1) [4].

Table 14.1 ASIA scores

ASIA score	Examination findings
A	Complete motor and sensory loss below the level of injury
B	Complete motor but incomplete sensory loss below the level of injury
C	Incomplete motor and sensory loss below the level of injury
D	Only incomplete sensory loss below the level of injury

Neurological impairment may be worse in the very early phase after the trauma because of a phenomenon known as spinal shock, manifested with flaccidity and areflexia. Neurogenic hypotension may also contribute to worsening neurological deficits. As spinal shock resolves and hypotension gets corrected, the findings on examination may improve. Consequently, serial reevaluation of neurological deficits and ASIA category is always necessary over the first few days after the injury. Resolution of the spinal shock is signaled by the reemergence of muscle tone—often progressing to spasticity—and deep tendon reflexes, sometimes with the appearance of Babinski signs and clonus.

Because of its frequency, it is worth making a separate mention of the central cord syndrome. This presentation typically occurs after transient cord compression caused by neck hyperextension. Preferential injury to the central tracts explains the clinical features: arms weaker than legs often accompanied by suspended sensory loss in lower cervical and upper thoracic dermatomes.

Radiological Evaluation

High-quality CT scanning of the cervical spine is indicated in all trauma patients with neck pain and when the patient is not fully alert (because of brain injury, intoxication, or another cause), and therefore it cannot be reliably established if symptoms suggestive of cervical cord injury may be present [5]. Cervical spine X-rays (anteroposterior, lateral, and odontoid views) should only be used as an alternative to CT scan when CT scan is not immediately available. When there is evidence of trauma to the thoracic spine or pain below the neck, CT scan of the thoracic spine is indicated. CT scanning is very useful to document bone fractures and spine alignment, but it provides more limited visualization of the intervertebral disks and may miss ligamentous injuries as compared to MRI.

MRI scanning is necessary to evaluate the cord itself. In the acute setting, MRI can show cord edema, hemorrhage, laceration, transection, and ischemia (Fig. 14.1). At later stages, it can demonstrate atrophy, myelomalacia, and syrinx.

Some patients, most often children, can have signs and symptoms of spinal cord injury despite a negative CT scan. This situation is known as spinal cord injury without radiological abnormalities (SCIWORA) [6]. Yet, careful review of spine MRI in these cases frequently discloses subtle abnormalities.

Fig. 14.1 MRI of the cervical spine (T2 sequence sagittal view) showing severe injury to the spinal cord from C3 to C6–7 with extensive cord swelling caused by compression from anterior subluxation of C5 on C6 related to major traumatic damage to the facet joints, longitudinal ligaments, and intervertebral disc

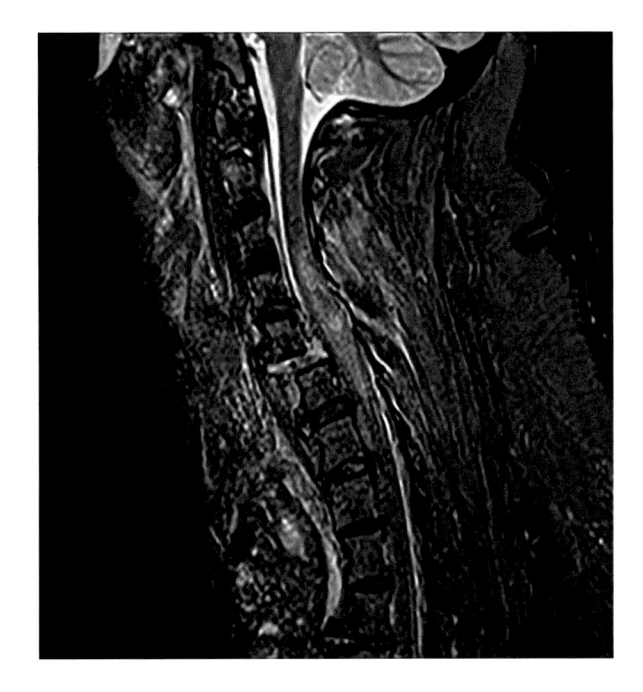

Treatment

Early immobilization of the potentially unstable spine is paramount to prevent additional cord injury from neck movements [5]. Ensuring adequate ventilation, oxygenation and perfusion, and excluding major injuries to the brain and to other organs constitute the other tenets of emergency management (Table 14.2) [7]. When possible, patients with severe traumatic spinal cord injury should be transferred to specialized centers with ample experience in treating these types of patients; data show that treatment at integrated, multidisciplinary, specialized spinal cord centers is associated with lower rates of complications, length of stay, and acute mortality [8].

There is some evidence that early (within 24 hours) surgical decompression and definite spine stabilization in the operating room is associated with better chances of recovery [9]. It is now being studied if surgery within 12 hours of the injury could further improve prognosis. Surgery may involve extensive fusion, and postoperative pain and worsening of the clinical deficits from swelling are frequently seen.

There is also weaker evidence supporting the common practice of inducing blood pressure augmentation for the first week, typically using intravenous catecholamines to keep a mean arterial pressure > 85 mmHg [10]. In patients who are not mechanically ventilated and otherwise stable, oral midodrine can represent a reasonable option to intravenous vasopressors. Monitoring spinal cord perfusion pressure (mean arterial pressure minus cerebrospinal fluid pressure as measured by an intrathecal catheter) is a strategy gaining attention. Maintaining a spinal cord

Table 14.2 Therapeutic priorities at different stages after a severe traumatic spinal cord injury

In the field
Spine immobilization
Ensure airway is secure
Treat hypotension
In the Emergency Department
Make sure the neck is well immobilized
Ensure adequate ventilation and oxygenation
Correct hypotension
Complete trauma survey, including spine imaging
Consult spine surgery/neurosurgery
In the ICU
Continue ensuring adequate ventilation and oxygenation
Surgical decompression within 24–36 hours when indicated (preceded by rapid closed reduction if fracture/dislocation)
Keep mean arterial pressure > 85 mmHg for 5–7 days (or spinal cord perfusion pressure > 50 mmHg if CSF pressure is monitored)
Analgesia
Nutrition
Weaning from mechanical ventilation
Prevent and treat secondary complications
Infections
Atelectasis
Bronchorrhea
Venous thromboembolism
Adynamic ileus
Temperature dysregulation
Urinary retention
Orthostatic hypotension
In rehabilitation
Physical and occupational therapy
Nutrition
Prevent and treat secondary complications (in addition to all of the above)
Autonomic dysreflexia
Spasticity
Constipation
Chronic pain
Depression
Sleep disturbances
Hypercalciuria with renal stones
Heterotopic ossification
Pressure sores

perfusion pressure greater than 50 mmHg during the first 7 days post-injury has been associated with better neurological recovery [11], and the value of cerebrospinal fluid drainage after acute spinal cord injury is being evaluated in an ongoing randomized controlled trial.

There is now general consensus against using high-dose intravenous methylprednisolone during the first day after spinal cord injury [5]. The trials evaluating this medication showed no consistent benefit (at most a very modest benefit in motor outcome only when treatment was started within 8 hours of the trauma) [12] and increased risk of various serious complications including sepsis, acute respiratory distress syndrome, and gastrointestinal bleeding.

Systemic complications are very common during the ICU course of patients with traumatic cervical spinal cord injury [13]. Apart from infections (pneumonia from aspiration or mechanical ventilation, urinary infection from indwelling catheter) and venous thromboembolism (from paralysis and immobility), adynamic ileus needs careful attention. In addition to the abdominal examination at the bedside, serial abdominal X-rays are often advisable to monitor the degree of intestinal dilatation (Fig. 14.2). Cathartics and rectal tube are sometimes insufficient and therapeutic colonoscopy may be necessary. If opiates may be contributing, methylnaltrexone is an option. Intravenous cholinergic agents to stimulate intestinal motility should be used very cautiously because they can dangerously exacerbate an ongoing bradycardia.

Neuropathic pain is a frequent problem and starting treatment with appropriate medications early is advisable. Gabapentin or pregabalin are often used, but duloxetine (also an antidepressant) is a good alternative in patients who are struggling to come to terms with the injury.

Fig. 14.2 Abdominal X-ray showing massive colonic dilatation without evidence of obstruction (i.e., consistent with adynamic ileus)

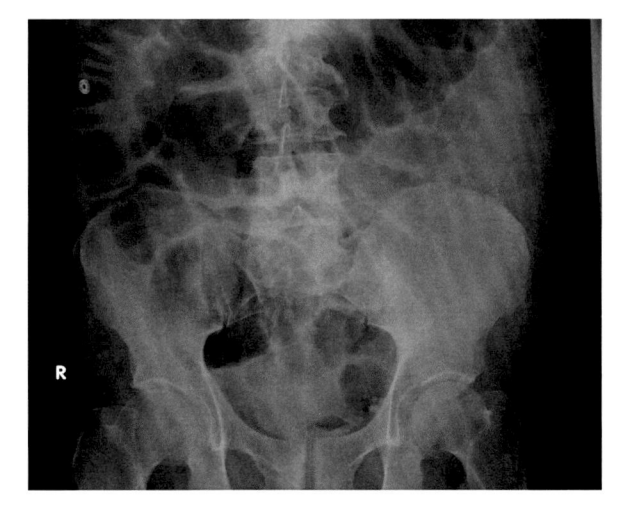

Spasticity becomes a major symptom as the initial phase of spinal shock resolves. Baclofen, diazepam, botulinum toxin injections, and physical therapy are used to control it. The most severe cases require implantation of an intrathecal baclofen pump.

Autonomic dysreflexia is another common complication in patients with severe cord injury at T6 or above. It generally appears after the acute phase but can be persistent. Because of this autonomic disorder, abrupt bouts of hypertension with either tachycardia or reflex bradycardia can be triggered by stimulation below the level of lesion. Common triggers include bladder or intestinal distension and mobilization of the legs during transfers. These stimuli produce an exaggerated sympathetic response [14]; yet, compensatory increase of vagal tone above the level of the lesion can produce parasympathetic manifestations in the upper body, such as flushing and increased oral and respiratory secretions. Patients often complain of acute headache. Recognizing and avoiding triggers is the best way of dealing with this problem. During an episode, it is advisable to act conservatively. Keeping the patient's trunk upright and, at most, administering a short-acting vasodilator are generally sufficient.

Prognosis

The ASIA grade (determined after resolution of the spinal shock), level of injury, and cord appearance on MRI are the strongest prognostic factors [15–17]. Early recovery of motor function is the best indicator that a favorable outcome is possible. Cervical injuries that remain complete after the acute phase generally have a poor prognosis. Yet, there is never a rush to prognosticate in these cases. While setting unrealistic expectations is deceiving and eventually counterproductive, telling a patient that she will not be able to walk again just a handful of days after the injury may plunge her into depression and detract from her participation in rehabilitation activities. In cases of high cervical cord injury, liberation from mechanical ventilation may not be possible. Yet, very gradual weaning can be successful in some instances with an early pessimistic outlook.

Multiple venues are being explored to promote neuroregeneration. Stem cell transplantation has captured most public attention, and various types of stem cells are being currently tested for this indication [18]. Direct electrical stimulation of the cord to reignite motor patterns of ambulation is another promising concept. Yet, these techniques remain entirely investigational at present.

Mortality continues to be increased for patients with severe cord injury throughout their life span [19]. Pulmonary embolism and sepsis remain common causes of death, but cardiovascular diseases are also more prevalent than in the general population.

Cardinal Messages
- Adequate emergency management can make the difference between severe disability and good functional recovery in victims of traumatic spinal cord injury.
- Immediate neck immobilization is crucial when spinal cord injury is considered possible.
- Examination should determine the level of injury and severity of motor and sensory deficits, and emergency CT scan is necessary to establish if there is ongoing cord compression that requires surgery.
- MRI can provide additional very useful information for treatment planning and for prognosis.
- When indicated for cord decompression and/or spine stabilization, it is better to proceed with surgery as soon as it is deemed safe, ideally within the first day.
- Take closely into account the level of injury when considering postoperative extubation.
- Based on the limited available evidence, supporting the blood pressure with vasopressors not just to treat the neurogenic shock but also to optimize cord perfusion through augmentation (i.e., targeting higher than normal values) is a reasonable strategy.
- In the acute phase, spinal shock and neurogenic hypotension can make the injury appear more complete than it really is. Thus, it is always prudent to wait until the acute phase is over before starting to estimate longer-term prognosis.

References

1. Devivo MJ. Epidemiology of traumatic spinal cord injury: trends and future implications. Spinal Cord. 2012;50(5):365–72.
2. Rabinstein AA. Traumatic spinal cord injury. Continuum (Minneap Minn). 2018;24(2., Spinal Cord Disorders):551–66.
3. Hadley MN, Walters BC, Grabb PA, et al. Clinical assessment after acute cervical spinal cord injury. Neurosurgery. 2002;50(3 Suppl):S21–9.
4. Maynard FM Jr, Bracken MB, Creasey G, et al. International standards for neurological and functional classification of spinal cord injury. American Spinal Injury Association. Spinal Cord. 1997;35(5):266–74.
5. Walters BC, Hadley MN, Hurlbert RJ, et al. Guidelines for the management of acute cervical spine and spinal cord injuries: 2013 update. Neurosurgery. 2013;60(CN_suppl_1):82–91.
6. Boese CK, Lechler P. Spinal cord injury without radiologic abnormalities in adults: a systematic review. J Trauma Acute Care Surg. 2013;75(2):320–30.

7. Shank CD, Walters BC, Hadley MN. Current topics in the management of acute traumatic spinal cord injury. Neurocrit Care. 2019;30(2):261–71.
8. Parent S, Barchi S, LeBreton M, Casha S, Fehlings MG. The impact of specialized centers of care for spinal cord injury on length of stay, complications, and mortality: a systematic review of the literature. J Neurotrauma. 2011;28(8):1363–70.
9. Fehlings MG, Vaccaro A, Wilson JR, et al. Early versus delayed decompression for traumatic cervical spinal cord injury: results of the Surgical Timing in Acute Spinal Cord Injury Study (STASCIS). PLoS One. 2012;7(2):e32037.
10. Ryken TC, Hurlbert RJ, Hadley MN, et al. The acute cardiopulmonary management of patients with cervical spinal cord injuries. Neurosurgery. 2013;72(Suppl 2):84–92.
11. Squair JW, Belanger LM, Tsang A, et al. Spinal cord perfusion pressure predicts neurologic recovery in acute spinal cord injury. Neurology. 2017;89(16):1660–7.
12. Bracken MB. Steroids for acute spinal cord injury. Cochrane Database Syst Rev. 2012;(1):CD001046.
13. Hagen EM. Acute complications of spinal cord injuries. World J Orthop. 2015;6(1):17–23.
14. Brown R, Burton AR, Macefield VG. Autonomic dysreflexia: Somatosympathetic and viscerosympathetic vasoconstrictor responses to innocuous and noxious sensory stimulation below lesion in human spinal cord injury. Auton Neurosci. 2018;209:71–8.
15. Wilson JR, Cadotte DW, Fehlings MG. Clinical predictors of neurological outcome, functional status, and survival after traumatic spinal cord injury: a systematic review. J Neurosurg Spine. 2012;17(1 Suppl):11–26.
16. Talbott JF, Whetstone WD, Readdy WJ, et al. The Brain and Spinal Injury Center score: a novel, simple, and reproducible method for assessing the severity of acute cervical spinal cord injury with axial T2-weighted MRI findings. J Neurosurg Spine. 2015;23(4):495–504.
17. Bozzo A, Marcoux J, Radhakrishna M, Pelletier J, Goulet B. The role of magnetic resonance imaging in the management of acute spinal cord injury. J Neurotrauma. 2011;28(8):1401–11.
18. Nagoshi N, Okano H. Applications of induced pluripotent stem cell technologies in spinal cord injury. J Neurochem. 2017;141(6):848–60.
19. Chamberlain JD, Meier S, Mader L, von Groote PM, Brinkhof MW. Mortality and longevity after a spinal cord injury: systematic review and meta-analysis. Neuroepidemiology. 2015;44(3):182–98.

Chapter 15
Neurologic Emergencies from Recreational Substances

Kaitlyn Barkley and Christopher P. Robinson

Introduction

Recreational substances have been part of human culture for thousands of years. Ephedra plants, which produce ephedrine and pseudoephedrine, were found at a burial site of a man who lived around 60,000 B.C. [1]. Residue from alcoholic drinks has been found on ceramics from 7000 B.C. [1]. The mid-twentieth century was ripe with the widespread use of recreational drugs, most specifically hallucinogens. Presently, a new generation of "designer drugs" has grown in popularity. These new drugs have unpredictable effects and create a diagnostic dilemma for physicians. It is estimated that 24.6 million Americans, 9.4% of the population, has used an illicit drug in the past month [2]. Marijuana is used by 19.8 million Americans, and prescription drugs with addiction potential (such as opiates) are used by 6.5 million Americans. Cocaine, hallucinogens, inhalants, and heroin are consumed by 1.5, 1.3, 0.5, and 0.3 million Americans, respectively.

Most sources divide recreational drugs into three main classes: those that stimulate the central nervous system, known simply as stimulants; those that depress the central nervous system, reciprocally called depressants; and those that are psychoactive, known as hallucinogens. In general, stimulants modulate the effect of the monoamine neurotransmitters norepinephrine and dopamine. Depressants

K. Barkley
Department of Neurosurgery, University of Florida, Gainesville, FL, USA

C. P. Robinson (✉)
Department of Neurology, University of Florida, Gainesville, FL, USA
e-mail: Christopher.robinson@neurology.ufl.edu

primarily enhance the activity of GABA or inhibit the activity of glutamate. Hallucinogens act on serotonergic and dopaminergic receptors to produce hallucinations that may be auditory, visual, or tactile. Figure 15.1 is a schematic depiction of the illicit substances commonly encountered by physicians that may cause a neurologic emergency. This chapter begins by discussing specific drugs and progresses to discussing management of the common neurologic emergencies that result from their use.

Stimulants

Colloquially referred to as uppers, stimulants are a class of drugs that stimulate the central nervous system. Most of these drugs act on monoamine neurotransmitters including dopamine, norepinephrine, and serotonin. In small doses, these drugs improve alertness, enhance mood, and combat fatigue. At higher doses, excessive activation results in paranoia and hallucinations and can lead to life-threatening neurological emergencies including intracerebral hemorrhage, aneurysmal rupture, ischemic stroke, and reversible cerebral vasoconstriction syndrome

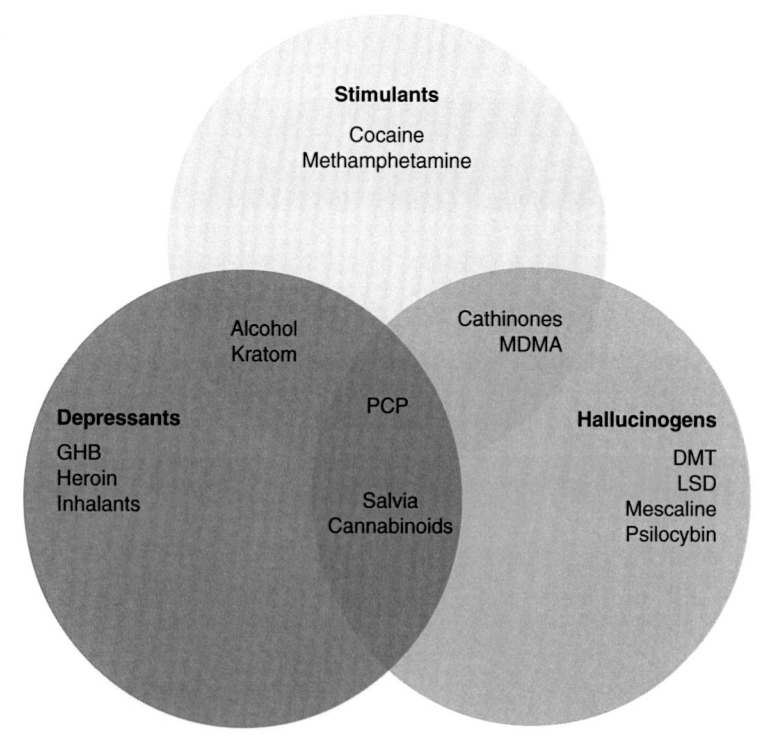

Fig. 15.1 Drugs of abuse based on class

(RCVS). This section discusses the most frequently encountered illicit stimulants: cocaine, methamphetamine, 3,4-methylenedioxymethamphetamine (MDMA), and cathinones.

Cocaine

Cocaine, extracted from the coca plant, can be insufflated, injected, or inhaled, with the latter referred to by the street name "crack." Other street names include blow, bump, coke, rock, and snow. Cocaine has a rapid onset resulting in mydriasis, euphoria, diaphoresis, tachycardia, and hypertension. At higher doses, agitation, paranoia, and psychosis may result. These effects last an hour or less depending on the route of administration. When taken with alcohol, a longer-lasting metabolite is formed and effects can last significantly longer [3].

Cocaine acts primarily by blocking the reuptake of synaptic monoamines. By increasing activity at α-adrenergic receptors, cocaine use results in abnormal cardiovascular physiology, inducing tachycardia and systemic vasoconstriction. Caution should be taken in the treatment of such patients, as use of beta-blockers result in unopposed alpha-adrenergic stimulation. Altogether, the use of cocaine predisposes patients to the secondary effects of unopposed vasoconstriction, including intracerebral hemorrhage, ischemic stroke, RCVS, myocardial ischemia, and rhabdomyolysis.

Methamphetamine

Methamphetamine is a synthetic substance made from multiple commercially available items including nasal decongestants. It can be used by insufflation (snorting), inhalation, or injection. Street names include crank, crystal meth, glass, ice, and speed. Similar to cocaine, euphoria, tachycardia, diaphoresis, and mydriasis occur. Agitation, hallucinations, and psychosis are common as well, perhaps more so than with cocaine intoxication. Management of acute intoxication is often focused on symptomatic treatment of hyperthermia and agitation.

MDMA

MDMA (3,4-methylenedioxy methamphetamine) is a modified amphetamine molecule that is often taken orally as a club drug under the street name ecstasy or molly. Growing in popularity in the 1970s, MDMA was touted as an amphetamine-like substance that did not result in the bothersome agitation and psychosis common to methamphetamine use. Like other amphetamines, MDMA produces euphoria, tachycardia, and hyperthermia. Effects more specific to MDMA include increased empathy and heightened sensation.

Cathinone Derivatives

Cathinone is a modified amphetamine that enhances release of dopamine and blocks reuptake of epinephrine and norepinephrine. One example of a pharmaceutically similar drug to cathinone is bupropion. These drugs act primarily as stimulants, but newer synthetic derivatives have strong hallucinogenic properties. Additionally, like bupropion, these substances can lower seizure threshold, and acute ingestion may present with status epilepticus. Pure cathinone is produced with the khat plant, and modified cathinone molecules are the major active ingredients in the street drug "bath salts."

Khat

Khat is a plant native to Africa, which has been cultivated for centuries and is either chewed or brewed into a tea. Still legal in many countries, khat is used as an appetite suppressant and mood enhancer. The active ingredient in khat is a cathinone and at higher doses can result in many of the effects common to amphetamine use.

Synthetic Cathinones (Bath Salts)

Synthetic cathinones, also known as "bath salts," are a derivative of the active ingredient in Khat and are often not scheduled by the Drug Enforcement Agency (DEA) [4]. New derivatives are continually being created and sold legally as incense and herbal supplements. Street names include bloom, cloud nine, cosmic blast, flakka, scarface, vanilla sky, and white lightning. The effects of these substances are similar to those of other amphetamines, including agitation, hyperthermia, euphoria, and profound rhabdomyolysis. Unlike standard amphetamines, synthetic cathinones have greater effects on serotonin pathways and may lead to serotonin syndrome [4]. In these patients, clonus and muscle rigidity may be the only distinguishing features.

Depressants

Depressants suppress the central nervous system by increasing the effects of inhibitory neurotransmitters (GABA, glycine) and decreasing the effects of excitatory neurotransmitters (glutamate). In general, these drugs result in confusion, poor coordination, decreased level of consciousness, and respiratory depression. Seizures can occur after withdrawal following prolonged use. This section will discuss the legal depressants alcohol and prescription opioids, the partially legal cannabinoids including marijuana and synthetic cannabinoids, and illegal substances including heroin, kratom, gamma-hydroxybutyric acid (GHB), and inhalants.

Alcohol

Humans have been using microbes to ferment alcohol for tens of thousands of years [1]. Although production and consumption of alcohol is legal, its overuse presents an ongoing major problem to society and public health. At small doses, alcohol acts as a stimulant, resulting in euphoria and disinhibition [5]. At higher doses, marked central nervous system depression results in impaired cognition and coordination, respiratory depression, and potentially stupor, coma, and death. The effects of alcohol at various blood concentrations are shown in Table 15.1.

Alcohol withdrawal can be lethal [5]. Within the first 24–36 hours, anxiety, tremor, agitation, and insomnia begin. Withdrawal seizures occur within the first 72 hours after cessation and can progress to status epilepticus. Delirium tremens occurs 3–10 days after cessation and is characterized by extreme autonomic dysregulation, delirium, hallucinations, and potentially death. Acute alcohol withdrawal should be treated with benzodiazepines under a symptoms triggered protocol such as the Clinical Institute Withdrawal Assessment (CIWA) or Richmond Agitation-Sedation Scale (RASS).

Cannabinoids

Marijuana

Marijuana is a psychoactive drug produced by the Cannabis plant that until recently was illegal in the United States. As of April 2019, 11 states have made marijuana legal for recreational use, and 34 states have laws making it legal for medical use.

Marijuana's chemical structure is composed of multiple compounds, most notably tetrahydrocannabinol (THC) and cannabidiol, which act on cannabinoid receptors. These substances stimulate the release of dopamine and in turn modulate opioid and glycine receptors. Street names for marijuana include blunt, bud, dope, ganja, grass, green, herb, joint, Mary Jane, pot, reefer, skunk, and weed. Acute

Table 15.1 Blood alcohol content and expected effects [5]

Blood alcohol content (mg/dL)	Effects
50	Relaxation, talkativeness
100	Impaired judgment, cognition, and motor function
200	Marked impairment in cognition and motor functions
300	Stupor
400	Severe respiratory depression, death (LD_{50})

LD_{50} lethal dose in 50% of the population

intoxication is manifested by euphoria, changes in perception, increased libido, dissociation, and pseudo-hallucinations.

One study attempted to quantify current evidence for marijuana use and long-term health effects [6]. With high levels of confidence, marijuana use was linked to subsequent use of other substances, diminished life achievement, motor vehicle accidents, and chronic bronchitis. With medium levels of confidence, marijuana use was linked to abnormal brain development, schizophrenia, depression, and anxiety. Therefore, marijuana use should be regarded as a major risk factor for abusing other drugs and may be associated with mental illness. As marijuana continues to be decriminalized, patients may be more forthcoming about using the drug, and healthcare professionals should consider screening for other drugs if there is concern.

Synthetic Cannabinoids

Sold legally in most states as herbal "incense," synthetic cannabinoids have variable composition and effects. There is a paucity of information about synthetic cannabinoids, as they are a newer designer drug, with their use beginning in early 2015. Although the DEA has criminalized the use of some of these compounds, overseas manufacturers continue to synthesize new derivatives. Street names include K2, spice, black mamba, bliss, bombay blue, crazy clown, genie, moon rocks, yucatan, and zohai. Preferred by drug users due to legal availability and absence of screening, synthetic cannabinoids have been linked to a series of patients presenting with seizures and death [7]. Other effects include delirium, acute kidney injury, psychosis, hallucinations, and cardiovascular collapse. It is unclear how to manage patients who present with synthetic cannabinoid intoxication. Current recommendations suggest seizure and agitation management with benzodiazepines and other supportive care until the drug is metabolized.

Opiates

Prescription Opiates

In recent years, the overuse of prescription opiates has reached epidemic proportions in the United States. Opiate-related emergency department visits and hospital admissions have more than doubled in the last two decades [8]. Rates of unintentional overdose and suicide in opiate users have also risen dramatically in recent years [9]. As a consequence, this "opiate crisis" has been called a national emergency. While heroine and synthetic opiates are major contributors to these figures, overuse of prescription opiates has become the leading culprit. Increasing the scrutiny of opiate prescription practices and emphasizing alternative strategies to manage acute and chronic pain are approaches being actively pursued to reverse the progression of this major healthcare problem. When a case of acute opiate intoxication is suspected, clear improvement naloxone can confirm the diagnosis.

Heroin

Heroin, a derivative of morphine (diamorphine), is the natural product of the opium plant. It was first synthesized in the nineteenth century in an attempt to create less addictive alternatives to morphine. Current street names for heroin include brown sugar, china white, dope, junk, smack, and white horse.

Major effects of acute intoxication include analgesia, euphoria, somnolence, and respiratory depression. The major mechanism of heroin overdose-related deaths is attributed to respiratory depression and can result in hypoxic cerebral ischemia and subsequent cerebral edema [10]. Secondary cerebral ischemia can also result from thromboembolism, vasculitis, septic emboli, and hypotension. Additional neurologic sequela of heroin use includes brain abscess formation. Skin and oropharyngeal flora are common culprits, but innumerable other rare bacteria, mycobacteria, fungi, and parasites have also been reported.

Kratom

Kratom is extracted from the Mitragyna plant, a member of the coffee family, and is native to South America. Street names include herbal speedball, biak-biak, ketum, and thom. Kratom acts primarily on opioid receptors but has some activity on serotonin and adrenergic receptors, resulting in paradoxical stimulant effects [11]. At low doses, stimulant effects predominate, whereas at high doses, the effects of analgesia and respiratory depression prevail. Kratom overdose should be treated as an opiate overdose with special attention to potential agitation upon reversal with naloxone.

Gamma-Hydroxybutyric Acid (GHB)

GHB, a chemical precursor of gamma-aminobutyric acid (GABA), activates GABA receptors. GHB is used recreationally and produces effects similar to alcohol. GHB gained popularity in the 1990s, being referred to as the "date rape" drug. GHB and its analogs have also been marketed as anabolic agents although there is limited evidence for their efficacy. Street names include Georgia home boy, goop, liquid ecstasy, liquid X, soap, and scoop. Acute GHB intoxication causes relaxation, disinhibition, euphoria, ataxia, and miosis [12]. Less common but fairly specific symptoms for GHB intoxication include myoclonus, nystagmus, bruxism, dystonia, and athetoid posturing. Seizures can occur both in intoxication and withdrawal states.

Treatment is focused on supportive care. There is no effective reversal agent for acute intoxication. Trials with antiepileptics, flumazenil, and naloxone have shown no effect.

Inhalants

Inhalants include glues, cleaning agents, organic solvents, aerosols, anesthetic gases, and nitrites [13]. Street names include poppers, snappers, whippets, and laughing gas. The effects of inhalants depend on the drug abused but, in general, cause euphoria, incoordination, stupor, and potentially coma and death. Inhalant intoxication is short-lived (5 minutes) so acute presentation to the healthcare setting is uncommon. Repeated use can cause damage to sensitive areas of the brain including the white matter, hippocampus, cerebellum, and basal ganglia [13]. These injuries can produce memory impairment, ataxia, and parkinsonism. The effects are usually permanent and do not respond well to any treatment.

Hallucinogens

The hallucinogens are a class of drugs in which the primary physiologic effects are auditory, visual, or tactile hallucinations. They may also have stimulant or depressant effects. Most of the hallucinogens exert their action on serotonin receptors. The synthetic hallucinogens are lysergic acid diethylamide (LSD) and phencyclidine (PCP), and the herbal hallucinogens are mescaline, psilocybin, and ayahuasca. The herbal hallucinogens are still commonly used in many cultures as part of spiritual ceremonies; however, globalization has made these drugs available to recreational drug users around the world.

Lysergic Acid Diethylamide (LSD)

LSD is a synthetic ergot that has effects on dopamine and serotonin receptors. It was synthesized in 1938 with the intention of creating a stimulant that counteracted tranquilizer overdose [14]. The drug was accidentally ingested and the hallucinogenic effects were quickly appreciated. LSD rapidly ascended in popularity in the 1960s for its mind-altering effects. Presently, street names include acid, blotter, blue heaven, cubes, microdot, and yellow sunshine.

LSD results in an emotional liability that usually favors positive moods, but severe anxiety and paranoia may occur instead [14]. Visual hallucinations, which can be elementary or complex, predominate. Blissfulness, disembodiment, and a sense of spirituality are also commonly reported. When users present in the healthcare setting, intoxication has usually resulted in a "bad trip," where hallucinations may be persecutory, delusions persist, and paranoia may be present. In this state, treatment is geared toward minimizing stimulation. Pharmacologic management with benzodiazepines and neuroleptics may be instituted if necessary. In high doses, LSD has been associated with serotonin syndrome.

Phencyclidine (PCP)

PCP is a dissociative anesthetic similar to ketamine that acts as an NMDA receptor antagonist [15]. Street names include angel dust, boat, love boat, and peace pill. PCP acts as a depressant, making it useful for anesthesia. However, during the wakeup phase, a paradoxical reaction can occur, resulting in agitation and psychosis. Additionally, users report significant hallucinations. Acute PCP intoxication mimics schizophrenia, to the point that PCP antagonists were investigated as a treatment for schizophrenia. PCP intoxication resulting in agitation should be treated by minimizing stimulation and managed pharmacologically with benzodiazepines and antipsychotics. The aggression associated with PCP has been widely associated with injury to healthcare workers; thus, PCP-intoxicated patients should be handled with great caution.

Mescaline (Peyote)

Mescaline is a naturally occurring hallucinogen from the peyote cactus that is native to Texas, Mexico, Central America, and South America [16]. Mescaline use is legal in the United States for members of the Native American Church. However, it has grown in popularity among drug users. Street names include buttons, cactus, and mesc. Like LSD, mescaline has the majority of its effects on serotonin receptors, and hallucinations may be simple, complex, or synesthetic. As with the other hallucinogens, agitation or paranoia associated with mescaline intoxication can be treated with benzodiazepines or antipsychotics.

Psilocybin

Psilocybin is a naturally occurring prodrug of psilocin, a powerful psychedelic drug. Psilocybin is produced by a large number of wild mushrooms lending to the street names magic mushroom and shrooms. The mushrooms are illegal to own or consume in the United States although they are used for ceremonies in Central and South America [16]. In contrast however, the spores are legal in all states except California, which makes the mushrooms easy to grow at home. Psilocybin intoxication may present in the same way as LSD or mescaline, with paranoia and persecutory delusions.

Ayahuasca

Ayahuasca is a tea brewed in South America that contains dimethyltryptamine (DMT), prepared from seeds of indigenous plants [16]. When smoked, DMT is a powerful hallucinogen, but ingestion of DMT alone produces no effects. Ayahuasca, however, incorporates a monoamine oxidase inhibitor that blocks metabolism of DMT in the gut and results in systemic absorption. DMT can also be extracted from grass species common to the United States, although its use is not widespread. The effects are characterized by hallucinations similar to those from LSD or psilocybin. Thus, acute intoxication should be handled in the same manner as the other hallucinogens.

Symptom-Based Approach

The final section in this chapter will discuss a symptom-based approach to recreational drug abuse. First, a differential diagnosis of altered mental status will be presented, including an algorithm to help identify the possible drug of abuse. Next, cerebrovascular events including stroke, intracranial hemorrhage, and RCVS will be discussed, followed by seizures and central nervous system (CNS) abscesses. Lastly, the management of drug-induced hyperthermia will be summarized.

Altered Mental Status

Altered mental status in the neurocritical care unit can be related to acute drug ingestion or acute drug withdrawal. Alternative diagnoses include metabolic dysfunction due to renal failure, liver failure, sepsis, electrolyte derangements, acidosis or alkalosis, and thyroid disease (see Chap. 1) [17]. Though the differential is broad, substance abuse should always be considered as a possible etiology of alteration in consciousness, because it represents a reversible form of encephalopathy. Figure 15.2 displays a simple approach to the diagnosis of altered mental status related to recreational substance abuse.

> **Diagnostic Keys**
> - When considering recreational substance abuse, categorizing a drug as a stimulant or depressant is key to diagnosis and prediction of complications.
> - Polysubstance abuse may result in unpredictable effects and should be considered in any case of drug abuse.

Treatment Priorities
- Stimulant and hallucinogen abuse may result in hyperactive delirium, posing a danger to the patient and others. Healthcare workers should be particularly careful when interacting with these patients. Benzodiazepines and antipsychotics should be employed to treat agitation.
- Ethanol abuse predisposes a patient to Wernicke's encephalopathy due to acquired dietary thiamine deficiency. Alcohol users should be given thiamine and dextrose on presentation to prevent this disease.
- Opiate intoxication is one of the few overdoses that has an antidote. If opiate overdose is suspected, naloxone should be administered, and any improvement in mental status should be considered

Prognosis at a Glance
- Encephalopathy or delirium from substance abuse often resolves when the substance is metabolized, with few exceptions.
- Supportive care through the acute intoxication most often affords good outcomes.

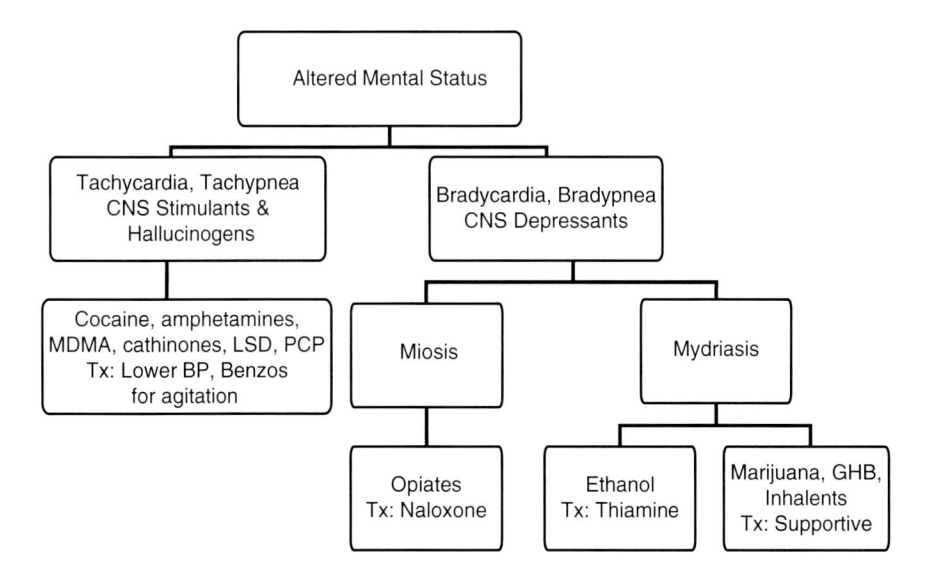

Fig. 15.2 Diagnostic algorithm for altered mental status in the setting of drug abuse

Ischemic Stroke

Stroke is a leading cause of morbidity and mortality in the United States (see Chap. 9). The vast majority of strokes in the United States are related to hypertension, diabetes, atrial fibrillation, carotid artery disease, and lifestyle choices. Yet, drug abuse may be a significant risk factor for stroke especially in certain populations. A recent review in a suburban stroke center showed that 11% of patients presenting with stroke had a positive urine toxicology, mostly for cocaine [18].

Drugs of abuse can cause ischemic strokes by a variety of mechanisms. Stimulants may predispose to cardiac arrhythmias like atrial fibrillation and result in cardioembolic infarctions. Stimulants and marijuana predispose patients to RCVS due to their vasoconstrictive properties. Drugs used intravenously like amphetamines, cocaine, and heroin can result in endocarditis and septic emboli. Drugs that result in significant cardiac depression, such as heroin and inhalants, may provoke hypoxic infarcts in watershed areas. Table 15.2 summarizes mechanisms of stroke related to specific drug use.

Regardless of the etiology, a stroke related to substance abuse should be treated using evidence-based guidelines by assessing eligibility for intravenous rt-PA or mechanical thrombectomy [19, 20]. Neurosurgical evaluation for decompressive craniectomy may be necessary for large territory infarctions or those involving the posterior fossa. Prognosis following stroke depends on the location and severity of the infarction.

Diagnostic Keys
- Identifying drug use as the etiology for the stroke is important in targeting treatment and prevention of future strokes.
- Reversible cerebral vasoconstriction syndrome (RCVS) is a clinical entity associated with cocaine and marijuana use as well as other medical diseases that presents with a thunderclap headache and can result in ischemic stroke, subarachnoid hemorrhage, or intracerebral hemorrhage.

Treatment Priorities
- Suspected drug intoxication is not a contraindication for intravenous thrombolysis [19].
- Prompt evaluation for mechanical thrombectomy should occur when an acute large artery occlusion is suspected [20].
- Large infarcts may result in cerebral edema and potential herniation. Neurosurgical consultation for hemicraniectomy should be considered in large territory infarcts especially in young patients or in posterior fossa infarcts.

> **Prognosis at a Glance**
> - Prognosis for ischemic stroke depends on the area and severity of the infarct.
> - Large infarcts will predispose to cerebral edema and may require hemicraniectomy which implies a significant morbidity.
> - Reversible cerebral vasoconstriction syndrome (RCVS) is usually a self-limited disease but can result in large areas of ischemia and lasting deficits.

Table 15.2 Drugs commonly associated with stroke

Drug	Proposed mechanism of stroke
Amphetamines	Cardioembolic, septic embolus, RCVS
Cocaine	Cardioembolic, septic embolus, RCVS
Heroin	Hypoxic, septic embolus
Inhalants	Cardioembolic, hypoxic
Marijuana	RCVS

RCVS reversible cerebral vasoconstriction syndrome

Intracranial Hemorrhage

Intracranial hemorrhage is a vast topic, covered in detail on Chap. 11. The most important aspect of intracranial hemorrhage related to recreational drugs is to recognize the risk factors associated with their use.

Intracranial hemorrhage occurs in one of five locations: epidural, subdural, subarachnoid, intraparenchymal, or intraventricular. Epidural and subdural hemorrhages are mostly associated with trauma, to which a person may be predisposed if abusing recreational drugs. Subarachnoid hemorrhage, aneurysmal or otherwise, occurs with greater incidence in drug users and may be associated with aneurysm (including mycotic), RCVS, or trauma. Cocaine users have higher risk of delayed vasospasm, but sometimes severe vasospasm may remain asymptomatic in these patients. Intraparenchymal hemorrhage is also known to occur in the setting of drug abuse. The majority of these incidents are associated with stimulants, including amphetamines and cocaine, and hypertension and vasoconstriction are the presumptive mechanisms. Table 15.3 provides a list of the most common types of intracranial hemorrhage by drug of abuse.

Regardless of etiology, intracranial hemorrhage should be managed using evidence-based guidelines. Subarachnoid hemorrhage may require neurosurgical management for external ventricular drain placement and aneurysm treatment. Likewise, subdural or epidural hemorrhage may require neurosurgical evaluation for craniectomy and evacuation. Intraparenchymal hemorrhage requires strict blood pressure control and monitoring for the development of symptomatic edema and mass effect.

Table 15.3 Drugs commonly associated with intracranial hemorrhage

Hemorrhage type	Mechanism	Key features	Drugs associated
Subarachnoid hemorrhage	Aneurysm	Cisternal blood	Alcohol, cocaine, nicotine
	Mycotic aneurysm	Associated with endocarditis	Amphetamines, cocaine, heroin
	RCVS	Along convexity	Cocaine, marijuana
	Traumatic	Along convexity	Any
Intracerebral hemorrhage	Hypertensive	Basal ganglia, pons	Amphetamines, cocaine
	RCVS	Associated with strokes or SAH	Cocaine, marijuana
	Trauma	Adjacent or contralateral skull fracture	Any
Subdural and epidural hemorrhage	Traumatic	Adjacent or contralateral skull fracture	Any

Diagnostic Keys
- Prompt evaluation with a CT scan is imperative to diagnose intracranial hemorrhage.
- If subarachnoid hemorrhage is present, consideration for aneurysmal source is important. CT angiogram should be obtained for subarachnoid hemorrhage with blood in the basal cisterns or Sylvian fissure.
- MRI should be considered in cases of intracerebral hemorrhage to assess cerebral amyloid angiopathy as an etiology.
- The presence of epidural or subdural hemorrhage should prompt immediate neurosurgical consultation.
- Intracranial hemorrhage in the setting of known intravenous drug abuse should prompt workup for endocarditis.

Treatment Priorities
- Subarachnoid hemorrhage and intracerebral hemorrhage can be associated with blood in the ventricles and may require a ventriculostomy to prevent obstructive hydrocephalus.
- Intracranial hemorrhage should be managed with strict blood pressure control to prevent worsening of the bleed.
- Osmotic therapy should be considered in cases of symptomatic cerebral edema.
- Emergent evacuation of subdural or epidural hemorrhages should be considered in the presence of impending herniation.

> **Prognosis at a Glance**
> - Intracerebral hemorrhage – prognosis depends mostly on severity of presentation and volume of the hematoma.
> - Subarachnoid hemorrhage – prognosis depends on symptom severity at presentation and whether the patient suffers parenchymal brain damage from the initial bleeding or subsequent delayed cerebral ischemia.
> - Epidural and subdural hemorrhage – prognosis dependent on severity and degree of herniation.

Seizure

Numerous drugs have been linked temporally to seizures including amphetamines, cocaine, heroin, and phencyclidine [21]. Newer agents like the synthetic cannabinoids have also been implicated as epileptogenic. Table 15.4 summarizes the features of drug-related seizures.

Treatment of seizures should be focused on their immediate termination with benzodiazepines and other antiseizure medications (see Chap. 2). Brain imaging is indicated in patients with focal onset because recreational drugs can also cause seizures through brain infarctions, intracranial hemorrhage, or cerebral abscesses. If there is concern for recurrence of seizures, antiseizure drugs with low abuse potential and street value should be chosen.

> **Diagnostic Keys**
> - Seizures from recreational drugs may be either convulsive or nonconvulsive.
> - EEG should be considered in a drug user with unexplained altered mental status.

> **Treatment Priorities**
> - Seizures should be treated acutely with benzodiazepines.
> - Status epilepticus should be managed according to evidence-based guidelines.
> - Alcohol withdrawal should be treated with a standardized protocol, which monitors symptoms and appropriately doses benzodiazepines to prevent florid withdrawal.

> **Prognosis at a Glance**
> - Seizures that occur under the influence of recreational substances are typically self-limited and do not necessarily predispose to epilepsy in the future.

Table 15.4 Drugs commonly associated with seizures

Drug	Other features
Drug intoxication	
Cocaine	May present with or without infarction or hemorrhage
Heroin	May present with or without infarction or infection
Methamphetamine	May present with or without infarction or infection
Phencyclidine	Interictal agitation common
Synthetic cannabinoids	Not detected on traditional drug screens
Synthetic cathinones	Not detected on traditional drug screens
Drug withdrawal	
Alcohol	May present with signs of Wernicke-Korsakoff syndrome
GHB	Myoclonus, nystagmus, bruxism, dystonia

CNS Abscesses

CNS infections, including intracranial and spinal epidural abscesses, frequently occur in patients who abuse drugs intravenously. Table 15.5 summarizes the drugs that are often injected. A more detailed discussion on CNS infections is presented on Chap. 7.

Spinal epidural abscesses occur almost exclusively in the setting of osteomyelitis and discitis. Presentation includes back pain, fever, and leukocytosis. Inflammatory markers including ESR and CRP are usually elevated. When severe, signs of spinal cord compression may also be evident. The imaging modality of choice is an MRI with and without contrast. In one series of intravenous drug users with osteomyelitis, the most commonly isolated microbe was methicillin-susceptible *Staphylococcus aureus* [22]. Treatment with long-term intravenous antibiotics is often necessary, which poses an ethical dilemma in patients who use intravenous drugs, as having a central line may promote increased drug abuse.

Cerebral abscesses may also occur in the setting of intravenous drug use. Cerebral abscesses often present with altered mental status and focal neurologic deficits. Up to 25% of cerebral abscess also manifest with seizures. Diffusion-weighted MRI sequences can be useful in distinguishing intracerebral abscess (which typically exhibits restricted diffusion at their core) from malignancy. Lumbar puncture can be helpful in diagnosing the causative organisms, though it may be contraindicated if the risk of herniation is deemed prohibitive. Neurosurgical management is necessary if the organism is not known or focal deficits persist. Antibiotic therapy should

15 Neurologic Emergencies from Recreational Substances

Table 15.5 Drugs that may be used intravenously

Drug	Routes of administration
Cocaine	Insufflation, inhalation, injection
DMT	Ingestion, inhalation, injection
Heroin	Injection, inhalation, insufflation
Methamphetamine	Ingestion, insufflation, inhalation, injection
PCP	Injection, insufflation, ingestion, inhalation
Synthetic cathinones	Ingestion, insufflation, injection

not be delayed in order to obtain culture of the intracranial abscess as treatment delays are associated with worse outcomes. Like with spinal epidural abscess, long-term management with intravenous antibiotics is often necessary. If ventriculitis is present, placement of an external ventricular drain may be necessary for CSF diversion and can be utilized for administration of intrathecal antibiotic therapy.

Rare infections such as those caused by mycobacterium, fungi, amoeba, and parasites can also occur, especially in immunocompromised hosts. Intravenous drug abuse predisposes users to contraction of HIV. Infections in this cohort carry a poor prognosis.

Diagnostic Keys
- Intracerebral abscesses present with focal neurologic symptoms.
- Spinal abscesses present with symptoms of acute cord or nerve root compression.

Treatment Priorities
- Urgent consideration for evacuation should be made in all cases presenting with focal deficits.
- Broad-spectrum antibiotics should be initiated in all patients following blood culture collection.
- In patients without focal deficits, attempts at culturing the abscess should be made.

Prognosis at a Glance
- Prognosis varies depending on extent of neurologic deficits and medical comorbidities.
- Infections with high mortality include ventriculitis, fungal organisms, and infections associated with HIV.

Hyperthermia

Hyperthermia associated with drug administration can be the result of hypothalamic dysfunction or muscle overactivity. In both circumstances, hyperthermia may carry significant risk due to disruption of the blood-brain barrier, neuronal cell death, and multisystem organ dysfunction. The drugs most commonly implicated in hyperthermia syndromes are amphetamines, cocaine, phencyclidine, and synthetic cathinones.

Typically, hyperthermia is not well controlled by antipyretics if it is a result of muscle overactivity. For this reason, sedation is usually the most effective treatment. Benzodiazepines should be titrated as needed for psychomotor agitation. Antipsychotics should be avoided as they can worsen hyperthermia through anticholinergic effects and propensity to cause neuroleptic malignant syndrome. If hyperthermia is refractory to sedation via benzodiazepines, paralytics can be used. Succinylcholine should be avoided if rhabdomyolysis is present because fatal hyperkalemia can result from its use. Cooling measures, such as cooled intravenous fluids, ice packs, and cooling blankets, can be utilized. Failure to adequately control hyperthermia can result in end-organ failure, including myocardial infarction, disseminated intravascular coagulation, rhabdomyolysis, and cerebral damage.

Diagnostic Keys
- Recognizing and correcting hyperthermia can prevent morbidity and mortality related to drug abuse.
- Hyperthermia in a drug user in the absence of leukocytosis or other signs of infection is likely due to muscle overactivity.

Treatment Priorities
- Hyperthermia from drug use may not respond to antipyretics. If hyperthermia is related to muscle overactivity, treatment should focus on sedation and potentially intubation and paralysis if severe.
- Antipsychotics may worsen hyperthermia and should be avoided if high fever is present.

Prognosis at a Glance
- If cooling measures are effective, hyperthermia usually has no long-term consequences.
- If cooling measures are ineffective, death due to organ failure may occur.

Conclusions

Recreational substances can cause various neurological emergencies and therefore it is important for clinicians to be keenly aware of the actions of various commonly used substances and the resulting toxidromes. Immediate recognition of the intoxication can be extremely valuable for making the correct therapeutic decisions, and sometimes it can even be life-saving.

> **Cardinal Messages**
> - Recreational substance use is widespread and may result in neurological emergencies.
> - Stimulants cause agitation and psychosis as well as tachyarrhythmias and vasoconstriction, which may predispose to stroke.
> - Depressants cause somnolence and potentially apnea, which may result in hypoxic ischemic events.
> - Stimulants, heroin, synthetic cannabinoids, and alcohol can present with seizures either from acute intoxication or withdrawal.
> - Central nervous system abscesses can cause permanent neurologic deficits or death if not promptly treated. Management often requires neurosurgical intervention and a long course of antibiotics.
> - A patient under the influence of hallucinogenic drugs may pose a risk to healthcare workers, and therefore these patients demand special care, sometimes in units dedicated to handle aggressive patients.

References

1. Guerra-Doce E. Psychoactive substances in prehistoric times: examining the archaeological evidence. Time and Mind. 2015;8(1):91–112.
2. NIDA. (2015). Nationwide trends. Retrieved from https://www.drugabuse.gov/publications/drugfacts/nationwide-trends on 2018, May 14.
3. Zimmerman JL. Cocaine intoxication. Crit Care Clin. 2012;28(4):517–26.
4. Banks ML, Worst TJ, Rusyniak DE, Sprague JE. Synthetic cathinones ("bath salts"). J Emerg Med. 2014;46(5):632–42.
5. Pohorecky LA, Brick J. Pharmacology of ethanol. Pharmacol Ther. 1988;36(2):335–427.
6. Volkow ND, Baler RD, Compton WM, Weiss SRB. Adverse health effects of marijuana use. N Engl J Med. 2014;370(23):2219–27.
7. Trecki J, Gerona RR, Schwartz MD. Synthetic cannabinoid–related illnesses and deaths. N Engl J Med. 2015;373(2):103–7.
8. Salzman M, Jones CW, Rafeq R, Gaughan J, Haroz R. Epidemiology of opioid-related visits to US Emergency Departments, 1999–2013: A retrospective study from the NHAMCS (National Hospital Ambulatory Medical Care Survey). Am J Emerg Med. 2019. pii: S0735-6757(19)30218-9. [Epub ahead of print].

9. Bohnert ASB, Ilgen MA. Understanding links among opioid use, overdose, and suicide. N Engl J Med. 2019;380(1):71–9.
10. Büttner A, Mall G, Penning R, Weis S. The neuropathology of heroin abuse. Forensic Sci Int. 2000;113(1):435–42.
11. Warner ML, Kaufman NC, Grundmann O. The pharmacology and toxicology of kratom: from traditional herb to drug of abuse. Int J Legal Med. 2016;130(1):127–38.
12. P Busardo F, W Jones A. GHB pharmacology and toxicology: acute intoxication, concentrations in blood and urine in forensic cases and treatment of the withdrawal syndrome. Curr Neuropharmacol. 2015;13(1):47–70.
13. Howard MO, Bowen SE, Garland EL, Perron BE, Vaughn MG. Inhalant use and inhalant use disorders in the United States. Addict Sci Clin Pract. 2011;6(1):18.
14. Carhart-Harris RL, Kaelen M, Bolstridge M, Williams TM, Williams LT, Underwood R, Feilding A, Nutt DJ. The paradoxical psychological effects of lysergic acid diethylamide (LSD). Psychol Med. 2016;46(7):1379–90.
15. Lodge D, Mercier MS. Ketamine and phencyclidine: the good, the bad and the unexpected. Br J Pharmacol. 2015;172(17):4254–76.
16. Halpern JH. Hallucinogens and dissociative agents naturally growing in the United States. Pharmacol Ther. 2004;102(2):131–8.
17. Behrouz R, Godoy DA, Azarpazhooh MR, Di Napoli M. Altered mental status in the neurocritical care unit. J Crit Care. 2015;30(6):1272–7.
18. Silver B, Miller D, Jankowski M, Murshed N, Garcia P, Penstone P, Straub M, Logan SP, Sinha A, Morris DC, Katramados A. Urine toxicology screening in an urban stroke and TIA population. Neurology. 2013;80(18):1702–9.17.
19. Jauch EC, Saver JL, Adams HP, Bruno A, Demaerschalk BM, Khatri P, McMullan PW, Qureshi AI, Rosenfield K, Scott PA, Summers DR. Guidelines for the early management of patients with acute ischemic stroke: a guideline for healthcare professionals from the American Heart Association/American Stroke Association. Stroke. 2013;44(3):870–947.
20. Powers WJ, Derdeyn CP, Biller J, Coffey CS, Hoh BL, Jauch EC, Johnston KC, Johnston SC, Khalessi AA, Kidwell CS, Meschia JF. 2015 American Heart Association/American Stroke Association focused update of the 2013 guidelines for the early management of patients with acute ischemic stroke regarding endovascular treatment: a guideline for healthcare professionals from the American Heart Association/American Stroke Association. Stroke. 2015;46(10):3020–35.
21. Alldredge BK, Lowenstein DH, Simon RP. Seizures associated with recreational drug abuse. Neurology. 1989;39(8):1037–1037.
22. Ziu M, Dengler B, CorDell D, Bartanusz V. Diagnosis and management of primary pyogenic spinal infections in intravenous recreational drug users. Neurosurg Focus. 2014;37(2):E3.

Chapter 16
Neurological Emergencies from Prescription Drugs

Sherri A. Braksick and Deena M. Nasr

Diagnostic Keys
- Ensure a careful and accurate medication reconciliation is completed on hospital admission.
- Determine timing of symptoms in relation to medication changes.
- Review the hospital medication administration record to identify new or omitted medications.

Treatment Priorities
- Ensure hemodynamic stability and determine if airway support is needed.
- Remove offending medications when possible.
- Reinstitute medications in the event of severe withdrawal.

Prognosis at a Glance
- In many cases discontinuation of an offending medication will result in clinical improvement.
- Provide adequate time for toxidromes or withdrawal symptoms to clear before assessing prognosis, particularly in patients with hepatic or renal impairment.

S. A. Braksick (✉) · D. M. Nasr
Department of Neurology, Mayo Clinic, Rochester, MN, USA

Introduction

The available treatments for most medical diagnoses have significantly increased over time, with new medications gaining approval for use from governmental agencies at a rapid rate. As with any therapy offered in medicine, the chances of benefit must be balanced with the risk of harm. All medications carry a risk of adverse events, many with neurologic effects, and some have also been found to have direct neurotoxicity, in therapeutic or toxic dosages. Additionally, sudden withdrawal of certain medications may also precipitate various neurologic sequelae, from benign symptoms to catastrophic or life-threatening complications. The presence of metabolic derangements, such as hepatic or renal injury, can precipitate or exaggerate adverse effects of medications due to impaired and prolonged clearance or metabolism.

In some medical diagnoses, such as multidrug-resistant infections or cancer, treatment options may be limited, and tolerating adverse effects or toxicities may sometimes be necessary so that the primary disease can continue to be treated. This can be a particularly challenging situation, which must be discussed with all involved physicians and the patient or their families to determine the best course of action.

This chapter should not be considered an all-inclusive list of adverse neurologic events associated with specific medications, but rather an emphasis on life-threatening toxicities or withdrawal syndromes and rare or under-recognized neurologic effects of these medications. Well-known and/or non-emergent side effects will largely be excluded from this text. Adverse effects, toxicities, and withdrawal phenomenon of particular interest will be discussed within the text, while other syndromes may be exclusively found in the tables within this chapter. Specific sources used within the chapter are cited as necessary within the text and tables (Table 16.1 and Table 16.2). Additional information was obtained from Micromedex, an online medication database [1].

Neurologic Emergencies and Specific Medication Classes

Anesthetic Agents

The administration of anesthesia is by and large neurologically safe when performed by experienced specialists, but anesthetic medications may rarely provoke neurologic events. The induction agent, etomidate, is known to occasionally precipitate myoclonus; however this effect is largely avoided with intravenous lidocaine pretreatment [2]. Propofol may also be associated with a movement disorder and encephalopathy during emergence from the medication. A recent case series demonstrated patients having paroxysms of abnormal, non-epileptic movements affecting the limbs, head, and eyes with associated encephalopathy and a variable

Table 16.1 Neurologic adverse effects/toxicities organized by medication and medication class

Medication/medication class	Neurologic adverse effect/syndrome	Targeted treatment
Analgesic medications		
Opioids	Miosis, hypopnea, myoclonus, encephalopathy	Removal of offending agent, airway protection in extreme toxicity, naloxone/naltrexone and/or expectant management
Ergots	RCVS, cerebral ischemia, serotonin syndrome	Discontinue medication, supportive care, consider angiography for directed therapy in RCVS
Triptans	RCVS, cerebral ischemia, serotonin syndrome	Discontinue medication, supportive care, consider angiography for directed therapy in RCVS
Anesthetic medications		
Etomidate	Myoclonus	Pretreatment with lidocaine [2]
Halothanes	Malignant hyperthermia (fever, rigidity, rhabdomyolysis, acidosis)	Convert to non-halothane anesthesia, hydration, dantrolene
Propofol	Abnormal movements (during emergence) [3]	Supportive care, resolves with time
Antiarrhythmics		
Lidocaine	Seizure, paresthesia, myoclonus	Discontinuation of medication, management of seizure
Antibiotics		
Aminoglycosides	Hearing loss, neuromuscular blockade (including exacerbation of myasthenia gravis)	Discontinuation of medication, supportive care, management of exacerbated myasthenia
Carbapenems	Seizure	Transition to different antibiotic; management of seizure
Cefepime[a]	Encephalopathy (may progress to coma), myoclonus, seizure	Transition to different antibiotic; management of seizure (if present), supportive care
Fluoroquinolones	Seizure, Guillain-Barre syndrome (rare)	Management of seizure, transition to different antibiotic if possible, GBS-specific treatment
Isoniazid	Peripheral neuropathy, seizure	Transition to different antibiotic if possible, management of seizure
Linezolid	Serotonin syndrome, seizure	Supportive care, avoid other serotoninergic agents, consider cyproheptadine or benzodiazepine, management of seizure, transition to different antibiotic if possible
Metronidazole [5]	Peripheral neuropathy, tremor, encephalopathy, dysarthria, ataxia	Withdrawal of medication and expectant management

(continued)

Table 16.1 (continued)

Medication/medication class	Neurologic adverse effect/syndrome	Targeted treatment
Anticholinergic medications		
Inhaled formulations	Unreactive mydriasis	Recovery expected with time, ensure mist does not escape mask during administration
Oral or transdermal (e.g., scopolamine)	Anticholinergic crisis—fever, hot and dry skin, myoclonus, encephalopathy, urinary retention, ileus, mydriasis, tachycardia	Discontinue medication, hydration, aggressive fever management, ensure bladder emptying, telemetry monitoring in severe cases
Antidepressants		
Bupropion	Seizure, tremor	Transition to a different medication, management of seizure
SNRI	Seizure	Discontinuation of medication, management of seizure
SSRI	Serotonin syndrome, RCVS, dystonia (rare) [6]	Serotonin syndrome: withdrawal of all serotoninergic medications (SSRI, ondansetron, fentanyl, etc.), supportive care RCVS: supportive care, consider angiography for directed therapy Dystonia: antihistamine, anticholinergic medications
TCA	RCVS, myoclonus, seizure	Discontinue medication; RCVS, consider angiography for directed therapy; seizure management, supportive care
Antiepileptic medications	Multiple medications: DRESS syndrome	Withdrawal of medication, supportive care, consider corticosteroids, subspecialty (dermatology) consultation
Carbamazepine	Hyponatremia, ataxia, encephalopathy; severe toxicity, coma, rhabdomyolysis	Discontinue medication, supportive care
Gabapentin[a]	Encephalopathy, dizziness, ataxia, myoclonus	Discontinue medication, supportive care
Lamotrigine	Hemophagocytic lymphohistiocytosis	Discontinue medication, hematology consultation
Oxcarbazepine	Hyponatremia	Hold medication, standard treatment for hyponatremia
Perampanel	Psychiatric symptoms	Transition to a different antiepileptic
Phenytoin	Ataxia, hemodynamic instability (during loading)	Ataxia, discontinue/hold medication, supportive care; hemodynamic issues, slow medication infusion rate, intravenous fluids

Table 16.1 (continued)

Medication/medication class	Neurologic adverse effect/syndrome	Targeted treatment
Valproic acid	Encephalopathy/coma (due to hyperammonemia), tremor, pancreatitis (rare)	Discontinue medication, treat elevated ammonia and pancreatitis
Antiemetics	Dystonia	Antihistamine or anticholinergic, discontinue offending medication
Ondansetron	Serotonin syndrome	Withdrawal of all serotoninergic medications (SSRI, ondansetron, fentanyl, etc.), supportive care, may consider cyproheptadine or benzodiazepines
Antipsychotics	Dyskinesia (tardive), neuroleptic malignant syndrome, dystonia	Discontinue medication; neuroleptic malignant syndrome: dantrolene, aggressive fever management and hydration; dystonia: antihistamine, anticholinergic
Lithium	Tremor, ataxia, seizure, cerebral edema (rare)	Discontinue medication, management of seizure, supportive care
Antirejection medications		
Cyclosporine [23]	Tremor, PRES—including seizure, encephalopathy (may progress to coma)	Transition to a different immunosuppressant, blood pressure management in PRES, supportive care
OKT-3 (muromonab-CD3) [23]	Headache, meningismus, psychosis, seizure	Targeted treatment of seizures, discontinue medication
Tacrolimus [23]	Tremor, PRES—including seizure, encephalopathy (may progress to coma)	Transition to a different immunosuppressant, blood pressure management in PRES, supportive care
Chemotherapy medications	PRES, peripheral neuropathy (multiple medications)	PRES: blood pressure control, discontinuation of medication, seizure management; neuropathy: discontinue medications (if possible)
Busulfan	Seizures	Discontinue medication (if possible), treat seizures
Carmustine (intracranial wafer implant)	Infection, cerebral edema, hydrocephalus, seizure, hemorrhage	Directed treatment of symptoms/syndrome
Cytarabine[a] [13]	Cerebellar toxicity, encephalopathy (may progress to coma)	Discontinue medication (if possible), supportive care
Ifosfamide [14]	Encephalopathy, seizure, tremor, myoclonus	Discontinue medication, methylene blue for severe cases

(continued)

Table 16.1 (continued)

Medication/medication class	Neurologic adverse effect/syndrome	Targeted treatment
L-Asparaginase	Coagulopathy, seizures, dural venous sinus thrombosis	Anticoagulation, management of seizures, transition to different medication, if possible
Methotrexate	Encephalopathy, seizures, aseptic meningitis (intrathecal administration), leukoencephalopathy	Discontinue medication, treat seizures, supportive care
VEGF/VEGF-R antagonists (e.g., bevacizumab)	PRES, intracerebral hemorrhage, ischemic stroke	PRES, blood pressure control, discontinuation of medication, seizure management; discontinuation of medication if possible. Management of hemorrhage/ischemic stroke
Cholesterol medications	Myopathy, rarely rhabdomyolysis	Discontinue medication, hydration; immunosuppression if HMG-CoA antibody is positive
Cholinesterase inhibitors (e.g., pyridostigmine)	Cholinergic excess (sialorrhea, diarrhea, miosis, blurred vision, diaphoresis, nausea/vomiting, bradycardia, hypotension)	Supportive care, atropine if bradycardic, vasopressors if hypotensive
Contraceptives	Thromboembolism (primarily estrogen-based compounds)	Management of thromboembolism (stroke, venous sinus thrombus, etc.)
Decongestant/sympathomimetic medications (e.g., ephedrine, pseudoephedrine)	RCVS	Discontinue medication, supportive care, consider angiography for directed therapy
Disease-modifying agents (MS, rheumatologic disease medications)	PML, opportunistic CNS infections (multiple medications)	Discontinue medication, infection-specific treatment, supportive care
TNF-α[alpha] inhibitors	Acute central or peripheral demyelination syndromes	Discontinue medication, treatment of cerebral edema, possible steroids
Dopaminergic medications (e.g., carbidopa-levodopa)	Dyskinesia, depression, hallucinations	Remove/decrease dose of drug (often not feasible), amantadine, clozapine
Immunotherapy		
CAR-T [16]	Encephalopathy (may progress to coma), cerebral edema, tremor	Tocilizumab or siltuximab, steroid therapy, management of cerebral edema and seizures
CTLA-4 inhibitors [17]	Guillain-Barre-type inflammatory syndrome, myasthenic syndrome, PRES, encephalitis, aseptic meningitis	Steroids, disease-specific therapy, supportive care, discontinuation of medication, if possible

Table 16.1 (continued)

Medication/medication class	Neurologic adverse effect/syndrome	Targeted treatment
PD-1 inhibitors [18, 19]	Myositis, Guillain-Barre-type inflammatory syndrome, ataxia, encephalopathy	Steroids, disease-specific therapy, supportive care, discontinuation of medication, if possible
IVIg [24]	Aseptic meningitis, headache, thrombotic events (e.g., stroke)	Nonsteroidal medications, steroids, migraine-directed therapy
Methylene blue	Serotonin syndrome	Withdrawal of all serotoninergic medications (SSRI, ondansetron, fentanyl, etc.), supportive care, may consider cyproheptadine or benzodiazepines
Muscle relaxants		
Baclofen[a] [20]	Weakness, ataxia, dyskinesia, encephalopathy, coma, seizure. In severe toxicity, may mimic brain death	Hold medication if toxicity (monitor for evidence of withdrawal); manage seizures, supportive care
Cyclobenzaprine	Encephalopathy, coma (in toxicity), seizures, anticholinergic crisis	Supportive care, treat seizures, fever control. Consider physostigmine in CNS toxicity/anticholinergic syndrome
Methocarbamol	Seizure, encephalopathy	Treat seizures, supportive care, discontinue medication
Paralytics		
Succinylcholine	Malignant hyperthermia (fever, rigidity, rhabdomyolysis, acidosis)	Hydration, consider dantrolene; discontinue medication
Steroids	Insomnia, psychosis, tremor	Discontinue when possible, antipsychotic medications for psychosis
Stimulants (e.g., methylphenidate, etc.)	Tremor, agitation, RCVS, seizure	Discontinue medication; RCVS, supportive care, consider angiography for directed therapy; directed therapy for seizure

CAR-T chimeric antigen receptor T-cell therapy, *CNS* central nervous system, *CTLA-4* cytotoxic T-lymphocyte-associated antigen 4, *DRESS* drug reaction with eosinophilia and systemic symptoms, *IVIg* intravenous immunoglobulin, *MS* multiple sclerosis, *PD-1* programmed cell death receptor-1, *PRES* posterior reversible encephalopathy syndrome, *PML* progressive multifocal leukoencephalopathy, *RCVS* reversible cerebral vasoconstriction syndrome, *SNRI* selective norepinephrine reuptake inhibitor, *SSRI* selective serotonin reuptake inhibitors, *TCA* tricyclic antidepressant, *TNF-α[alpha]* tumor necrosis factor-alpha, *VEGF* vascular endothelial growth factor
[a]Typically in the presence of impaired clearance

degree of recollection of the spells. Supportive care and avoidance of additional propofol resulted in full recovery [3].

The risk of malignant hyperthermia due to halothane anesthesia is a well-characterized syndrome, occurring in rare patients with ryanodine receptor mutations. It is important for all providers to be aware of this complication as symptom

Table 16.2 Neurologic emergencies due to medication withdrawal

Medication	Neurologic withdrawal symptoms	Targeted treatment
Antipsychotic medications	Recurrent psychosis	Reinitiation of medication
Antidepressant medications	Serotonin discontinuation syndrome (dizziness, fatigue, headache) [7]	Supportive care for mild symptoms. Severe symptoms: reinitiate medication and perform a prolonged taper
Baclofen	Increased spasticity, encephalopathy, seizure, fever, anxiety, restlessness, rhabdomyolysis, death	Reinstitution of medication, supportive care
Benzodiazepines	Seizure or status epilepticus, anxiety, tremor	Reinstitution of medication and slow taper when discontinuing
Dopaminergic medications (e.g., carbidopa-levodopa)	Parkinsonism-hyperpyrexia syndrome (fever, rigidity, encephalopathy, autonomic instability)	Reinstitution of medication; dantrolene for severe presentations, fever control, hydration
Opioid medications	Agitation	Slow taper, supportive care. Complex cases will require pain management service consultation

development may occur up to 24 hours following anesthesia. Management includes immediate withdrawal of gas anesthesia, hydration, and dantrolene administration.

Antibiotics

Antimicrobial use is common in hospitalized patients, and most tolerate it without complication. Yet, several antimicrobial medications and medication classes have been associated with neurologic symptoms, and balancing the need for a particular antibiotic (e.g., in patients with multidrug-resistant organisms where medication choices are particularly limited) against the potential neurologic risk can be difficult.

Cefepime is a fourth-generation cephalosporin used to treat multiple organisms in the hospitalized patient and is generally well-tolerated. A syndrome of encephalopathy, myoclonus, and seizures (cefepime neurotoxicity) has been described in patients receiving this medication, with renal impairment being a known risk factor [4]. Improvement is common but not guaranteed, and clinical improvement may be delayed once the medication is removed, necessitating a period of supportive care and observation in these patients prior to prognostication.

Antibiotics in the carbapenem class (e.g., ertapenem and meropenem) and fluoroquinolone classes (e.g., levofloxacin, ciprofloxacin) can lower the seizure threshold. Caution should be exercised when using these medications in patients with a history of seizures. As previously mentioned, the increasing development of multi-drug-resistant organisms sometimes limits a clinician's ability to transition to other antimicrobial agents, and if a breakthrough seizure occurs, increasing the antiepileptic regimen during the treatment period may be necessary to allow the patient to tolerate and complete antimicrobial therapy.

An uncommon neurologic syndrome may rarely happen in patients treated with metronidazole. Cerebellar symptoms, particularly ataxia, are common, as well as encephalopathy and seizures. Imaging frequently shows hyperintensity of the cerebellar dentate nuclei (Fig. 16.1). After drug discontinuation, symptoms and imaging abnormalities improve in most patients, though ataxia may be persistent in some cases [5].

Antidepressant Medications

The use of antidepressant medications is common and generally safe. That said, many medications in this category lower the seizure threshold, particularly bupropion, selective norepinephrine reuptake inhibitors, and tricyclic antidepressants. Transitioning to a different drug class (e.g., selective serotonin reuptake inhibitors (SSRI)) is warranted if the patient suffers a seizure after initiation of these medications.

SSRI medications, as the name implies, prevent the reuptake of serotonin by neuronal cells, leading to an increased risk of serotonin syndrome, particularly when this medication is combined with other serotoninergic medications (see the separate section within this chapter regarding the clinical presentation and implicated medications in this syndrome).

Antidepressants, particularly when used concurrently with antipsychotics, have also been associated with the development of dystonia. In cases of acute dystonic reaction, the causal medication(s) should be held, and treatment includes either anticholinergic or antihistamine medications [6].

Patients who have been on long-term SSRI medications are also at risk for serotonin discontinuation syndrome if the drug is abruptly stopped. These patients develop increased anxiety, restlessness, fatigue, and headache. Symptoms are often uncomfortable, but not life-threatening (except for the possibility of acute exacerbation of depression resulting in suicide). In patients with severe symptoms, the medication may need to be reinitiated and then tapered more slowly [7].

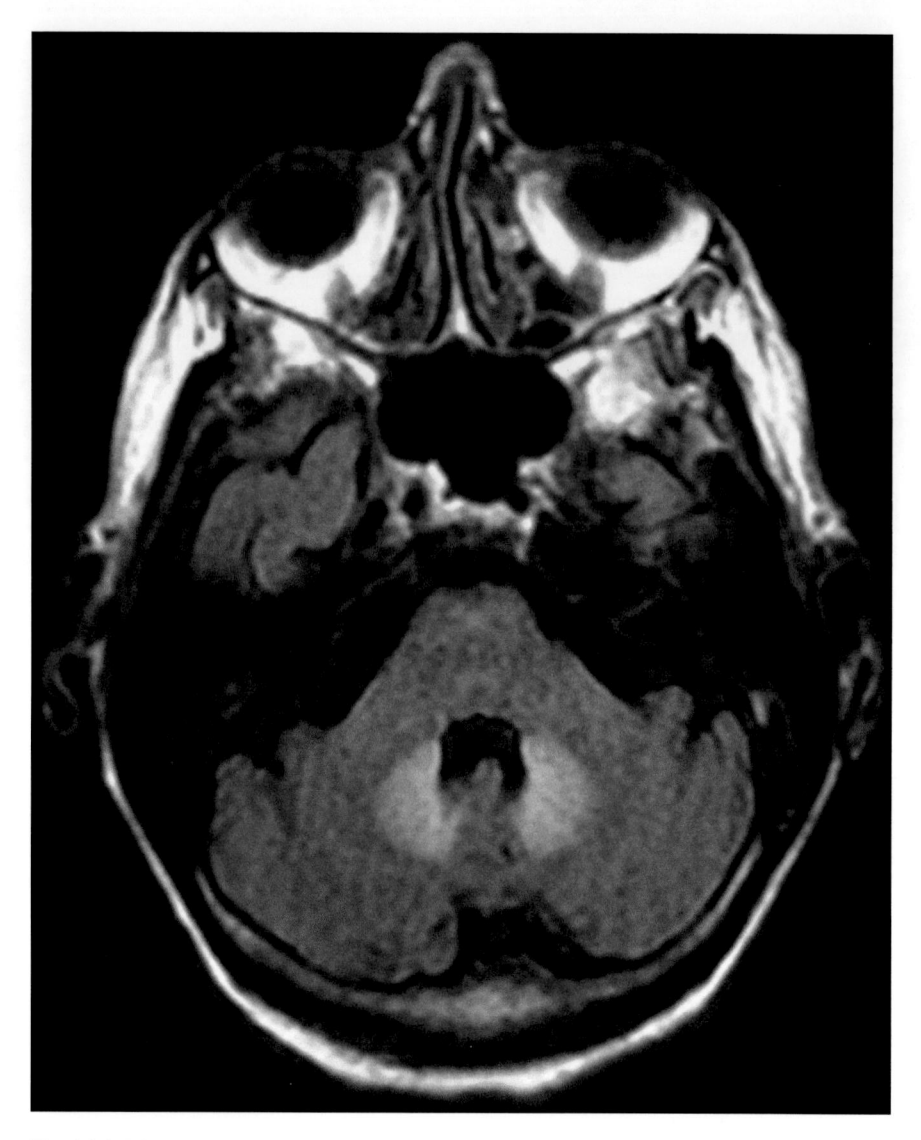

Fig. 16.1 T2 FLAIR brain magnetic resonance image demonstrating hyperintensity of the bilateral dentate nuclei in a patient with metronidazole-induced neurologic symptoms. With drug discontinuation and supportive care, the patient's symptoms resolved and imaging returned to normal

Antiepileptic Medications

Antiepileptics have a long list of adverse reactions, with few directly affecting the nervous system. Many different antiepileptics (in addition to medications from other drug classes) can predispose patients to an uncommon, but life-threatening systemic condition—drug reaction with eosinophilia and systemic symptoms

(DRESS) syndrome. Symptoms typically occur weeks after the medications are initiated, and they involve the skin and various other organ systems. The instigating medication must be stopped and corticosteroids (topical or oral) are commonly used. Subspecialty consultation with dermatology is warranted to help determine the appropriate diagnosis and guide management [8].

Carbamazepine and oxcarbazepine can cause chronic hyponatremia. A minority of patients will develop severe, symptomatic hyponatremia and require hospitalization as a result [9]. The implicated medication must be discontinued when hyponatremia is symptomatic, unless an additional factor precipitated transient worsening of a chronic, drug-induced, mild hyponatremia.

The Food and Drug Administration (FDA) recently released a warning implicating lamotrigine as a causal agent in a hematologic disorder known as hemophagocytic lymphohistiocytosis (HLH). Diagnosis and management requires the assistance of hematology subspecialists, and the instigating medication must be discontinued immediately.

In patients requiring a loading dose of phenytoin (or fosphenytoin) or those who are otherwise supratherapeutic, a transient and potentially severe ataxia may develop. With time, as the medication is metabolized, symptoms gradually improve and the medication can often be continued. Hypotension is common during phenytoin loading, which should be supported with intravenous fluids and/or vasopressor agents. Decreasing the rate of infusion often results in stabilization of the patient as well.

Hyperammonemia, elevated transaminases, and, rarely, pancreatitis have all been attributed to valproic acid use, which may result in asterixis, encephalopathy, or a depressed level of consciousness. Hyperammonemia and pancreatitis are managed according to usual standards, and valproic acid is usually discontinued in these cases.

Gabapentin is a commonly used medication as an adjuvant for epilepsy and one of the first-line options for neuropathic pain. Toxicity from this medication can occur with excessive intake and also in the setting of acute renal impairment resulting in decreased medication clearance. Patients will present with encephalopathy, myoclonus, and ataxia. With supportive care and discontinuation of the medication, symptoms will improve.

Antirejection Medications

Solid organ transplantation necessitates the long-term use of immunosuppressive agents in organ recipients to prevent organ rejection. Calcineurin inhibitors, particularly cyclosporine and tacrolimus, can cause neurotoxicity. Neurotoxicity is more frequent in the early posttransplant phase, but symptoms can occur at any time following transplantation. Sirolimus has a lower risk of neurotoxicity [10]. The most common symptom is tremor, with more severe symptoms including encephalopathy or psychosis, hallucinations, and seizures, often consistent with the diagnosis of posterior reversible encephalopathy syndrome (PRES). Blood pressure is usually not elevated in these patients, however. Serum drug levels do not seem to correlate with symptom onset, as patients may develop symptoms of neurotoxicity when appropriately therapeutic. Toxic leukoencephalopathy with status epilepticus after months of therapy with tacrolimus has been described, with resolution of symptoms following discontinuation of the medication [11].

In patients with severe symptoms, transitioning to an alternative immunosuppressant medication may be necessary, and recovery often occurs but may not be complete. In cases of mild symptoms (e.g., tremor), discussion among the transplant team, patient, and neurologist may be necessary to weigh the risks and benefits of discontinuing or remaining on an otherwise effective medication.

Chemotherapeutic Agents

The use of chemotherapy medications places patients at risk for multiple complications, including those involving the nervous system. Many different medications, particularly platinum-based therapy, taxane, and vinca alkaloids, predispose patients to chronic peripheral neuropathy that is likely to present to the outpatient setting for evaluation.

More acutely, patients may develop abrupt mental status changes from a number of different reasons. PRES (with symptoms of encephalopathy, seizures, variable degrees of cortical vision loss, and posterior vasogenic edema on head imaging) has been reported with many different chemotherapeutic agents, even in the absence of hypertension or labile blood pressure, similar to that seen with antirejection medications (Fig. 16.2) [12]. Supportive care, correction of any blood pressure abnormalities, and discontinuation of the implicated medication (if possible) will improve symptoms.

Other chemotherapeutic agents have been associated with specific neurologic complications. Busulfan predisposes to seizures, and therefore patients are often given prophylactic antiepileptics when receiving this medication [13]. Carmustine is occasionally used for intracranial tumors as an implant during surgical procedures and may therefore predispose to complications similar to those of the surgical procedures themselves—infection, seizure, cerebral edema, or intracranial hemorrhage.

Methotrexate is commonly well-tolerated from a neurologic standpoint but rarely may cause a dramatic clinical presentation with altered mental status and diffuse leukoencephalopathy, necessitating discontinuation of the medication with a variable and uncertain degree of clinical improvement. More acutely, seizures and nonspecific encephalopathy may occur shortly after treatment with improvement expected over time. Intrathecal methotrexate has been associated with aseptic meningitis, which also improves with supportive care [13].

Cytarabine (also known as Ara-C) is used in hematologic malignancies and may cause a fulminant cerebellar syndrome with severe ataxia, and intrathecal adminis-

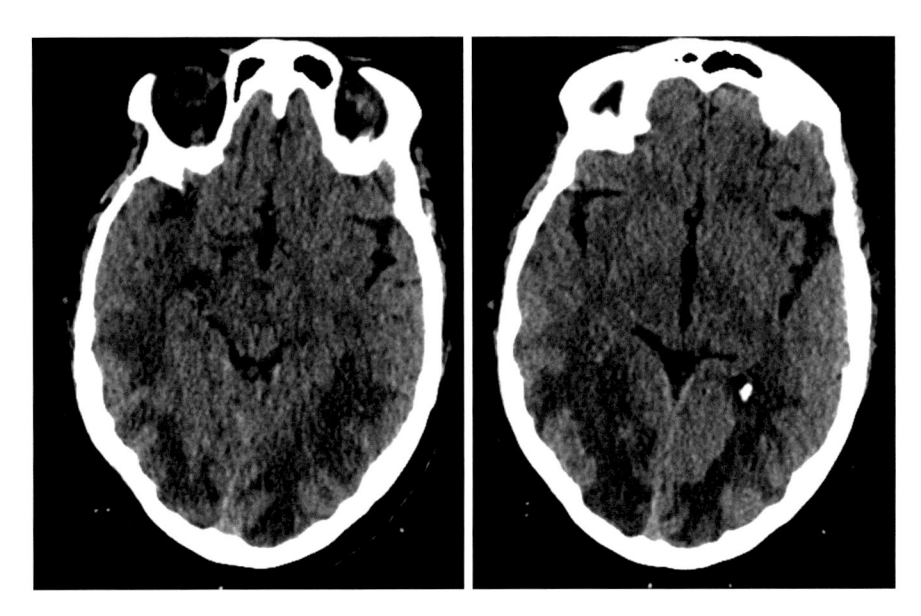

Fig. 16.2 Non-contrast CT scan demonstrating posterior-predominant vasogenic edema, consistent with PRES, in a cancer patient who had received platinum-based chemotherapy several days prior to presentation. Her examination demonstrated encephalopathy with poor attention and cortical blindness. With time and careful blood pressure control, her symptoms gradually resolved

tration may rarely cause aseptic meningitis or myelopathy. The medication must be immediately discontinued when symptoms develop. There is no specific treatment for reversal, and with time some patients may improve, while others remain disabled [13].

The use of ifosfamide may result in a severe encephalopathy syndrome and seizures within hours to days of administration. Fortunately this is a self-limiting and transient phenomenon if the medication is discontinued [14]. There are reports of methylene blue being used for directed treatment, though it is uncertain if the medication, or simply time, is responsible for the clinical improvement [15].

L-Asparaginase is used primarily for treatment of leukemia and is associated with seizures and thrombogenesis, including dural venous sinus thrombosis. If either event occurs, directed treatment (antiepileptics or anticoagulation) is warranted, and the medication should be discontinued, if possible. Occasionally L-asparaginase may be continued once the adverse effects are adequately treated [13].

Bevacizumab, an antagonist to vascular endothelial growth factor (anti-VEGF), is used in multiple cancer types and also as an intraocular injection for macular degeneration. Due to its mechanism of action, it has been associated with both ischemic and hemorrhagic strokes, as well as PRES [12, 13].

Cholinesterase Inhibitors

Cholinesterase-inhibiting medications, such as those used in patients with myasthenia gravis, are often well-tolerated when given in proper doses. Clinical symptoms of cholinergic excess include sialorrhea, diarrhea, and miosis. Severe cases may also have concomitant bradycardia and/or hypotension. Sialorrhea may occur in a myasthenic patient due to excessive use of pyridostigmine, which patients may increase when they perceive worsening myasthenic symptoms; however, sialorrhea may also occur as a result of orofacial weakness and dysphagia when an exacerbation occurs. A careful history will frequently allow the clinician to distinguish between cholinergic excess and uncontrolled myasthenia, as management for the two entities differs. For patients with uncontrolled myasthenia gravis, continuation and titration of the anticholinesterase medication or additional immunosuppressive agents are often necessary. In patients with a syndrome of true cholinergic excess, supportive care and withdrawal of the offending medication is often all that is needed. When severe and associated with hemodynamic instability, atropine or vasopressor agents may also be required.

Dopaminergic Medications

The use of dopaminergic medications is common in patients with hypoactive movement disorders, particularly Parkinson disease, where patients have a primary loss of dopaminergic neurons in the substantia nigra. These medications require ongoing titration and over time can produce dyskinesias and psychiatric symptoms, including depression or hallucinations. Additionally, dopamine agonists, such as ropinirole or pramipexole, have been associated with impulse-control disorders (e.g., hypersexuality, gambling, etc.) and sleep attacks that may be particularly dangerous in patients who are still driving.

An uncommon but easily overlooked consequence of dopaminergics is a syndrome caused by sudden medication withdrawal. The abrupt loss of dopamine can precipitate a dopamine-depletion syndrome that appears identical to neuroleptic malignant syndrome but is termed parkinsonism-hyperpyrexia syndrome. Management includes reinitiation of the dopaminergic medication, hydration, fever control, monitoring for rhabdomyolysis (rare and only seen in severe cases), and consideration of dantrolene in patients with severe clinical presentations. Reinitiation of the medication is often the only treatment necessary.

Immunotherapy

Numerous advances in directed therapies for cancer have occurred in the last decade and include the development of immunotherapy, treatments targeting specific cell surface receptors to activate the patient's immune response to the abnormal tumor cells. Additional immune-mediated adverse events, many affecting the nervous system, have been observed with the increasing use of these medications.

A recently approved treatment, chimeric antigen receptor T-cell therapy (CAR-T), is used primarily in refractory B-cell lymphoma, but indications will likely grow rapidly. Neurotoxicity is commonly seen as part of the cytokine release syndrome induced by this therapy. Because of this, a standardized cognitive screen should be completed during routine nursing checks following drug administration. Signs and symptoms of neurotoxicity include tremor, encephalopathy, speech abnormality or aphasia, seizure, and cerebral edema. Directed rescue therapy includes steroids and/or tocilizumab or siltuximab to decrease the immune-driven response [16]. Standard treatment for seizures, elevated intracranial pressure, and other neurologic symptoms should occur simultaneous to the administration of rescue therapies. Prophylactic antiepileptics are sometimes included in CAR-T protocols, but the risk-benefit of this strategy is unclear.

Cytotoxic T-lymphocyte-associated protein 4 (CTLA-4) therapies (e.g., ipilimumab) are approved for use in several solid tumors and lymphoma. Reported neurologic events include myasthenic syndrome, a painful Guillain-Barre-type syndrome, encephalitis, and aseptic meningitis. Steroid therapy often improves symptoms, though directed therapy for myasthenia or Guillain-Barre may also be necessary [17].

Programmed cell death receptor 1 (PD-1) inhibitors (e.g., pembrolizumab or nivolumab) are used in multiple tumor types and have also been associated with a Guillain-Barre are presentation, myasthenic syndrome, necrotizing myopathy, and ataxia [18]. Given the immune-mediated nature of symptoms, steroids are often given, with immunoglobulin and plasma exchange occasionally being used as well [19].

As our experience with these relatively new medications increases, further clinical characterization and optimal treatment regimens will likely develop.

Muscle Relaxants

The use of muscle relaxants can generally cause somnolence and, particularly in elderly patients, confusion or encephalopathy. Rarely, anticholinergic crisis may occur and requires prompt treatment.

One particular medication, baclofen, can cause severe effects when taken in inappropriately high doses or after sudden withdrawal. When this medication is intentionally or inadvertently taken in large amounts, patients may develop ataxia, alterations of consciousness (including coma), seizures and, in rare cases, may mimic brain death. Supportive care and management of any seizures is necessary, and recovery generally occurs with time. The presence of renal impairment may potentiate the effects of baclofen, and hemodialysis may aid in medication clearance in these patients [20].

In sudden baclofen withdrawal, patients may become very agitated or anxious, suffer seizures, and develop hyperthermia and/or encephalopathy. If the medication is not reinitiated, the syndrome can progress to severe rhabdomyolysis and multi-organ dysfunction. For this reason, in patients admitted for baclofen overdose, reinitiation of low-dose baclofen under careful monitoring is advisable once improvement is seen. Of note, the risk of serious baclofen withdrawal is much more common in patients with intrathecal baclofen pumps.

Bismuth Toxicity

An uncommon but important toxicity to recognize is excessive bismuth intake (as may be seen in patients who have severe irritable bowel disease or esophageal reflux). These patients may present either to the inpatient or outpatient setting with rapidly progressive encephalopathy, memory loss, tremor, and myoclonus, similar to Creutzfeldt-Jakob disease. A careful history and medication reconciliation will divulge the excessive use of this over-the-counter medication, and bismuth discontinuation and supportive care results in symptom improvement [21].

Vitamin Deficiencies

Vitamin deficiencies often do not happen in isolation and may be due to poor dietary intake or gastrointestinal malabsorption. Bariatric surgery has become more commonplace over the recent past, and these patients may have preexisting or postoperative nutritional deficiencies, some of which are summarized in Table 16.3. Many of these deficiencies do not precipitate neurological emergencies, though they may be an underlying and/or undiagnosed reason for hospitalization.

Of particular concern is thiamine deficiency, which may produce Wernicke encephalopathy, characterized by altered mental status, ophthalmoplegia, and ataxia. If left untreated, thiamine deficiency may ultimately lead to Korsakoff syndrome—a disabling dysfunction of anterograde memory. Patients who present to emergency rooms with hypoglycemia that will receive dextrose-containing solutions should first or simultaneously receive thiamine to prevent this serious complication.

Table 16.3 Neurologic emergencies due to vitamin/supplementation toxicity [25]

Bismuth toxicity	Rapidly progressive syndrome with cognitive changes and myoclonus—may mimic Creutzfeldt-Jakob disease	Withdrawal of medication, supportive care
Thiamine deficiency	Wernicke-Korsakoff syndrome	High-dose thiamine (prior to dextrose administration), supportive care
Vitamin A toxicity	Pseudotumor cerebri	Discontinue supplement, supportive care

Serotonin Syndrome

Serotonin syndrome is an uncommon syndrome with many potential precipitants. It is characterized by hypertension, diaphoresis, tachycardia, mydriasis, variable degrees of encephalopathy, prominent bowel sounds or diarrhea, and rigidity, hyperreflexia, and clonus preferentially affecting the legs.

Hospitalized patients often receive multiple medications that may precipitate this syndrome, particularly if they are receiving serotoninergic medications prior to admission (e.g., antidepressant medications). Known medication triggers of serotonin syndrome include antidepressants, fentanyl, 5-HT$_3$ antagonists (e.g., ondansetron), muscle relaxants, migraine therapies, and linezolid, among others. Management involves removal of all serotoninergic medications and supportive care. Benzodiazepines, if needed, may be used for sedation. There is limited data for the use of cyproheptadine, though this is often not necessary as supportive care will result in improvement over time. There are reports of a similar syndrome of serotoninergic excess occurring following cardiac arrest, and management in these patients is identical to those with serotonin syndrome due to medication effects [22].

Conclusion

Medications, in isolation or when given in combination, may result in emergent neurologic syndromes, and a high index of suspicion is required to identify a causal relationship. Providers must have an understanding of potential adverse effects when prescribing medications to their patients. Additionally, withdrawal syndromes cannot be overlooked, and a careful history and medication reconciliation may lead the clinician to the proper diagnosis.

Cardinal Messages
- Adverse effects of medications are common and may result from direct toxicity or drug-drug interactions.
- An accurate clinical and medication history is imperative to identify a causal relationship between symptoms and medication administration.
- Patients with hepatic or renal impairment may have prolonged medication metabolism and clearance times, and are more prone to supratherapeutic levels and toxicity.
- Withdrawal syndromes may be easily overlooked and must be deliberately considered by medical providers.
- Patients may omit vitamins or supplements from their home medication list, and this must be specifically addressed when taking a medication history.
- While most neurotoxic effects of medications are reversible, major complications can occur if the neurotoxicity is not promptly recognized.

References

1. Micromedex [Internet]. Truven Health Analytics [cited October 23, 2019].
2. Gultop F, Akkaya T, Bedirli N, Gumus H. Lidocaine pretreatment reduces the frequency and severity of myoclonus induced by etomidate. J Anesth. 2010;24(2):300–2.
3. Carvalho DZ, Townley RA, Burkle CM, Rabinstein AA, Wijdicks EFM. Propofol frenzy: clinical spectrum in 3 patients. Mayo Clin Proc. 2017;92(11):1682–7.
4. Garces EO, Andrade de Anzambuja MF, da Silva D, Bragatti JA, Jacoby T, Saldanha Thome F. Renal failure is a risk factor for cefepime-induced encephalopathy. J Nephrol. 2008;21(4):526–34.
5. Kuriyama A, Jackson JL, Doi A, Kamiya T. Metronidazole-induced central nervous system toxicity: a systematic review. Clin Neuropharmacol. 2011;34(6):241–7.
6. van Harten PN, Hoek HW, Kahn RS. Acute dystonia induced by drug treatment. BMJ. 1999;319(7210):623–6.
7. Bainum TB, Fike DS, Mechelay D, Haase KK. Effect of abrupt discontinuation of antidepressants in critically ill hospitalized adults. Pharmacotherapy. 2017;37(10):1231–40.
8. Cacoub P, Musette P, Descamps V, Meyer O, Speirs C, Finzi L, et al. The DRESS syndrome: a literature review. Am J Med. 2011;124(7):588–97.
9. Berghuis B, van der Palen J, de Haan GJ, Lindhout D, Koeleman BPC, Sander JW, et al. Carbamazepine- and oxcarbazepine-induced hyponatremia in people with epilepsy. Epilepsia. 2017;58(7):1227–33.
10. Maramattom BV, Wijdicks EF. Sirolimus may not cause neurotoxicity in kidney and liver transplant recipients. Neurology. 2004;63(10):1958–9.
11. Junna MR, Rabinstein AA. Tacrolimus induced leukoencephalopathy presenting with status epilepticus and prolonged coma. J Neurol Neurosurg Psychiatry. 2007;78(12):1410–1.
12. Singer S, Grommes C, Reiner AS, Rosenblum MK, DeAngelis LM. Posterior reversible encephalopathy syndrome in patients with cancer. Oncologist. 2015;20(7):806–11.
13. Lee EQ, Arrillaga-Romany IC, Wen PY. Neurologic complications of cancer drug therapies. Continuum (Minneap Minn). 2012;18(2):355–65.
14. Savica R, Rabinstein AA, Josephs KA. Ifosfamide associated myoclonus-encephalopathy syndrome. J Neurol. 2011;258(9):1729–31.
15. Patel PN. Methylene blue for management of Ifosfamide-induced encephalopathy. Ann Pharmacother. 2006;40(2):299–303.
16. Neelapu SS, Tummala S, Kebriaei P, Wierda W, Gutierrez C, Locke FL, et al. Chimeric antigen receptor T-cell therapy—assessment and management of toxicities. Nat Rev Clin Oncol. 2018;15(1):47–62.
17. Fellner A, Makranz C, Lotem M, Bokstein F, Taliansky A, Rosenberg S, et al. Neurologic complications of immune checkpoint inhibitors. J Neuro-Oncol. 2018;137:601.
18. Haddox CL, Shenoy N, Shah KK, Kao JC, Jain S, Halfdanarson TR, et al. Pembrolizumab induced bulbar myopathy and respiratory failure with necrotizing myositis of the diaphragm. Ann Oncol. 2017;28(3):673–5.
19. Kao JC, Liao B, Markovic SN, Klein CJ, Naddaf E, Staff NP, et al. Neurological complications associated with anti-programmed death 1 (PD-1) antibodies. JAMA Neurol. 2017;74(10):1216–22.
20. Porter LM, Merrick SS, Katz KD. Baclofen toxicity in a patient with hemodialysis-dependent end-stage renal disease. J Emerg Med. 2017;52(4):e99–e100.
21. Jungreis AC, Schaumburg HH. Encephalopathy from abuse of bismuth subsalicylate (Pepto-Bismol). Neurology. 1993;43(6):1265.
22. Fugate JE, White RD, Rabinstein AA. Serotonin syndrome after therapeutic hypothermia for cardiac arrest: a case series. Resuscitation. 2014;85(6):774–7.
23. Wijdicks EF. Neurotoxicity of immunosuppressive drugs. Liver Transpl. 2001;7(11):937–42.
24. Duhem C, Dicato MA, Ries F. Side-effects of intravenous immune globulins. Clin Exp Immunol. 1994;97(Suppl 1):79–83.
25. NIH Office of Dietary Supplements [Internet]. National Institutes of Health. [cited October 23, 2019]. Available from: https://ods.od.nih.gov/.

Acute Disseminated Encephalomyelitis

Acute disseminated encephalomyelitis (ADEM) and its hyper-acute form known as acute necrotizing hemorrhagic encephalopathy (ANHE) are acute immune-mediated inflammatory demyelinating illnesses. ADEM typically manifests as a monophasic illness due to diffuse or multifocal CNS inflammation and presents with an abrupt onset of symptoms and signs days to weeks after certain viral infection, immunization, or vaccination (influenza, DPT, varicella, polio, rabies, measles, and hepatitis B). In pediatric patients, ADEM is usually associated with systemic viral infections, including herpes simplex, cytomegalovirus, Epstein-Barr virus, influenza A and B, rubella, HIV, and coxsackievirus [2]. The incidence rate of ADEM is approximately 0.4–0.8/100,000 population without gender or ethnic preference. ADEM is encountered more often in winter and spring seasons.

Although encephalopathy may be present in acute MS, presence of encephalopathy is characteristic of ADEM. Systemic symptoms including fever, headache, nausea, vomiting, malaise, and myalgia may occur before the appearance of neurological symptoms [4]. Although the symptoms and signs typically depend on the areas of CNS involvement, the most common are altered mentation, bowel/bladder incontinence, hemiparesis, ataxia, cranial nerve(s) palsy, stupor, and coma. In pediatric cases, fever, headache, seizure, and signs of meningeal irritation are more frequently observed. ADEM can also present with symptoms of optic neuritis (impaired vision) and transverse myelitis including breathing difficulty, bowel/bladder dysfunction, weakness or paralysis, spasticity, and paresthesia [2, 5]. Sensory deficits are more common in adults, and seizures are more frequent in children [3]. Less common manifestations of ADEM include ataxia, myoclonus, and memory loss [5].

ADEM is diagnosed based on clinical features and neuroimaging characteristics (Figure 17.1) [5, 6]. Presently, no specific biomarker exists to establish the diagnosis. Laboratory studies are usually performed to exclude viral and bacterial infections. Cerebrospinal fluid (CSF) analysis may show increased inflammatory cells and protein concentration. MRI of the brain and spine are very useful to establish the diagnosis of ADEM. Lesions in ADEM are usually large (5 mm to 5 cm in length), bilateral, multifocal, and located in deep and subcortical white matter. Lesions are also observed in the brainstem and spinal cord [6]. In the spinal cord, lesions typically extend over multiple segments of the cord. Except for neuropathology, there is no means for definitive diagnosis of ADEM. Perivenular infiltration of lymphocytes, macrophages, and occasional plasma cells with edematous white matter and demyelination are noted in brain biopsy. In addition, perivascular hemorrhage and some axonal fragmentation also have been observed.

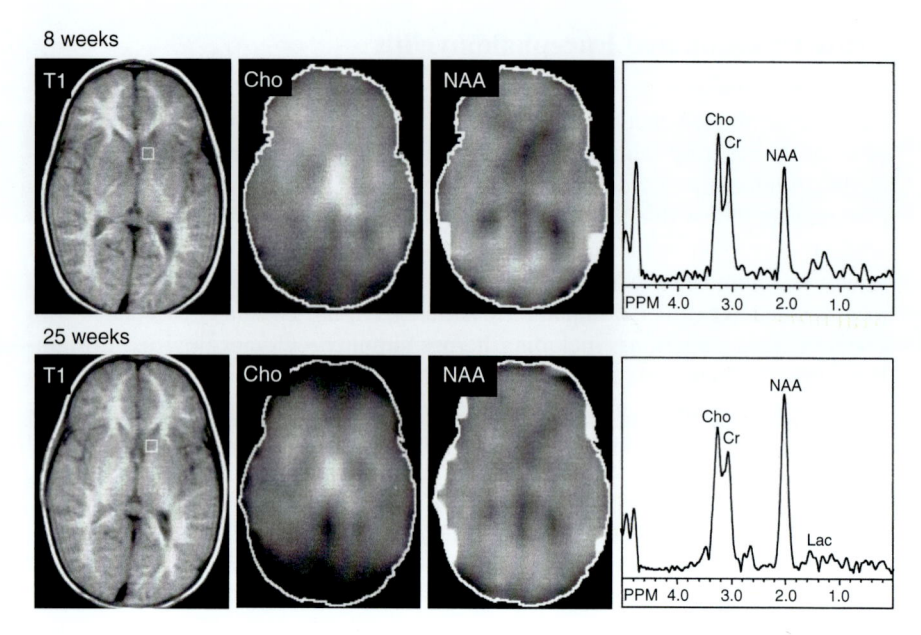

Fig. 17.1 Acute disseminated encephalomyelitis. Proton MRSI at 8 (top) and 25 (bottom) weeks after initial symptom onset. Localizer T1-weighted MR images at 300/13/1 (TR/TE/excitation) and metabolic images at 2300/280/1 (TR/TE/excitation) of choline and NAA from the second of four sections shown. Selected spectrum from left caudatum shown at both time points (voxel location indicated on T1-weighted images). At 8 weeks, NAA image shows decreased levels in left caudatum, lenticular nuclei, and right internal capsule, corresponding to lesions seen in T2-weighted MR images. Choline signals within normal limits; note high choline signal in thalamic region is normal for these regions. By 25 weeks, NAA recovered to normal levels in all these regions, whereas creatine and choline levels remain stable. (From: Bizzi et al. [23]; used with permission)

Multiple Sclerosis

Multiple sclerosis (MS) is a chronic immune-mediated demyelinating and neurodegenerative disease of the central nervous system, which usually affects young adults (peak age of onset, 29 years). The prevalence of MS is approximately 2.5 million worldwide with 400,000 cases in the United States [7], and the relapsing form of MS is more common in females. Neuropathology of MS has two components: inflammatory demyelination with loss of oligodendrocytes and neuronal and axonal loss (neurodegeneration). Clinical manifestations of MS are protean and depend on the areas of CNS involvement. MS commonly manifests with weakness, numbness/tingling, visual impairment, double vision, falls, fatigue, ataxia, neuralgias, urinary and fecal incontinence, and cognitive decline. Uncommonly, MS patients develop seizures and dementia. Such clinical deficits, either alone or in combination, cause significant disability.

An acute attack of MS (also known as relapse or exacerbation) is defined as an episode of focal neurological deficit(s) lasting more than 24 hours without an alternate explanation and with a preceding period of stabilization of clinical symptoms for at least 30 days. An attack could manifest with new MS symptoms or worsening of previously stable symptoms. Infection, fever, stress, and extreme heat are the potential triggers of MS attacks [8].

Marburg Disease

Marburg variant of MS is a malignant form of demyelination, which typically leads to death within 1 year of the onset of clinical signs. It is distinguishable from classical MS by the presence of encephalopathy, rapidly progressive course, and development of numerous large and destructive demyelinating lesions in deep white matter. Clinically, Marburg disease presents with hemiplegia, hemianopsia, aphasia, seizure, and confusion. Brainstem involvement manifests with quadriparesis, ophthalmoplegia, dysarthria, ataxia, and bulbar dysfunction. Death can occur from cerebral herniation or aspiration pneumonia. Neuroradiologically, demyelinating lesions of Marburg disease demonstrate cerebral edema with mass effect and may overlap with radiological findings observed in Balo disease or tumefactive MS. The distribution of demyelinating lesions in Marburg disease is relatively unique because of the simultaneous appearance of lesions at multiple levels of the CNS. These lesions are not only more widespread but also more destructive than in traditional MS. CSF analysis may reveal slight increase in mononuclear cells and elevated protein levels [9]. On neuropathology, Marburg disease lesions are characterized by severe axonal injury, edema, and necrosis.

Balo Concentric Sclerosis

Balo concentric sclerosis (BCS) is considered as a variant of tumefactive MS with rapidly progressive and often lethal course and with distinctive neuroimaging and neuropathological features. BCS is also known as leukoencephalitis and concentric sclerosis [3]. The term "concentric sclerosis" is utilized to describe the typical circular bands of demyelination alternating with partial remyelination. It usually appears as a solitary tumorlike lesion, either in the cerebrum or the brainstem. BCS typically affects young adults and presents with a monophasic course similar to the Marburg variant of MS. Death may occur in weeks to months. It also may follow a rapidly progressive and relapsing course [9]. A lesion in the cerebral hemisphere can cause hemiparesis, hemisensory loss, or aphasia. A brainstem lesion may result in quadriparesis, ophthalmoplegia, dysarthria, ataxia, and bulbar dysfunction. Headache, seizures, and cognitive decline are also common symptoms [3]. The diagnosis is mainly based on MRI features which include the presence of concentric ring or a whorled appearance on T2-weighted and contrast-enhanced T1-weighted images [10]. Supportive evidence includes the presence of mononuclear cells along with the presence of oligoclonal bands in the CSF. Treatment of BCS includes supportive therapy, intravenous methylprednisone, adrenocorticotropic hormone, azathioprine, and cyclophosphamide [10]. Death can be caused by cerebral herniation or aspiration pneumonia from bulbar dysfunction.

Tumefactive Multiple Sclerosis

Tumefactive MS (TMS) is defined as a solitary demyelinating lesion with atypical neuroimaging features. The characteristics of TMS include more than 2 cm in size, accompanying vasogenic edema along with mass effect, and contrast enhancement (particularly partial open-ring enhancement) [11]. Such neuroimaging features of mass effect and ring enhancement make the lesion difficult to distinguish from certain neoplasms, such as high-grade glioma, primary CNS lymphoma, and metastatic tumor; hence, this form of MS is sometimes called demyelinating pseudotumor. The symptoms of TMS also mimic those of tumor, stroke, or brain abscess. Although symptoms vary with the size and location of the lesion, common symptoms include cognitive issues (learning, memorizing, and organizing), aphasia apraxia, mental confusion, cortical blindness, seizure, and headache [11]. Stupor, coma, and even death can occur if there is transtentorial herniation from mass effect. Lesions involving the brainstem can cause quadriplegia, ophthalmoplegia, and bulbar dysfunction [3]. On MR imaging, TMS usually shows mass-like lesion with ill-defined borders, central necrosis, mass effect with midline shift and transtentorial herniation, perilesional edema, and ring enhancement (Fig. 17.2a–d). MR spectroscopy or stereotactic biopsy may be useful to distinguish TMS from brain tumor [3]. If present, the presence of open-ring enhancement signals the diagnosis of TMS. When the diagnosis is inconclusive, brain biopsy is indicated.

Neuromyelitis Optica

Neuromyelitis optica (NMO) is characterized by severe attacks of bilateral optic neuritis and transverse myelitis from inflammation and demyelination of the central nervous system (CNS). NMO was previously known as Devic disease [12]. The incidence and prevalence rate of NMO and its spectrum are not definitively established, but available data estimates NMO incidence and prevalence rates to be 0.053–0.4/100,000 and 0.52–4.4 /100,000, respectively. The prevalence is 3–9 times higher in females and the median age of onset is 35–45 years in adults. Patients with NMO may experience a monophasic or a relapsing course. Detection of a unique antibody (NMO-immunoglobulin G) specifically reactive to the aquaporin-4 (a water channel protein on astrocytes) sets NMO apart from MS.

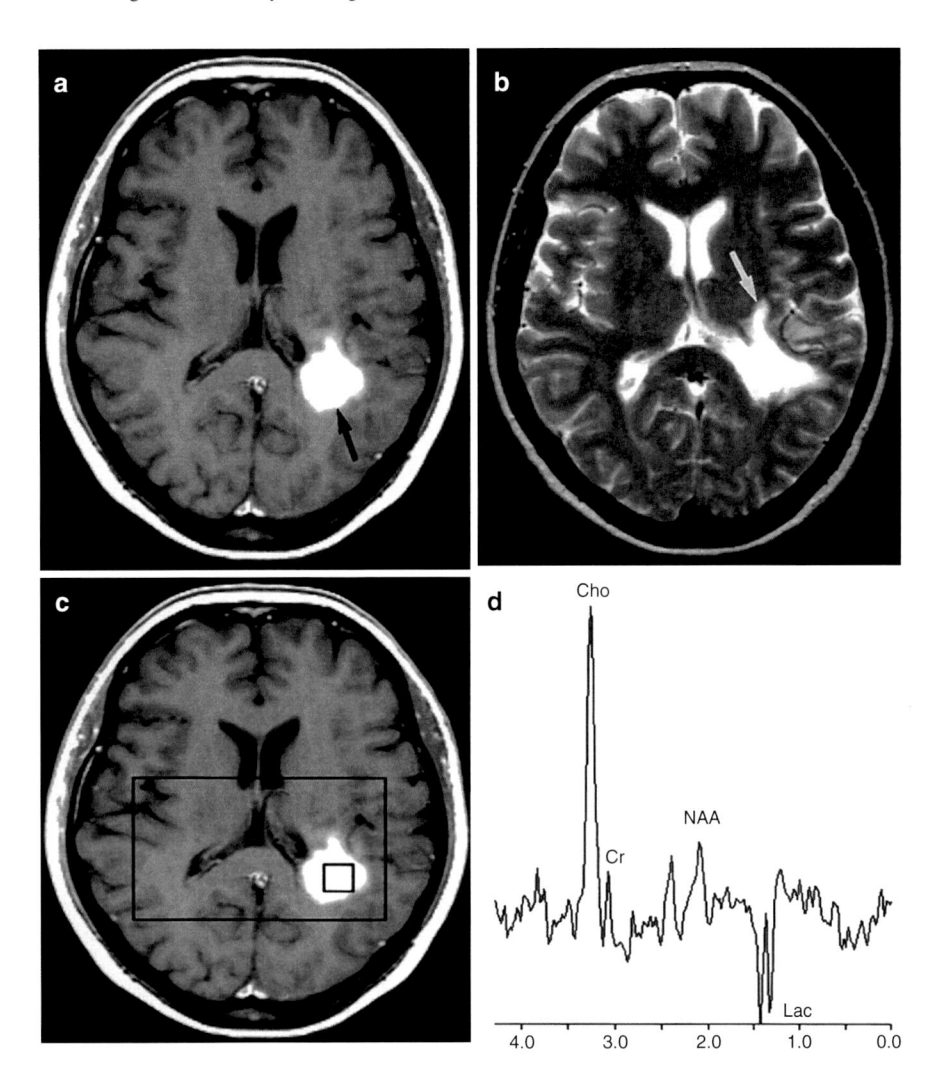

Fig. 17.2 Tumefactive multiple sclerosis images in a 50-year-old woman with biopsy-proven tumefactive demyelinating lesion. (**a**) Contrast-enhanced axial T1-weighted image (600/14/1) demonstrates an ill-defined enhancing mass (arrow) in the left frontoparietal periventricular white matter. (**b**) Axial T2-weighted image (3400/119/1) shows increased signal intensity (arrow) around the lesion. (**c**) Localizing image (600/14/1) for proton MR spectroscopy displays a voxel in the central portion of the lesion. (**d**) Proton MR spectrum obtained by using PRESS (1500/144) demonstrates an elevated Cho value, a decreased NAA value, and a Lac doublet. (From: Saindane [24]; used with permission)

Predictors for NMO relapse include older age at onset, female gender, prolonged interval between the first two attacks, and preexisting autoimmune disease. Concurrent or simultaneous optic neuritis and transverse myelitis are the usual features of NMO. Optic neuritis is most often associated with unilateral ocular pain (upon movement of the eye in the eye socket) and transient vision loss; however, ocular involvement can be bilateral. In fact, sequential or concurrent bilateral ocular involvement with rapid progression and severe visual impairment should be considered strongly suspicious of NMO rather than MS. Spinal cord involvement presents with complete transverse myelitis resulting in paraplegia or tetraplegia, well-defined sensory level, sphincter dysfunction, pain, and spasm of the trunk and extremities. Abnormal sensation, radicular pain, and the presence of Lhermitte's sign are common. In addition, if the neuropathologic process extends into the brainstem, patients may develop hiccups, intractable nausea, respiratory failure, vertigo, hearing loss, facial weakness, trigeminal neuralgia, nystagmus, diplopia, and ptosis. Hypothalamic involvement can cause hypothermia and narcolepsy with somnolence. NMO spectrum disorder can also manifest with posterior reversible encephalopathy syndrome (Fig. 17.3a–d). International consensus diagnostic criteria for NMO include optic neuritis and myelitis along with two out of the three following: (1) contiguous spinal MRI lesion extending ≥3 vertebral segments, (2) MRI criteria not meeting the revised McDonald criteria of MS, and (3) presence of serum NMO immunoglobulin G (Fig. 17.4a, b).

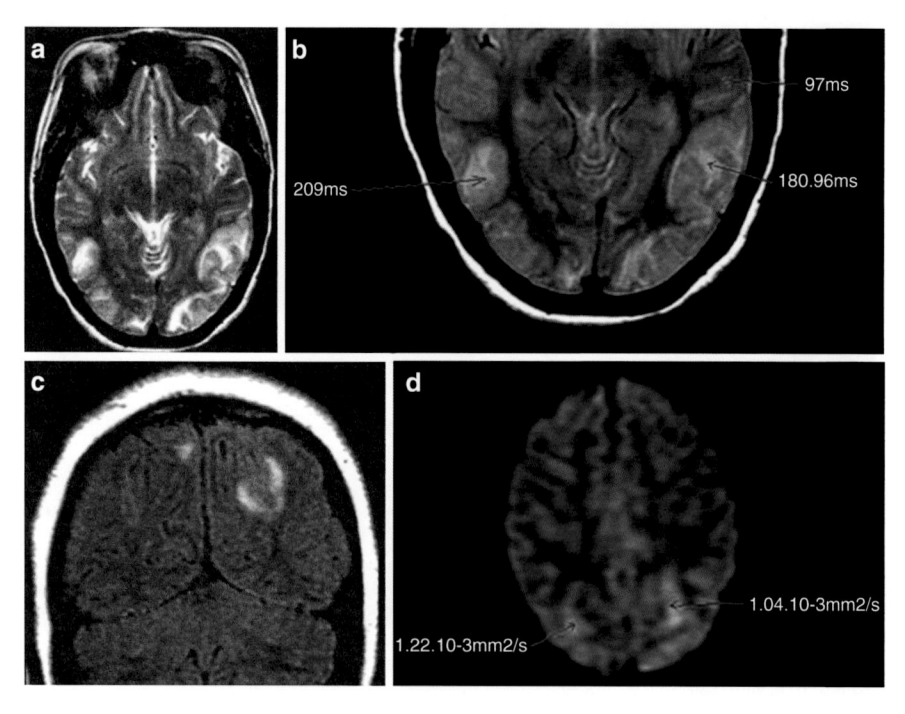

Fig. 17.3 Posterior reversible leukoencephalopathy syndrome. (**a**) Axial T2WI. Hyperintensities in the posterior white matter. Most of the cases also have some lesions in frontal lobes. (**b**) Proton density axial slice showing increased values of T2 in the lesions. (**c**) Coronal FLAIR. Subcortical hyperintensities. (**d**) High diffusion values. There is no restriction

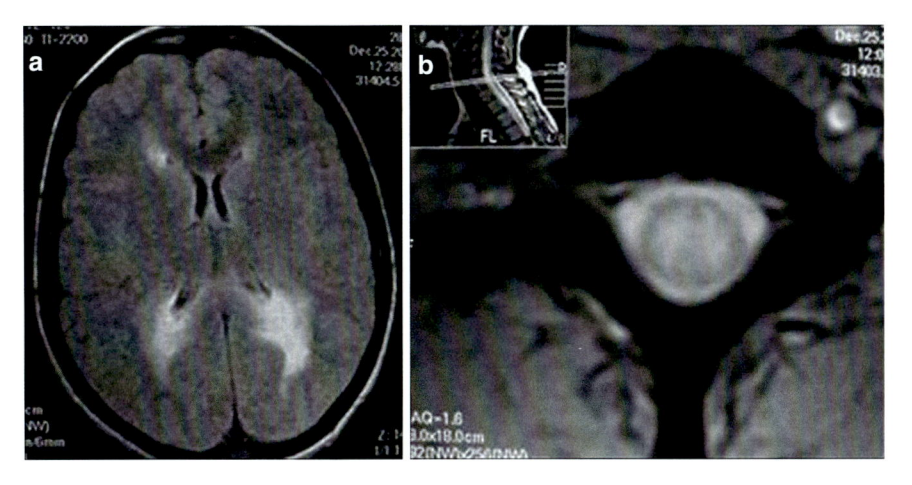

Fig. 17.4 Neuromyelitis optica. (**a**) Axial FLAIR sequence. Prominent irregular hyperintensities. (**b**) Axial MERGE (Multiple Echo Recombined Gradient Echo) sequence. Spinal cord swollen and hyperintense (demyelination). Patient was seropositive for AQP4 antibodies

Optic Neuritis

Optic neuritis (ON) implies inflammation of the optic nerve. However, inflammation of the optic nerve may occur with or without demyelination [13, 14]. The terms optic papillitis or retrobulbar neuritis are used to indicate inflammation in the head (anterior part) and posterior part of the optic nerve, respectively. The incidence rate of ON is 5.1/100,000. Optic neuritis is more predominant in females (F:M 3:1) and Caucasians (85%) [13].

Clinically, ON manifests with eye pain (92%) which worsens with eye movements, uni- or bilateral visual loss which may progress over hours or days, visual field defects, loss of color vision, and flashing or flickering on eye movement [13]. Visual acuity varies widely from minimal impairment to nearly complete blindness. Dyschromatopsia is a common feature, which presents with less intense perception of red color with dimmer light. Common visual field defects in optic neuritis can be altitudinal, quadrantanopia, centrocecal, or hemianopia. Funduscopic examination may reveal edema in cases of papillitis, with occasional presence of retinal hemorrhage and exudates. However, edema presents only in one-third of cases of retrobulbar neuritis. Severe papilledema (sometimes with hemorrhage) is a common feature of idiopathic ON. ON can be the initial presentation of MS. However, the presence of the following features argues against a diagnosis of MS: painless eye, severe edema and hemorrhage on the optic disc, macular scars, and absent light perception [13].

Diagnosis of ON rests on obtaining a detailed medical history, a complete ophthalmologic examination, use of brain and optic nerves MR imaging (searching for typical MS lesions and enhancement of the optic nerve sheath), and CSF analysis [15]. CSF typically shows oligoclonal bands, increased IgG index, and inflammatory mononuclear cells. Visual evoked potential reveals delayed visual evoked response. Quantification of retinal nerve fiber layer thickness using optic coherence tomography is useful to evaluate the severity of the disease and may also be used to monitor its progression. Patients with ON associated with MS usually have loss of retinal nerve fiber layer thickness, while the thickness may be preserved in patients with isolated ON [16].

Transverse Myelitis

Transverse myelitis (TM) is an inflammatory disorder of the spinal cord causing damage to myelin and impairment of nerve conduction. It manifests with acute or subacute spinal cord dysfunction resulting in paresis, a sensory level and autonomic impairment including the bowel/bladder, or sexual dysfunction [17]. The annual incidence of TM ranges from 1.34 to 4.60 cases per million, but rate is higher when considered in conjunction with MS (24.6 cases/million). It can occur at any age, but a bimodal distribution is observed with a peak incidence of 10–19 and 30–39 years [17].

There are numerous causes of TM, which are broadly categorized as immune-mediated illnesses (e.g., MS, NMO, postinfectious, or postimmunization autoimmune phenomenon and abnormal immune response to underlying cancer), viral infections (including varicella zoster, cytomegalovirus, Epstein-Barr, influenza, echovirus, and West Nile), bacterial infections (syphilis, tuberculosis, *Actinomyces*, pertussis, tetanus, diphtheria, and Lyme disease), fungal infections (*Aspergillus*, *Blastomyces*, *Coccidioides*, and *Cryptococcus*), parasitic infections (toxoplasmosis, cysticercosis, schistosomiasis), and other inflammatory disorders including sarcoidosis, lupus, Sjogren syndrome, drugs/toxins, and paraneoplastic syndromes [17]. Despite extensive etiological search, TM may remain unexplained and such cases are termed idiopathic.

TM can be classified based on the extent of disease. Acute complete TM indicates total loss of motor and sensory function as well as sphincter and autonomic impairment below the level of the lesion. Acute partial TM is defined as asymmetric neurologic impairment localizable to the spinal cord or deficits attributable to a specific anatomic tract. Longitudinally extensive TM is a spinal cord lesion that extends over three or more vertebral segments and, on cross section, involves the center of the cord over more than two-thirds of the spinal cord area.

Symptoms and signs of TM include acute or rapidly progressive weakness (involving legs with or without the arms depending on the level of the lesion); neuropathic pain affecting the limbs, genital region, and torso; paresthesia in the legs; sensory level and bowel/bladder dysfunction variably expressed as increased frequency or urge to void; incontinence; difficulty voiding; and constipation [17, 18].

Diagnosis of TM mostly hinges on a detailed medical history, neurologic examination, MR imaging, and blood and CSF studies [17]. Spinal cord MRI typically shows the cord lesion, whereas a brain MRI may provide clues to other underlying causes, especially MS [19]. Blood test is performed to rule out viral or bacterial infections and to assess for the presence of autoantibodies [17, 19]. Serology for NMO antibody (anti-aquaporin-4 antibody) should be ordered. CSF analysis shows an inflammatory profile with mononuclear pleocytosis and increased protein concentration [17].

Imitators of Acute Demyelinating Disease

A large number of acute and subacute diseases that cause acute leukoencephalopathy should be included in the differential diagnosis of acute demyelination. Such illnesses can cause leukoencephalopathy, myelopathy, or both (Table 17.1) [3]. When a clinician has to assess a patient with acute leukoencephalopathy, particular attention should be paid to accompanying manifestations. For example, risk factors for stroke, recent diagnosis of cancer, medications (biological agents, chemotherapy), immune-mediated diseases (such as sarcoidosis or systemic lupus erythematosus), presence of oral or genital ulcers (suggestive of Behcet disease), and toxic exposures can suggest an alternative diagnosis.

The diagnosis of acute demyelination comes to mind when optic nerves or long tract neuroanatomic pathways are affected, while acute leukoencephalopathies present more often with gray matter involvement and manifest with seizures, cognitive decline, or

Table 17.1 Differential diagnosis of patients with acute leukoencephalopathy

Infections
Human immunodeficiency virus and opportunistic infections
Neurosyphilis
Whipple disease
Progressive multifocal leukoencephalopathy
Postinfectious
Radiation-induced syndromes
Medication and toxic causes
Methotrexate
Nitrous oxide
Carbon monoxide
Methanol
Genetic diseases
Cerebral autosomal dominant arteriopathy with subcortical infarcts and leukoencephalopathy (CADASIL)
Mitochondrial encephalopathy
Neoplasms

(continued)

Table 17.1 (continued)

Glioma of the central nervous system
Primary lymphoma of the central nervous system
Glioblastoma cerebri
Paraneoplastic and autoimmune encephalitis
Metabolic and nutritional abnormalities
B12 deficiency
Central pontine myelinolysis
Radiation-caused leukoencephalopathy
Vascular diseases
Thromboembolic ischemic strokes
CADASIL
Moyamoya disease
Primary central nervous system vasculitis
Drug-induced vasculitis
Systemic vasculitis
Infection-associated vasculitis
Immune-mediated and inflammatory diseases
Neurosarcoidosis
Behcet syndrome
Systemic lupus erythematosus
Sjogren syndrome
Drug-induced acute demyelinating syndrome (5FU and monoclonal antibodies against TNF-α[alpha])
Posterior reversible encephalopathy syndrome (PRES)
Chronic lymphocytic inflammation with pontine perivascular enhancement responsive to steroids (CLIPPERS)

depressed level of consciousness (Fig. 17.5). MRI can therefore be invaluable in the discrimination of demyelination from other pathologies. The presence of multiple acute demyelinating lesions with limited mass effect and particularly the presence of an open-ring pattern of contrast enhancement suggest the diagnosis of demyelination. Instead, the presence of a large single lesion with substantial mass effect raises the possibility of TMS, malignant tumor, or brain abscess. Multiple lesions without contrast enhancement may point toward diagnoses of progressive multifocal leukoencephalopathy, ischemic infarctions, or autoimmune encephalitis [3].

Management of Acute Inflammatory Demyelinating Diseases

Management and treatment of acute demyelinating diseases consists of three components: supportive therapy, immunosuppressive therapies to induce rapid remission, and treatment of other medical complications.

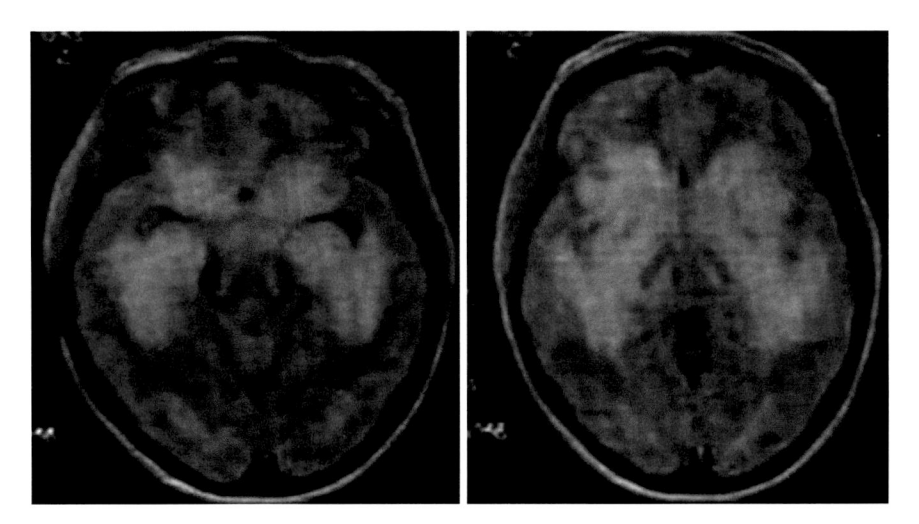

Fig. 17.5 Axial FLAIR. Intoxication with methanol. Patient presented with blindness and confusion

General supportive therapy is heavily focused on airway support and mechanical ventilation, intravenous fluid replacement, treatment of respiratory and urinary tract infections, and prevention of deep vein thrombosis and pressure ulcers [3].

Treatment of acute demyelinating diseases includes treatment with intravenous corticosteroids and plasma exchange. The recommended regimen for acute demyelinating events is high-dose methylprednisolone (1000 mg intravenously daily) for a course of 5 days followed by tapering oral steroids. While treatment with corticosteroids may improve the patient's condition in the short term, their effect on long-term prognosis is less clear [2, 3].

Plasma exchange is another effective treatment for acute demyelinating illnesses. In fact, the use of plasma exchange to treat acute demyelinating conditions (such as ADEM, transverse myelitis, neuromyelitis optica, and acute relapses of MS) is supported by randomized trial data [20]. Adverse events of plasma exchange may include hypotension, venous access complications, and transfusion reactions. Some centers use intravenous immunoglobulin instead of plasma exchange, but evidence supporting the usefulness of intravenous immunoglobulin for this indication is scant.

Immunosuppressive therapy with agents such as cyclophosphamide is reserved for the most fulminant cases and based solely on anecdotal data. Rituximab has been reported to be helpful in individual case reports.

Disease-modifying therapy should be administered to patients with MS [21]. Medications used for relapse prevention in patients with NMO spectrum disorders include azathioprine, rituximab, and mycophenolate mofetil; in these patients it is recommended to avoid natalizumab, alemtuzumab, and fingolimod because these drugs could actually exacerbate the disease [22].

Prognosis of Acute Demyelinating Diseases

The prognosis of acute demyelinating disease is highly variable depending on the specific diagnosis and type of presentation. ADEM is monophasic and usually carries a favorable prognosis. However, other forms of fulminant demyelination (such as TMS, BCS, and Marburg disease) can follow an unrelenting course despite aggressive treatment with immunosuppression.

MS and NMO spectrum disorders are typically recurrent and often become progressive. Disease-modifying therapy can improve short-term prognosis in patients with MS. As compared to typical MS, patients with NMO spectrum disorder tend to accumulate disability faster over recurrent attacks. Greater frequency of attacks, greater severity of attacks, and older age at onset are associated with worse prognosis.

A summary of the diagnostic, therapeutic, and prognostic features of acute demyelinating diseases is presented in Table 17.2.

Table 17.2 Diagnostic, therapeutic, and prognostic features of acute demyelinating disease

Disease	Diagnostic keys	Treatment priorities	Prognosis
ADEM	MRI of the brain and spine CSF study	IV methylprednisolone IVIg Plasma exchange	Acute: shorten duration of acute symptoms with treatment Long term: half of the patient may recover completely, others may have lifelong neurological impairment or could be fatal in severe cases
Acute attack of MS, BCS, and tumefactive sclerosis	MRI of the brain and spine CSF study	IV methylprednisolone IVIg Plasma exchange	Two-thirds of the patients have normal life Some may need cane or wheelchair for ambulation No cure
Neuromyelitis optica	MRI of the brain and spine Seropositivity for AQP4	IV methylprednisolone IVIg Plasma exchange	Most of the patients may have permanent weakness in limbs or vision loss Respiratory muscle weakness leads to breathing difficulty
Optic neuritis	MRI of the brain CSF study RNFL measurement	IV methylprednisolone IVIg Plasma exchange	Ninety percent of patients will recover most of their vision within 6 months
Transverse myelitis	MRI of the spine CSF study	IV methylprednisolone IVIg Plasma exchange	Partial TM: complete or near-complete recovery within several months Longitudinally extensive individual TM: recovery ranges from complete to none (permanent and severe motor and sensory deficits)

Cardinal Messages
- Acute demyelinating diseases can represent as medical emergencies.
- Multiple forms of acute demyelination can present emergently, including ADEM, TMS, NMO, and TM.
- MRI scanning of the brain and the spianl cord can be invaluable in the diagnostic evaluation of patients with suspected acute demyelination.
- Acute demyelinating diseases have an extensive differential diagnosis. Careful attention to details from the history and examination and refined interpretation of neuroimaging findings are necessary to reach the correct diagnosis.
- Acute demyelinating disorders should ideally be treated with pulse-dose intravenous steroid and plasma exchange.
- Prognosis of acute demyelinating diseases varies depending on the particular underlying cause. Severe presentations can be followed by excellent recovery in some instances (e.g., ADEM), but severe sequelae and even death are possible with fulminant forms of demyelination.

References

1. Lucchinetti CF, Mandler RN, McGavern D, Bruck W, Gleich G, Ransohoff RM, Trebst C, Weinshenker B, Wingerchuk D, Parisi JE, Lassmann H. A role for humoral mechanisms in the pathogenesis of Devic's neuromyelitis optica. Brain. 2002;125:1450–61.
2. Karussis D. The diagnosis of multiple sclerosis and the various related demyelinating syndromes: a critical review. J Autoimmun. 2014;48–49:134–42.
3. Bunyan RF, Tang J, Weinshenker B. Acute demyelinating disorders: emergencies and management. Neurol Clin. 2012;30:285–307.. ix-x
4. Sonneville R, Klein I, de Broucker T, Wolff M. Post-infectious encephalitis in adults: diagnosis and management. J Infect. 2009;58:321–8.
5. Noorbakhsh F, Johnson RT, Emery D, Power C. Acute disseminated encephalomyelitis: clinical and pathogenesis features. Neurol Clin. 2008;26:759–80.. ix
6. San Pedro EC, Mountz JM, Liu HG, Deutsch G. Postinfectious cerebellitis: clinical significance of Tc-99m HMPAO brain SPECT compared with MRI. Clin Nucl Med. 1998;23:212–6.
7. Brass SD, Duquette P, Proulx-Therrien J, Auerbach S. Sleep disorders in patients with multiple sclerosis. Sleep Med Rev. 2010;14:121–9.
8. Leary SM, Porter B, Thompson AJ. Multiple sclerosis: diagnosis and the management of acute relapses. Postgrad Med J. 2005;81:302–8.
9. Capello E, Mancardi GL. Marburg type and Balo's concentric sclerosis: rare and acute variants of multiple sclerosis. Neurol Sci. 2004;25(Suppl 4):S361–3.
10. Darke M, Bahador FM, Miller DC, Litofsky NS, Ahsan H. Balo's concentric sclerosis: imaging findings and pathological correlation. J Radiol Case Rep. 2013;7:1–8.
11. Lucchinetti CF, Gavrilova RH, Metz I, Parisi JE, Scheithauer BW, Weigand S, Thomsen K, Mandrekar J, Altintas A, Erickson BJ, Konig F, Giannini C, Lassmann H, Linbo L, Pittock SJ, Bruck W. Clinical and radiographic spectrum of pathologically confirmed tumefactive multiple sclerosis. Brain. 2008;131:1759–75.

12. Marignier R, Confavreux C. Devic's neuromyelitis optica and related neurological disorders. Presse Med. 2010;39:371–80.
13. Clark D, Kebede W, Eggenberger E. Optic neuritis. Neurol Clin. 2010;28:573–80.
14. Atkins EJ, Biousse V, Newman NJ. The natural history of optic neuritis. Rev Neurol Dis. 2006;3:45–56.
15. Wilhelm H, Schabet M. The diagnosis and treatment of optic neuritis. Dtsch Arztebl Int. 2015;112:616–25.. quiz 626
16. Costello F, Hodge W, Pan YI, Metz L, Kardon RH. Retinal nerve fiber layer and future risk of multiple sclerosis. Can J Neurol Sci. 2008;35:482–7.
17. Beh SC, Greenberg BM, Frohman T, Frohman EM. Transverse myelitis. Neurol Clin. 2013;31:79–138.
18. Scott TF, Frohman EM, De Seze J, Gronseth GS, Weinshenker BG. Therapeutics and Technology Assessment Subcommittee of American Academy of N. Evidence-based guideline: clinical evaluation and treatment of transverse myelitis: report of the Therapeutics and Technology Assessment Subcommittee of the American Academy of Neurology. Neurology. 2011;77:2128–34.
19. Campi A, Pontesilli S, Gerevini S, Scotti G. Comparison of MRI pulse sequences for investigation of lesions of the cervical spinal cord. Neuroradiology. 2000;42:669–75.
20. Weinshenker BG. Therapeutic plasma exchange for acute inflammatory demyelinating syndromes of the central nervous system. J Clin Apher. 1999;14:144–8.
21. Rae-Grant A, Day GS, Marrie RA, Rabinstein A, Cree BAC, Gronseth GS, Haboubi M, Halper J, Hosey JP, Jones DE, Lisak R, Pelletier D, Potrebic S, Sitcov C, Sommers R, Stachowiak J, Getchius TSD, Merillat SA, Pringsheim T. Practice guideline recommendations summary: disease-modifying therapies for adults with multiple sclerosis: report of the guideline development, dissemination, and implementation Subcommittee of the American Academy of Neurology. Neurology. 2018;90(17):777–88.
22. Wu Y, Zhong L, Geng J. Neuromyelitis optica spectrum disorder: pathogenesis, treatment, and experimental models. Mult Scler Relat Disord. 2019;27:412–8.
23. Bizzi A, Ulug AM, Crawford TO, Pase T, Bugiani M, Bryan RN, Barke PB. Quantitative proton MR spectroscopic imaging in acute disseminated encephalomyelitis. Am J Neuroradiol. 2001;22(6):1125–30.
24. Saindane AM. Proton MR spectroscopy of tumefactive demyelinating lesions. Am J Neuroradiol. 2002;23(8):1378–86.

Chapter 18
Emergencies in Movement Disorders

Julieta E. Arena

Diagnostic Keys
- History of previous medical conditions and medication intake is of utmost importance for identification of possible causes of movement disorders emergencies.
- Drug-induced movement disorders are among the most frequent causes of medical emergencies in movement disorders.
- Imaging can aid the diagnosis when physical examination points to a specific brain area.

Treatment Priorities
- Always secure proper ventilation and hemodynamic stability, and correct metabolic derangements.
- Treatment of the movement itself is not always mandatory.
- Some movement disorders may be self-limited and treatment of the underlying cause should be the priority.

J. E. Arena (✉)
Movement Disorders Section, Neurology Department, Fleni, Buenos Aires, Argentina
e-mail: jarena@fleni.org.ar

> **Prognosis at a Glance**
> - Prognosis in movement disorders emergencies is very variable.
> - Some conditions such as neuroleptic malignant syndrome can be life-threatening.
> - Acute chorea after stroke can be socially uncomfortable, but typically self-limited.
> - Drug-induced movement disorders can improve with time. Attempts to taper treatment drugs should be done whenever possible.

Introduction

Movement disorders are typically insidious, and this is not an area known to have many clinical emergencies. However, being able to recognize them is important, since there are some circumstances under which urgent care might be needed to prevent severe and even life-threatening complications.

A movement disorders emergency (MDE) has been defined as "any neurological disorder evolving acutely or subacutely in which the clinical presentation is dominated by a primary movement disorder, and in which failure to accurately diagnose and manage the patient may result in significant morbidity or even mortality" [1].

For practical purposes, as it has been done classically for the study of movement disorders, we can divide MDEs as being either hyperkinetic or hypokinetic. Although complications in patients with Parkinson disease (PD) do not necessarily occur in an acute manner, they can be the reason for an Emergency Department consultation [2]. For practical purposes, these will be included under hypokinetic MDEs (Table 18.1).

Table 18.1 Summary of movement disorders emergencies

Hypokinetic emergencies	Hyperkinetic emergencies
Acute parkinsonism	Acute chorea
Neuroleptic malignant syndrome	Acute dystonia-status dystonicus
Serotonin syndrome	Myoclonus

Parkinson disease complications:
  Acute psychosis-impulse control disorders
  Dopamine agonist withdrawal syndrome
	Tic status

Hypokinetic Movement Disorders Emergencies

Acute Parkinsonism

When parkinsonian symptoms appear and progress rapidly over the course of hours or days, secondary causes should always be ruled out. Acute parkinsonism is generally the akinetic-rigid type (and not tremor dominant).

The most common cause of acute parkinsonism is exposure to dopamine-blocking drugs, such as neuroleptics or antiemetics. Differential diagnoses include toxic exposure (consider 1-methyl-4-phenyl-1,2,3,6-tetrahydropyridine [MPTP], organophosphate pesticides, carbon monoxide, carbon disulfide, cyanide, and methanol) [1], viral infections, and structural lesions with damage to the nigrostriatal pathway. Structural damage due to mechanical compression can also be secondary to acute hydrocephalus or rapid hydrocephalus correction (Table 18.2). It is appropriate to consider obtaining a brain MRI to rule out structural causes in the cases of acute parkinsonism, particularly when the presentation is rapid, atypical, or asymmetrical.

Treatment will depend on the identified cause. Dopamine-blocking agents should be discontinued, exposure to toxic agents stopped, and structural causes resolved if possible. The use of levodopa or dopamine agonists may also be necessary.

Drug-Induced Movement Disorders

Neuroleptic Malignant Syndrome

Neuroleptic malignant syndrome (NMS) is a rare condition, with an estimated incidence of 0.2% [3]. Despite its low incidence, its importance cannot be underestimated because it can be life-threatening.

Table 18.2 Causes of acute parkinsonism

	Etiology
Structural	Basal ganglia stroke, hydrocephalus or its rapid correction, subdural hematoma
Drug induced	Neuroleptics, antiemetics (metoclopramide, sulpiride), antidepressants, amiodarone, lithium, antiepileptics (valproic acid), calcium channel blockers (flunarizine, cinnarizine)
Metabolic	Central pontine myelinolysis (fast hyponatremia correction)
Toxic	MPTP, carbon monoxide, manganese, cyanide, methanol
Infectious	Viral encephalitis, HIV, Whipple disease, postinfectious
Psychiatric	Catatonia, psychogenic parkinsonism
Hereditary	Rapid-onset dystonia-parkinsonism (ATP1A3 gene), Wilson's disease

NMS is caused by treatment with neuroleptic drugs, being more common with typical antipsychotics (e.g., haloperidol) than with the newer atypical neuroleptics. NMS characteristically occurs or starts within the first week of introduction of the neuroleptic agent, and it can take up to a week until the full-blown syndrome emerges. It can also occur when neuroleptic dose is escalated fast or one neuroleptic is changed for another. Nonetheless, it is important to remember that NMS usually occurs with neuroleptic doses that are within the therapeutic range [4]. Taking this into account, along with its low incidence, it is reasonable to hypothesize that an underlying individual predisposition is necessary for this complication to happen.

NMS is characterized by the combination of acute-onset severe parkinsonism, dysautonomia, and sometimes alteration of mental status. There is generalized rigidity, often combined with akinesia; dysphagia is common. Rhabdomyolysis with consequent renal failure can be a major complication of extreme rigidity. Dysautonomia can present with fever, fluctuations in blood pressure, sweating, tachypnea, and tachycardia. In severe cases admission to ICU becomes necessary for hemodynamic monitoring and stabilization.

Diagnosis is made on clinical grounds, but some laboratory results, such as elevation of serum creatine phosphokinase (CPK), can aid the diagnosis. If CPK levels are high, renal function should be monitored. Since leukocytosis may be present, NMS can be misdiagnosed as sepsis.

Treatment requires withdrawing all neuroleptic medications. Secondary metabolic abnormalities are common and should be corrected. For more severe cases, dopamine agonists may be required. Bromocriptine is the most widely used, with doses ranging from 2.5 to 15 mg per day, administered three times daily. If needed, muscle relaxation can be achieved by using dantrolene with a dose ranging from 25 mg per day to 75 mg per day or higher, administered three times daily. These treatments may need to be continued for several weeks.

Electroconvulsive therapy has been used, especially in cases of severe psychosis or lack of response to the conventional treatment [5]. Usefulness of benzodiazepines as muscle relaxants is controversial.

Serotonin Syndrome

Serotonin syndrome is a condition secondary to serotonin toxicity, which is generally caused by drug interactions, intentional overdose, or even therapeutic medication use, causing excessive enhancement of serotonin transmission [6]. It is always a consequence of excess serotoninergic activation on the central nervous system (CNS) and peripheral serotonin receptors [7, 8].

The syndrome can occur with multiple drugs (Table 18.3) and has been reported to occur in 14 to 16% of people who overdose on SSRIs [9]. Used in therapeutic doses, an incidence of 0.4 cases per 1000 patient-months was reported in patients taking nefazodone [10].

The spectrum of clinical manifestations is very broad. Clinical symptoms often begin with tremor, akathisia, and diarrhea, followed by myoclonus and possible

Table 18.3 Drugs reported to cause serotonin syndrome

Category	Drug
Inhibitors of serotonin reuptake	SSRIs, serotonin-norepinephrine reuptake inhibitors, tricyclic antidepressants, cocaine, opiates (except morphine), dextromethorphan, dexamphetamine
Inhibitors of serotonin metabolism	MAO-B inhibitors (selegiline, rasagiline), MAO inhibitors antidepressants
Enhancers of serotonin synthesis and release	L-Tryptophan, MDMA (3,4-methylenedioxymethamphetamine-ecstasy), amphetamines, cocaine
Serotonin agonists	Triptans, ergotamines, buspirone, lysergic acid diethylamide (LSD)
Enhancers of serotonin activity	Lithium, valproic acid, linezolid, electroconvulsive therapy

SSRI, selective serotonin reuptake inhibitors; MAO, monoamine oxidase

alteration of mental status, that can finally lead to muscle rigidity (characteristically greater in the legs and in the arms) and hyperthermia; the most severe cases can become life-threatening [6]. Early detection of mild clinical symptoms is of utmost importance to prevent clinical deterioration.

It is interesting to note that clinical symptoms of serotonin syndrome may resemble NMS, but the former can take more time for full clinical symptoms to present and generally takes less time to improve. Alteration of consciousness, muscle rigidity, autonomic dysfunction, and CK elevation are more common with NMS.

Drug interactions are common precipitants of serotonin syndrome. For movement disorders specialists, there is frequent combination of drugs in patients with PD that should not be overlooked. It is still very frequent nowadays that patients with PD will receive monoamine oxidase inhibitors (MAOIs) at the beginning of their disease and SSRIs for the treatment of previous or subsequent depression. The combination of these two is very frequent and increases the risk for developing serotonin syndrome.

Complications of Parkinson Disease

Acute Psychosis-Impulse Control Disorders

Many times, the combination of dopaminergic medication with other drugs that can potentiate their action, such as MAO and catechol-O-methyltransferase (COMT) inhibitors, can precipitate acute psychotic states. Some have proposed that patients with PD and mild cognitive impairment or dementia are more prone to this kind of reactions. This phenomenon is more prominent with the use of dopamine agonists (DAs) frequently used for the treatment of PD, such as pramipexole or ropinirole. Psychotic symptoms may present in the form of hallucinations, mostly visual.

Another phenomenon precipitated by DAs (and more rarely by levodopa) is the impulse control disorders (ICD), including compulsive gambling, eating, shopping, hoarding, and sexual behaviors. It is believed that younger patients are the most prone to suffer from ICD (it is important to note that this group of patients is the one that receives DAs more frequently) and that it has a dose-effect relationship with DAs. Its cumulative 5-year incidence is estimated to be 46% for patients on treatment with DAs [11].

The treatment of acute psychosis in a patient with PD should start with ruling out conditions that could have triggered the symptoms, such as infections or metabolic disturbances. The next step for the treatment of acute psychosis is evaluating the need to lower the dose(s) of dopaminergic agents. In some cases, this is all that is needed for the symptoms to subside. It is important to remember that anticholinergic drugs (often used for the treatment of tremor or urinary incontinence) or amantadine can also precipitate psychotic symptoms. Sometimes it is necessary to introduce antipsychotic medications. Using atypical neuroleptics, such as clozapine or quetiapine, is advisable because they have lower potential to worsen the motor symptoms of PD.

For the treatment of ICD, tapering or even discontinuing DAs is mandatory. If the patient is only on DAs, a switch to levodopa can be attempted.

Dopamine Agonist Withdrawal Syndrome (DAWS)

Some patients develop a DAWS when a DA is tapered. Symptoms of DAWS are highly variable, resembling those of any other drug withdrawal. They include anxiety, panic attacks, dysphoria, severe depression, agitation, irritability, suicidal ideation, fatigue, orthostatic hypotension, nausea, vomiting, diaphoresis, and generalized pain. The severity and prognosis are also variable. It has been proposed that patients with ICD are more prone to suffering DAWS when tapered from dopaminergic medications, but they are also the ones that benefit the most from their withdrawal. Incidence has been estimated at 19% [12].

There is currently no specific treatment for DAWS. Therefore patients should be warned about possible DAs side effects and risk of DAWS before treatment initiation. DAs should be tapered slowly and DAWS symptoms should be closely monitored. When a more rapid DA withdrawal is needed, admission to the hospital for close monitoring should be considered.

Hyperkinetic Movement Disorders Emergencies

Acute Chorea

Chorea is a movement disorder characterized by brief, irregular, non-rhythmic movements, that appear to flow from one muscle to the next. Sometimes they accompany voluntary movements; hence the patient looks clumsy and fidgety.

When chorea presents in an acute fashion, it may be secondary to toxic/metabolic imbalances or lesions that may result from vascular or infectious disorders. In children, Sydenham chorea, manifestation of rheumatic fever, is the most common cause of acquired chorea. Symptoms may begin from 1 to 6 months after streptococcal pharyngitis and its diagnosis is clinical, but supported by elevated antistreptolysin O antibody titers. Treatment includes penicillin (to prevent other complications), and chorea can be treated with valproic acid or carbamazepine, if needed [13]. Sometimes dopamine depleters, such as pimozide, might be needed.

In adults, acute chorea more commonly manifests as a unilateral phenomenon (hemichorea), associated with hemiballism (with large amplitude, flinging movements). Structural lesions of the basal ganglia (specifically the contralateral subthalamic nucleus) should be investigated with a brain MRI, stroke being the most frequent cause. Treatment of the movement disorder is generally not needed, since symptoms are self-limited.

The second most common cause of hemichorea/hemiballismus is acute nonketotic hyperglycemia. MRI can demonstrate T1-hyperintense signal in the putamen, caudate nucleus, and globus pallidus [14]. In some cases, stabilization of glucose levels is all that is needed for symptoms to subside, but sometimes dopamine depleters, such as tetrabenazine, are used until symptoms resolve by themselves over time. Therefore, tapering of the medication should be attempted after a few weeks to months. Other metabolic causes such as hyperthyroidism and antiphospholipid antibody syndrome should also be ruled out.

Although it usually does not present acutely, chorea gravidarum is a cause of chorea in pregnant women which neurologists can encounter in the Emergency Department. It typically starts in the first trimester and disappears by the third or immediately after delivery.

Acute Dystonia-Status Dystonicus

Dystonia is a movement disorder characterized by repetitive muscle contractions leading to twisting or abnormal posturing of different parts of the body. There are several causes of acute dystonic reactions (Table 18.4).

Table 18.4 Causes of acute dystonia

Cause	Comments
Drug induced	Dopamine D2 receptor antagonism (neuroleptics or antiemetics)
Toxic	Carbon monoxide, methanol, cyanide, pesticides
Metabolic	Inherited metabolic disorders, not always acute presentation: Leigh disease, aminoacidurias, and urea cycle disorders. (More common in children and seen in association with other manifestations)
Vascular or structural	Basal ganglia stroke (putamen), posterior fossa or spinal cord lesions
Infectious	Retropharyngeal abscess (more common in children), tonsillitis, mastoiditis, or as part of encephalitis of other causes (also more common in children)
Genetic	Rapid-onset dystonia-parkinsonism (ATP1A3 gene)

Drugs are the most common cause of acute focal dystonic reactions, which are generally associated with the use of neuroleptics, either when treatment is initiated or when dose is escalated. Dopamine-blocking antiemetics are also a common cause. Less frequently, dopamine agonists, phenytoin, carbamazepine, SSRIs, tricyclic antidepressants, and cocaine have been implicated in the pathogenesis of acute dystonic reactions.

Drug-induced dystonia can affect different parts of the body, being either focal, multifocal, segmental, or generalized. Oculogyric crises, laryngeal dystonia, blepharospasm, torticollis, focal limb dystonia, tongue protrusion dystonia, and trismus have been described.

Discontinuation of the drug can be enough in some cases and other times treatment with anticholinergics is needed. Intravenous benztropine (1–2 mg) or diphenhydramine (25–50 mg) followed by a short course of oral anticholinergics is very effective.

Status dystonicus or dystonic storm can happen in patients with previous primary or secondary dystonia. Patients experience acute generalized or focal unremitting dystonic spasms secondary to changes in medication, infection, metabolic imbalances, or trauma. These spasms can lead to hyperpyrexia, dehydration, respiratory insufficiency, and rhabdomyolysis with subsequent renal failure [15]. When this occurs, management in the ICU is generally warranted to control and correct metabolic derangements. Treatment involves a combination of anticholinergics (trihexyphenidyl), benzodiazepines (clonazepam, diazepam), catecholamine-depleting agents, dopamine receptor blockers (tetrabenazine, pimozide, haloperidol), and muscle relaxants (baclofen). Refractory or very severe cases may require general anesthesia with mechanical ventilation. Surgery (pallidotomy or deep brain stimulation of the globus pallidus interna) can be the measure of last resort if symptoms do not respond to any of the previous treatments.

Myoclonus

Myoclonus consists of brief, shock-like movements that can be due to sudden muscle contraction (positive myoclonus) or sudden loss of muscle tone (negative myoclonus, also known as asterixis). It is frequently encountered in an acute fashion in patients that have been admitted to the hospital for other reasons and is usually associated with toxic-metabolic derangements, such as hepatic failure, uremia, or drugs.

Myoclonus can also present itself as an isolated manifestation of diverse causes. There are several drugs that can cause myoclonus such as SSRIs, tricyclic antidepressants, opiates, levodopa, gabapentin, triptans, and recreational drugs such as lysergic acid diethylamide (LSD), amphetamines, cocaine, and 3,4-methylenedioxy methamphetamine (MDMA or ecstasy). Metabolic imbalance correction or drug withdrawal is usually enough in these cases to solve the problem.

Acute myoclonus can also be a manifestation of hypoxic brain damage, either as myoclonic status epilepticus or postanoxic myoclonus. The former can occur in the hours immediately following a cerebral anoxic event and manifests as generalized multifocal myoclonus involving the face, limbs, and axial musculature in comatose patients. It generally carries a poor prognosis [16], but not uniformly [17, 18]. Postanoxic myoclonus, also called Lance-Adams syndrome, typically occurs after recovery from an anoxic event. As it is characteristic of cortical myoclonus, it will occur whenever movement is attempted, manifesting as an action myoclonus involving any part of the body, including the muscles control in the vocal cords. Treatment typically requires multiple combined drugs to obtain a good response. Drugs used for the treatment of myoclonus are anticonvulsants such as levetiracetam and valproic acid, benzodiazepines such as clonazepam; and piracetam (where available). Drug tapering should be attempted over months to years, since this syndrome may improve with time.

Tic Status

Tics are brief paroxysmal movements, sometimes accompanied by a premonitory urge, which can be voluntarily suppressed, even if it is for a short period of time. The term tic status can be used when there is an exacerbation of the condition with an increase in the severity of tics or an inability to suppress them for more than a few seconds. This condition can be quite alarming and patients may present to the Emergency Department. The approach to this situation should be to reduce medications that can exacerbate tics first, such as stimulants and antidepressants. If further treatment is needed, dopamine-depleting agents can be used, such as haloperidol, risperidone, or tetrabenazine.

> **Cardinal Messages**
> - A very frequent cause of emergencies in movement disorders is drug adverse reactions.
> - Patients should be warned about possible adverse reactions when given a medication that can cause movement disorders as an adverse effect.
> - Treatment of the movement itself is not always necessary.
> - Attention should be paid to the cause of the movement disorder to offer the correct treatment and prevent further complications.

References

1. Poston KL, Frucht SJ. Movement disorder emergencies. J Neurol. 2008;255(Suppl 4):2–13.
2. Munhoz RP, Scorr LM, Factor SA. Movement disorders emergencies. Curr Opin Neurol. 2015;28(4):406–12.3.

3. Caroff SN, Mann SC. Neuroleptic malignant syndrome. Med Clin North Am. 1993;77(1):185–202.
4. Shalev A, Munitz H. The neuroleptic malignant syndrome: agent and host interaction. Acta Psychiatr Scand. 1986;73:337–47.
5. Hashim H, Zeb-un-Nisa ASA, Al Madani AA. Drug resistant neuroleptic malignant syndrome and the role of electroconvulsive therapy. J Pak Med Assoc. 2014 Apr;64(4):471–3.
6. Boyer EW, Shannon M. The serotonin syndrome. N Engl J Med. 2005;352:1112.
7. Sternbach H. The serotonin syndrome. Am J Psychiatry. 1991;148:705–13.
8. Dunkley EJ, Isbister GK, Sibbritt D, Dawson AH, Whyte IM. The Hunter Serotonin Toxicity Criteria: simple and accurate diagnostic decision rules for serotonin toxicity. QJM. 2003;96:635–42.
9. Isbister GK, Bowe SJ, Dawson A, Whyte IM. Relative toxicity of selective serotonin reuptake inhibitors (SSRIs) in overdose. J Toxicol Clin Toxicol. 2004;42:277–85.
10. Mackay FJ, Dunn NR, Mann RD. Antidepressants and the serotonin syndrome in general practice. Br J Gen Pract. 1999;49:871–4.
11. Corvol JC, Artaud F, Cormier-Dequaire F, Rascol O, Durif F, Derkinderen P, Marques AR, Bourdain F, Brandel JP, Pico F, Lacomblez L, Bonnet C, Brefel-Courbon C, Ory-Magne F, Grabli D, Klebe S, Mangone G, You H, Mesnage V, Lee PC, Brice A, Vidailhet M, Elbaz A, DIGPD Study Group. Longitudinal analysis of impulse control disorders in Parkinson disease. Neurology. 2018. [Epub ahead of print].
12. Rabinak CA, Nirenberg MJ. Dopamine Agonist Withdrawal Syndrome in Parkinson Disease. Arch Neurol. 2010;67(1):58–63.
13. Genel F, Arslanoglu S, Uran N, Saylan B. Sydenham's chorea: clinical findings and comparison of the efficacies of sodium valproate and carbamazepine regimens. Brain and Development. 2002;24(2):73–6.
14. Oh SH, Lee KY, Im JH, Lee MS. Chorea associated with non-ketotic hyperglycemia and hyperintensity basal ganglia lesion on T1-weighted brain MRI study: meta-analysis of 53 cases including four present cases. J Neurol Sci. 2002;200(1–2):57–62.
15. Manji H, Howard RS, Miller DH, et al. Status dystonicus: the syndrome and its management [published correction appears in Brain. 2000;123(pt 2):419]. Brain. 1998;121(pt 2):243–52.
16. Wijdicks EFM, Hijdra A, Young GB, Bassetti CL, Wiebe S. Quality Standards Subcommittee of the American Academy of Neurology. Practice parameter: prediction of outcome in comatose survivors after cardiopulmonary resuscitation (an evidence-based review): report of the Quality Standards Subcommittee of the American Academy of Neurology. Neurology. 2006;67(2):203–10.
17. Braksick SA, Rabinstein AA, Wijdicks EF, Fugate JE, Hocker S. Post-ischemic myoclonic status following cardiac arrest in young drug users. Neurocrit Care. 2017;26(2):280–3.
18. Dalic LJ, Fennessy G, Edmonds M, Carney P, Opdam H, Archer J. Early electroencephalogram does not reliably differentiate outcomes in post-hypoxic myoclonus. Crit Care Resusc. 2019;21(1):45–52.

Chapter 19
Neurologic Emergencies in Transplant Patients

Jeffrey Brent Peel and Lauren K. Ng

> **Diagnostic Keys**
> - Careful review of medication history is crucial when evaluating encephalopathy in a transplant patient.
> - When possible, MRI of the brain should be obtained in transplant patients with acute neurological symptoms because of the increased risk of posterior reversible encephalopathy syndrome (PRES), stroke, and central nervous system (CNS) infections.
> - Due to an impaired inflammatory response because of immunosuppression, the clinical manifestations of CNS infections can be diminished.
> - Lumbar puncture is imperative for diagnosis of a CNS infection.
> - Electroencephalography (EEG) should be considered in encephalopathic patients because of the increased risk for seizures, which may be nonconvulsive.

J. B. Peel
Department of Neurology, Mayo Clinic, Jacksonville, FL, USA

L. K. Ng (✉)
Department of Critical Care Medicine, Neurology, and Neurosurgery, Mayo Clinic, Jacksonville, FL, USA
e-mail: Ng.lauren@Mayo.edu

Treatment Priorities
- When neurotoxicity from immunosuppressive medications is suspected, consider dose reduction of the offending medication and close monitoring of therapeutic drug levels.
- In cases of PRES, replacement of the calcineurin inhibitor with a different immunosuppressant may be indispensable to allow recovery.
- Providers should have a low threshold for initiating empiric antimicrobials in transplant recipients with headache and unexplained fever.
- Seizures and status epilepticus should be treated according to established algorithms but with attention to the metabolic impairments of the transplant patient.
- While recent surgery will exclude a patient from receiving intravenous thrombolysis, endovascular intervention should be considered for acute cerebral ischemia secondary to a large vessel occlusion.
- Cerebral edema in fulminant liver failure should be treated emergently, and placement of an intracranial pressure (ICP) monitoring device should be considered to help guide management in the perioperative phase.

Prognosis at a Glance
- PRES usually has a favorable prognosis, but drug-related cases usually do not improve until the responsible drug is discontinued.
- CNS infections can increase mortality significantly after solid organ transplantation, especially if initiation of appropriate antimicrobial therapy is delayed.
- CNS fungal infections after solid organ transplantation have a particularly high mortality (greater than 90%).
- Osmotic demyelination is a serious complication after liver transplantation, but even patients with severe presentations may improve meaningfully over time.
- Perioperative stroke after heart transplant is associated with a higher 1-year mortality compared with most other neurological complications.

Introduction

Advances in perioperative care, surgical techniques, and postoperative management have reduced morbidity and mortality in transplant recipients. Despite improvements in care, approximately one-third of patients receiving solid organ transplantation will develop neurological symptoms. Neurological symptoms can arise during both the pre- and postoperative time period with most occurring within 30 days of

Table 19.1 Common neurological complications/emergencies related to transplant type

Transplant type	Common complications
Liver	Cerebral edema (fulminant liver failure), osmotic demyelination, encephalopathy, seizures
Heart	Stroke, hyperperfusion syndrome
Lung	Encephalopathy, stroke
Kidney	Stroke, PRES

transplantation [1]. Some complications are inherent to all transplanted patients, such as increased risk of central nervous system infections secondary to immunosuppressant medication, while most others are specific to the type of organ transplanted (Table 19.1). For example, heart transplant patients tend to have a higher risk of ischemic stroke, and liver transplant patients have a higher prevalence of osmotic demyelination syndrome compared to other types of organ transplantation. A wide array of neurological complications, ranging from altered cognition to tremor, can be seen after solid organ transplantation; however, this chapter is limited to acute neurological emergencies associated with solid organ transplantation including the neurotoxicity of immunosuppressive agents, opportunistic infections, seizures, encephalopathy, and cerebrovascular events.

General Principles

Neurotoxicity of Immunosuppressant Medications

Much of the posttransplant neurological complications are associated with immunosuppressive medications. Fortunately, over time, experience with administration and dosing of these drugs has reduced extreme manifestations of neurotoxicity. Corticosteroids, mycophenolate mofetil, calcineurin inhibitors, and non-calcineurin inhibitors are the most commonly used immunosuppressant medications, and each has potential neurotoxic effects (Table 19.2). Protocols for the induction and maintenance of immunosuppression may vary according to centers, and the clinician should become familiar with the common regimens used at their institution.

Neurological complications of corticosteroids often involve neurocognitive symptoms, such as psychosis and delirium. A thorough review of the patient's medical record to evaluate for contributing factors should be performed prior to dose reductions. In many cases, multiple contributing factors are present, and in such instances, it is a mistake to attribute the altered mentation solely to corticosteroids.

Calcineurin inhibitors, such cyclosporine and tacrolimus, can cause neurotoxic effects in multiple areas of the central nervous system (CNS), such as the cerebral cortex, cerebellum, hippocampus, striatum, and substantia nigra [2]. The main emergency associated with neurotoxicity from calcineurin inhibitors is posterior

Table 19.2 Neurological complications associated with immunosuppressive medications

Class	Common neurotoxic effects
Corticosteroids	Insomnia, behavior and mood changes, psychosis, encephalopathy, myopathy
Calcineurin inhibitors (cyclosporine, tacrolimus)	PRES, seizures, akinetic mutism, headache, encephalopathy, mood changes, paresthesias, tremor
mTOR inhibitors (sirolimus, everolimus)	Confusion, headache, tremor, paresthesias
Mycophenolate mofetil	Headache, psychiatric disturbances
Monoclonal antibodies	Aseptic meningitis, encephalopathy, headache, seizures

mTOR mammalian target of rapamycin

reversible encephalopathy syndrome (PRES); other forms of encephalopathy and seizures are also possible. Risk factors for neurotoxicity include hypocholesterolemia, hypertension, hypomagnesemia, uremia, concomitant high-dose steroids, and beta-lactam antibiotics [3, 4]. Serum levels of cyclosporine or tacrolimus do not correlate with the risk of PRES.

The presentation of PRES can have a variable spectrum but often includes a combination of encephalopathy, seizure, headache, visual disturbances, focal neurological deficits, and status epilepticus [5]. Diagnosis relies on the presence of these clinical findings on the appropriate scenario and radiographic imaging. While some evidence may be seen on noncontract CT, an MRI is more sensitive for diagnosis. Typical findings of PRES on MRI are hyperintensities on T2 or fluid-attenuated inversion recovery sequences in the occipital and parietal regions. The posterior predominance of vasogenic edema in PRES may be related to a paucity of sympathetic innervations in the posterior fossa; however, it is now well known that PRES often involves other areas of the brain, such as the frontal region [6]. Failure to recognize the wide clinical and radiographic spectrum of PRES may lead to misdiagnosis and inadequate management. The calcineurin inhibitor should be stopped or replaced if at all possible, regardless of what is the serum level of the drug. Additional treatment measures include correction of electrolyte abnormalities, treating hypertension and renal failure, and supportive care. Antiepileptic drugs (AEDs) are required if the patient has seizures or status epilepticus, but a short course of approximately one month is typically sufficient.

Encephalopathy presenting as an alteration in awareness, arousal, and confusion within the first 30 days after transplantation in the absence of PRES-like changes on MRI is sometimes attributed to initiation or supratherapeutic serum levels of calcineurin inhibitors [7]. In this setting, other causes of encephalopathy must be excluded, such organ failure/rejection, infection, nutritional deficiencies, metabolic derangements, and nonconvulsive seizures. Treatment often requires dose reduction of the offending medication and close monitoring of therapeutic drug levels.

Seizures due to calcineurin inhibitors tend to be generalized, and serum levels of calcineurin inhibitors are often within the therapeutic range. Monitoring with electroencephalography (EEG) is often necessary to exclude nonconvulsive seizures or nonconvulsive status epilepticus after clinical seizure activity has ceased.

Table 19.3 Common organisms responsible for CNS infections and treatment

Organism	Antimicrobial medication
Bacterial	
Listeria monocytogenes	Ampicillin+gentamicin, ampicillin+ceftriaxone+vancomycin
Nocardia asteroides	Trimethoprim/sulfamethoxazole
Toxoplasma gondii	Pyrimethamine, sulfadiazine+folinic acid
Mycobacterium tuberculosis	Rifampicin, isoniazid, ethambutol+pyridoxine, amikacin,
Viral	
Varicella *zoster*	Acyclovir
Herpes *simplex*	Acyclovir
Cytomegalovirus	Ganciclovir/foscarnet
Human herpesvirus 6	Ganciclovir
Fungal	
Aspergillus fumigatus	Amphotericin B/fluconazole
Cryptococcus neoformans	Amphotericin B + fluconazole/flucytosine

CNS Infections

CNS infections are frequent and one of the leading causes of morbidity and mortality after solid organ transplantation (Table 19.3) [3]. Headache with an unexplained fever is the most reliable symptom complex suggesting a CNS infection in the transplant patient. Unfortunately, due to an impaired inflammatory response because of immunosuppression, the clinical manifestations of CNS infections can be diminished. Therefore, it is imperative to consider CNS infections in the setting of fever, headache, and altered mental status even in the absence of other manifestations [8].

MRI with and without contrast is often crucial for diagnosis. The differential diagnosis can usually be developed by characteristic findings on MRI. Aspergillus and toxoplasmosis commonly present as mass lesions with ring enhancement, and CNS aspergillosis is often associated with hemorrhagic cerebral infarction. Lumbar puncture is imperative for diagnosis and should include measurements of opening and closing pressures. CSF analysis should include cultures, glucose (serum should also be obtained at approximately the same time), protein, viral PCRs, cytology, cryptococcal antigen, tuberculosis PCR, and additional fluid for storage in case further testing is needed.

Critically ill or deteriorating patients should be started on empiric antimicrobial therapy as soon as possible. A suggested empiric regimen of ceftriaxone, vancomycin, ampicillin, and acyclovir should be administered before initial test results are available. In many cases, a discussion or consultation with an infectious disease specialist will be helpful.

CNS infections can be stratified by time course after transplantation and then further into bacterial, fungal, viral, and protozoal (Table 19.4). In the first month after transplantation, CNS infections are rare; however, when they do occur, they are usually donor transmitted, nosocomial, or exacerbation of infections already present

Table 19.4 Common CNS infections by time course posttransplant

Time course	Infections
First 30 days	Pretransplant colonization Nosocomial Infections (MRSA, *Candida*, *Aspergillus*) Donor-derived transmission
30 days to 6 months	Viral infections (HSV, CMV, EBV) Opportunistic infections (*Nocardia*, *Toxoplasma*, *Listeria*)
Over 6 months	Opportunistic infections Community-acquired infections Reactivation of previous infections

before transplantation. The 30-day to six-month posttransplant period is when patients are at the greatest risk for infection, predominately from viral and opportunistic pathogens. Varicella zoster virus (VZV), Epstein-Barr virus (EBV), and cytomegalovirus (CMV) are the most commonly implicated viral pathogens. Compared with immunocompetent persons, transplant recipients have herpes simplex virus (HSV) reactivation more frequently, have more severe clinical manifestations, and may be less responsive to antiviral therapy [9]. Opportunistic infections can be caused by *Nocardia*, *Aspergillus*, *Toxoplasma*, *Listeria*, and *Cryptococcus*. After 6 months, infections are stratified into three different categories: reactivation of previous infections, opportunistic infections secondary to chronic immunosuppression, and community-acquired infections, also seen in non-immunocompromised patients.

Seizures

Seizures can be divided into generalized and focal seizures (with and without alterations in awareness). Most seizures after transplantation are due to drug toxicity and present clinically as generalized seizures. Generalized seizures can also be due to metabolic derangements, most notably hyponatremia, hypomagnesemia, hypoglycemia, and hyperammonemia. Focal seizures may be due to focal structural abnormalities such as intracranial hemorrhage, abscess, malignancy such as posttransplant lymphoproliferative disorder (PTLD), and PRES.

Lumbar puncture and CSF analysis should be conducted if there are signs of infection associated with seizures. Neuroimaging is indicated in any transplant patient presenting with a first-time seizure. A noncontrast head CT can be obtained in the emergency setting to exclude catastrophic conditions; however, brain MRI is usually more informative. If no provoking factors can be identified and corrected, then seizures should be treated using established algorithms (see Chap. 2). EEG monitoring should be pursued to monitor for nonconvulsive seizures/nonconvulsive status epilepticus in the poorly responsive or encephalopathic patient. Of note, posttransplant patients can also have adventitious movements (tremors, myoclonus, asterixis) from drug toxicity or metabolic derangements. These abnormal movements need to be differentiated from seizures, and EEG can be extremely valuable in facilitating this discrimination.

If seizures are recurrent, an intracranial structural abnormality is identified, or if the EEG demonstrates epileptogenic abnormalities, AED therapy should be started. AED therapy should be tailored depending on the patient's metabolic condition. Phenytoin, valproic acid, phenobarbital, and carbamazepine undergo hepatic metabolism and often affect the metabolism of other medications. Given the adverse effects of older AEDs, levetiracetam has become the drug of choice for posttransplant seizures. Lacosamide is another good choice for treatment of focal seizures given identical bioavailability between intravenous and enteral formulations and favorable safety profile.

Encephalopathy

An acute confusional state is perhaps the most common reason for neurological consultation in transplant units. Encephalopathy can present with symptoms of altered mental status, such as disorientation, alterations in alertness and awareness, agitation, and hallucinations. Encephalopathy usually occurs within the first 30 days after transplantation and can be attributed to medication toxicity (especially from calcineurin inhibitors), metabolic derangements (hypoglycemia, hyponatremia or hypernatremia, hyperammonemia, hypercalcemia, or hypermagnesemia), systemic or CNS infections, PRES, and stroke [10].

Among the metabolic derangements, hyperammonemia is frequently associated with hepatic transplantation and very rarely associated with lung transplantation. The threshold for obtaining an EEG in an encephalopathic patient after organ transplantation should be very low in order to evaluate for possible nonconvulsive seizures or nonconvulsive status epilepticus. Encephalopathy is often multifactorial and should include a thorough review of the patient's past medical history, medications (both home and hospital), and social history (alcohol and substance use). A complete review of the anesthesia history should be performed in the acute postoperative period. Particular attention should be paid to all potential sedative, and CNS-acting drugs should be performed. Administration of reversal agents such as flumazenil or naloxone can be considered. Laboratory investigations should be tailored to the type of transplant and clinical situation. Common blood tests to consider include complete cell counts, complete metabolic panel, arterial blood gases, TSH, hepatic enzymes, and ammonia. Established treatment protocols for electrolyte replacement should be followed. Correction of chronic hyponatremia should be gradual (not faster than 10 mmol/L per day) to avoid the risk of inducing osmotic demyelination. Typical treatment of hyperammonemia involves varying combinations of protein restriction, bowel decontamination, amino acids, nitrogen scavengers, and dialysis.

Organ-Specific Emergencies

Liver Transplant

Most neurological complications after liver transplant are forms of encephalopathy. During the initial 30 days after transplantation, metabolic encephalopathy is most common; causes include calcineurin inhibitors, hyponatremia, and osmotic demyelination (central pontine and extrapontine myelinolysis) [11]. Seizures are also common after liver transplantation, and EEG is essential to evaluate for nonconvulsive seizures/nonconvulsive status epilepticus in liver transplant patients with encephalopathy.

Perhaps the most challenging scenario in liver transplantation is management of cerebral edema in patients who received a liver after fulminant hepatic failure. Management often begins during the pretransplant phase but carries over into the postoperative phase. Brain edema can occur rapidly, and management of elevated intracranial pressure is essential. MRI is the imaging modality of choice but may not be feasible in the most critical cases. CT scans do not always correlate with the degree of cerebral edema but may still be useful to characterize the severity of the edema and exclude hemorrhage. Features to evaluate on CT include visibility of cortical sulci, white matter, and basal cisterns [12]. Placement of an ICP monitoring device should be considered to help guide management in the perioperative phase [13]. Risk of hemorrhage is increased in relation to the severity of thrombocytopenia and INR elevation [14].

Osmotic drugs are typically used in the treatment of elevated ICP [15]. Hypertonic saline is a good option especially in patients who have developed hepatorenal syndrome because the use of mannitol may exacerbate the renal function impairment. Hypothermia and high-dose propofol or barbiturates can be considered in cases of refractory elevated ICP; however, there are no data supporting better outcomes with these exceptional rescue measures.

Osmotic demyelination (central pontine and extrapontine myelinolysis) is a serious neurological complication that characteristically affects liver transplant recipients in the first 1–2 weeks after transplantation. Central pontine myelinolysis was initially described in alcoholic patients after rapid correction of hyponatremia; however, there is no consistent link between hyponatremia and the development of osmotic demyelination in liver transplant patients, and its cause and pathophysiology in these cases remain unknown [16, 17]. Risk factors for development include severe hyponatremia, multiple transfusions, hemorrhagic complications, diabetes, malnutrition, chronic hyponatremia, and cyclosporine use. Clinical manifestations include progressive confusion, decreased alertness, dysarthria, dysphagia, pseudobulbar palsy, ophthalmoplegia, and quadriplegia; tremor, catatonia, ataxia, mutism, and myoclonus can be seen with extrapontine involvement [16]. MRI is the imaging modality of choice and demonstrates T2 hyperintensities in the pons and often in various extrapontine locations. There is no treatment available. In the setting of hyponatremia, established protocols for treatment should be followed. Meaningful functional recovery is possible even in very severe cases [18].

Lung Transplant

Lung transplant patients have the highest mortality of any solid organ transplant recipients [19]. Encephalopathy is the most common neurological complication, and calcineurin inhibitor toxicity is often involved [20]. The most severe complications are related to postoperative stroke. An acute hyperammonemia without a completely elucidated mechanism can also be seen in these patients. It is theorized that lung transplant recipients are susceptible to neurological complications because of "decreased brain reserve" from chronic hypoxia [21].

Heart Transplant

Neurological complications are among the most common adverse events after heart transplantation. Stroke is the most common neurological complication associated with heart transplantation and often represents a neurological emergency [22]. Most strokes are due to ischemic infarctions, but hemorrhagic strokes can also occur. Cardiovascular risk factors for ischemic stroke are found in many heart transplant patients, including hypertension, hyperlipidemia, atrial fibrillation, and diabetes mellitus. Technical and surgical complications of heart transplantation, such as preoperative use of intra-aortic balloon pump or left ventricular assist device, prolonged cardiopulmonary bypass, intraoperative hypotension, or perioperative hemodynamic instability, can contribute to increase the risk of cerebral infarction [23]. Acute neurological changes in a heart transplant patient warrant emergent neurological consultation. Emergency head CT scan should be performed to evaluate for hemorrhage or early ischemic changes. While recent surgery will exclude a patient from receiving intravenous thrombolysis, endovascular intervention could still be considered in the setting of a large vessel occlusion (see Chap. 9). Hyperperfusion syndrome can also be seen after cardiopulmonary bypass [24]. Strict postoperative blood pressure control is essential in these cases, and improvement of symptoms over days to weeks is the rule.

Kidney Transplant

Kidneys are the most commonly transplanted solid organ, and recipients have a high rate of neurological complications [25]. The most common neurological complications after renal transplant are cerebrovascular events. This is mostly due to advanced atherosclerosis from preexisting conditions, such as diabetes and hypertension, which are very prevalent in patients with end-stage renal disease. Cerebral hemorrhage is also seen in renal transplant patients because of risk factors such as hypertension and polycystic kidney disease. While the risk of cerebrovascular events after renal transplantation is high, this risk diminishes over time because transplantation is often associated with improvement in vascular risk factors when compared to patients who remain on dialysis [26].

Cardinal Messages
- Neurotoxicity from immunosuppressive medications and CNS infections are inherent risks after all types of organ transplantation.
- Consider CNS infections in the setting of fever, headache, and altered mental status even in the absence of other manifestations.
- There should be a low threshold to obtain additional investigations—neuroimaging, EEG, and CSF analysis—in immunosuppressed patients with severe neurological symptoms after organ transplant.
- CNS infections can be stratified into early (1 month), intermediate (1–6 months), and late (after 6 months) time periods, and each has specific risk for certain organisms.
- Cerebral edema is common in fulminant hepatic failure and requires prompt ICP monitoring and management.
- Stroke is the most common complication after heart and kidney transplantations.

References

1. Shah M. Inpatient neurologic consultation in solid organ transplant patients. Semin Neurol. 2015;35(6):699–707.
2. Asai A, Qiu J, Narita Y, et al. High level calcineurin activity predisposes neuronal cells to apoptosis. J Biol Chem. 1999;274(48):34450–8.
3. Patchell RA. Neurological complications of organ transplantation. Ann Neurol. 1994;36(5):688–703.
4. Pustavoitau A, Bhardwaj A, Stevens R. Neurological complications of transplantation. J Intensive Care Med. 2011;26(4):209–22.
5. Fugate JE, Rabinstein AA. Posterior reversible encephalopathy syndrome: clinical and radiological manifestations, pathophysiology, and outstanding questions. Lancet Neurol. 2015;14(9):914–25.
6. Burnett MM, Hess CP, Roberts JP, et al. Presentation of reversible posterior leukoencephalopathy syndrome in patients on calcineurin inhibitors. Clin Neurol Neurosurg. 2010;112(10):886–91.
7. Dhar R, Human T. Central nervous system complications after transplantation. Neurol Clin. 2011;29(4):943–72.
8. Conti DJ, Rubin RH. Infection of the central nervous system in organ transplant recipients. Neurol Clin. 1988;6(2):241–60.
9. Lee DH, Zuckerman RA, AST Infectious Diseases Community of Practice. Herpes simplex virus infections in solid organ transplantation: guidelines from the American Society of Transplantation Infectious Diseases Community of Practice. Clin Transpl. 2019;12:e13526. [Epub ahead of print].

10. Senzolo M, Ferronato C, Burra P. Neurologic complications after solid organ transplantation. Transpl Int. 2009;22(3):269–78.
11. Kim JM, Jung KH, Lee ST, et al. Central nervous system complications after liver transplantation. J Clin Neurosci. 2015;22(8):1355–9.
12. EFm W, Plevak DJ, Rakela J, Wiesner RH. Clinical and radiologic features of cerebral edema in fulminant hepatic failure. Mayo Clin Proc. 1995;70:119–24.
13. Brandsaeter B, Hockerstedt K, Friman S, et al. Fulminant hepatic failure: outcome after listing for highly urgent liver transplantation: 12 years experience in the Nordic countries. Liver Transpl. 2002;8:1055–62.
14. O'grady J. Modern management of acute liver failure. Clin Liver Dis. 2007;11:291–303.
15. Maloney PR, Mallory GW, Atkinson JL, Wijdicks EF, Rabinstein AA, Van Gompel JJ. Intracranial pressure monitoring in acute liver failure: institutional case series. Neurocrit Care. 2016;25(1):86–93.
16. Pizzi M, Ng L. Neurologic complications of solid organ transplantation. Neurol Clin. 2017;35:809–23.
17. Singh TD, Fugate JE, Rabinstein AA. Central pontine and extrapontine myelinolysis: a systematic review. Eur J Neurol. 2014;21(12):1443–50. Epub 2014 Sep 15.
18. Graff-Radford J, Fugate JE, Kaufmann TJ, Mandrekar JN, Rabinstein AA. Clinical and radiologic correlations of central pontine myelinolysis syndrome. Mayo Clin Proc. 2011;86(11):1063–7. Epub 2011 Oct 13.
19. Christie JD, Edwards LB, Kucheryavaya AY, et al. The registry of the International Society for Heart and Lung Transplantation: twenty-eighth adult heart and heart- lung transplant report–2011. J Heart Lung Transplant. 2011;30(10):1104–22.
20. Shigemura N, Sclabassi RJ, Bhama JK, et al. Early major neurologic complications after lung transplantation: incidence, risk factors, and outcome. Transplantation. 2013;95(6):866–71.
21. Pierson DJ. Pathophysiology and clinical effects of chronic hypoxia. Respir Care. 2000;45(1):39–51.. [discussion: 51–3].
22. Zierer A, Melby SJ, Voeller RK, et al. Significance of neurologic complications in the modern era of cardiac transplantation. Ann Thorac Surg. 2007;83(5):1684–90.
23. Acampa M, Lazzerini PE, Guideri F, et al. Ischemic stroke after heart transplantation. J Stroke. 2016;18(2):157–68.
24. Wijdicks EF, Campeau N, Sundt T. Reversible unilateral brain edema presenting with major neurologic deficit after valve repair. Ann Thorac Surg. 2008;86(2):634–7.
25. Potluri K, Holt D, Hou S. Neurologic complications in renal transplantation. Handb Clin Neurol. 2014;121:1245–55.
26. Lentine KL, Rocca Rey LA, Kollis S, et al. Variations in the risk for cerebrovascular events after kidney transplant compared with experience on the waiting list and after graft failure. Clin J Am Soc Nephrol. 2008;3:1090–101.

Chapter 20
Neurological Emergencies in Pregnant Patients

Jason Siegel

> **Diagnostic Keys**
> - The differential diagnosis for neurological symptoms in pregnant patients is wide, including conditions common in the general population, in addition to conditions unique to pregnancy.
> - Detailed history and exam should be promptly conducted, with detailed description of all neurological and systemic features.
> - CT and MRI should not be withheld if clinically indicated, but unnecessary use should be minimized. Contrast administration should also be minimized.

> **Treatment Priorities**
> - The typical treatments used in the nonpregnant population often lack strong supporting evidence on safety and efficacy in the pregnant population.
> - For acute ischemic stroke, tissue plasminogen activator (tPA) and mechanical thrombectomy are not contraindicated in most cases.
> - Plasma exchange and IVIg are used safely in immunologic conditions.
> - Many anti-seizure medications are contraindicated in pregnancy; midazolam, levetiracetam, fosphenytoin, and propofol are used most commonly.

J. Siegel (✉)
Departments of Neurology, Neurosurgery, and Critical Care Medicine, Mayo Clinic Florida, Jacksonville, FL, USA
e-mail: Siegel.jason@mayo.edu

> **Prognosis at a Glance**
> - A multidisciplinary team of neurology/neurocritical care, obstetrics, neonatology, and, when pertinent, neurosurgery is necessary to manage these high-risk patients.
> - For most diseases, prognosis is similar to that of the general population, but for some diagnoses, it may vary from it.
> - Pregnancy termination is not typically indicated, but induction of labor or cesarean section can be considered and often done at term.

Introduction

Pregnancy is associated with several anatomical and physiological changes to the carrying mother. Unfortunately, these changes can be accompanied by neurological or systemic disease. Only about 0.1–1.3% of all pregnancies require intensive care unit admission [1]. But due to the delicate nature of pregnancy, including two lives being at risk, neurological emergencies must be quickly and accurately diagnosed and managed. Neurological emergencies in pregnant patients span the spectrum of neurology and include autoimmune, neuromuscular, cerebrovascular, movement disorders, and epilepsy. In this chapter, we discuss several neurological emergencies, with practical tables and algorithms for workup and management. We also discuss limitations and special circumstances in working up and treating a pregnant patient with a neurological emergency.

Initial Assessment

The workup of acute neurological changes in a pregnant patient should be guided by presenting symptoms and clinical findings. There is significant overlap, however, in the clinical presentation of several of these conditions.

Headache is the most common neurological problem in pregnancy [2–4]. Headache in pregnant patients could represent benign cephalalgias or life-threatening conditions. Important characteristics include the following:

- Location – holocephalic, frontal, unilateral, occipital, associated with neck pain
- Severity
- Character – throbbing, stabbing, sharp, shooting, dull
- Onset – rapid or gradual
- Previous history of headaches and any notable differences
- Positional change – avoids lying flat or standing up
- Red flags that suggest emergency diagnoses include the following:

- Thunderclap (reaches maximum intensity immediately), "worst headache of my life"
- Drowsiness or depressed level of consciousness
- Papilledema, retinal hemorrhages
- Worse with straining and Valsalva
- Stiff neck, meningismus
- Accompanied by other neurological symptoms – seizures, weakness, vision loss, history of cerebrovascular disease
- Accompanied by other systemic symptoms – hypertension, peripheral edema
- A change in features from previous headaches

Headache description helps generate a differential diagnosis (Table 20.1).

Visual change is also common in pregnant patients and has a wide differential. The ophthalmologic exam should include visual acuity (with pinhole exam), visual fields, Amsler grid testing, swinging light test (looking for a relative afferent pupillary

Table 20.1 Common headache emergencies in pregnant patients

Description	Possible diagnosis
Unilateral, throbbing, photophobia, phonophobia, osmophobia, nausea/vomiting, improved with sleep	Migraine[a]
Nonspecific and unremitting seizures, focal neurological symptoms, signs of raised ICP	Cerebral venous sinus thrombosis
Headache refractory to analgesia Hypertension, proteinuria	Preeclampsia/eclampsia (headache can be sentinel feature to eclampsia)
Blurred vision, scotoma, flashing lights	PRES from hypertension
Thunderclap, fluctuating neurological deficits, seizures	Reversible cerebral vasoconstriction syndrome (postpartum vasculopathy)
Thunderclap, orbitofrontal or diffuse Nausea, vomiting, hypotension, vision loss (bitemporal hemianopia), altered consciousness	Pituitary apoplexy
Thunderclap, often unilateral Nausea, vomiting, neck stiffness, altered consciousness	Subarachnoid hemorrhage
Diffuse, neck pain, meningismus, possibly thunderclap Cranial neuropathies, fever	Meningitis/meningoencephalitis
Diffuse, worse with coughing or Valsalva Papilledema, sixth nerve palsy	Space-occupying lesion or other causes of increased intracranial pressure (including idiopathic intracranial hypertension)
Nonspecific quality, moderate intensity Focal neurologic symptoms	Acute ischemic stroke

ICP intracranial pressure, *PRES* posterior reversible encephalopathy syndrome
[a]Migraine is a common headache experienced in pregnant patients and typically does not represent an emergency. But recognizing the symptoms can help the clinician rule out other conditions

defect), ocular motility testing for full ductions, alignment and convergence testing, and a fundoscopic exam.

Important features include the following:

- Negative phenomena – vision loss, blackening, blurriness, black scotoma, "shade falling," visual field loss
- Positive phenomena – scintillating scotoma, fortification spectra, hallucination
- Monocular – eye or optic nerve pathology
- Binocular – retro-chiasm pathology

Note that patients often report a homonymous hemianopia as monocular visual loss because they appreciate the large defect in the temporal field, but not the nasal defect of the contralateral eye.

Red flags regarding visual change include the following:

- Papilledema
- Acute monocular or binocular vision loss
- Accompanying neurological or systemic symptoms

Pregnancy induces a relative hypercoagulable state that can promote thrombosis at various sites throughout the body and central nervous system, including the eye. These events predominantly lead to negative symptoms. Posterior reversible encephalopathy syndrome (PRES) and migraine can cause both positive and negative visual phenomena.

Pregnancy may induce or worsen malnourished states, especially in the first trimester when nausea, food aversion, and hyperemesis gravidarum are at their peaks. The combination of nutrient depletion and increased demand for thiamine can precipitate Wernicke encephalopathy. Patients can present with diplopia, nystagmus, ptosis, ataxia, and confusion. Emergency replenishment with high-dose IV thiamine is necessary to avoid a potentially irreversible amnestic state.

Description of visual loss helps generate a differential diagnosis (Table 20.2).

Weakness, when severe, should always prompt immediate workup. Important descriptors include the following:

- Onset – acute vs progressive
- Unilateral vs bilateral
- Course – fluctuating, progressive, or fixed

For most etiologies of weakness, the presentation in pregnant patients is similar to what is expected in the general population. Like in the general patient population, the first step in characterizing weakness is to localize it as a central or peripheral process.

Many peripheral causes of weakness occur frequently in pregnancy and do not represent neurological emergencies. These include median neuropathy of the wrist (carpal tunnel syndrome), ulnar and radial neuropathies, femoral and obturator neuropathies, fibular neuropathy, lateral femoral cutaneous neuropathy, lumbosacral plexopathy, lumbosacral radiculopathy, and polyneuropathy.

Table 20.2 Common presenting symptoms and possible diagnoses of visual change

Visual change	Possible diagnosis
Negative symptoms (blurry vision, vision loss, scotoma)	
Corrects with pinhole and near card	Refractory error (progesterone-induced lens and cornea edema)[a]
"Shade being pulled down"	Retinal ischemia
High serum glucose and blood pressure (correlates with degree of injury) Fundoscopic exam: microaneurysms, nerve fiber layer and intraretinal hemorrhages, macular edema, cotton wool spots, exudates, retinal vascular changes, disc edema [13, 14]	Diabetic retinopathy in pregnancy
Fundoscopic exam: retinal whitening [15–17]	Retinal arteriolar occlusion from cardioembolic source, hypercoagulable state, inflammatory vasculitis, amniotic embolism
Fundoscopic exam: hemorrhages	Venous occlusions
Mild vision loss without RAPD Fundoscopic exam: accumulation of fluid underneath retinal pigmented epithelium	Central serous chorioretinopathy (typically resolves without treatment)
Homonymous visual field defect (hemianopia, quadrantanopia)	Acute ischemic or hemorrhagic stroke involving the thalamus, optic radiations, or occipital lobe
Bitemporal hemianopia	Pituitary enlargement or macroadenoma or apoplexy (especially with thunderclap headache)
Alexia (with or without agraphia), Balint syndrome (simultanagnosia, oculomotor apraxia, optic ataxia), cerebral blindness. Intact pupillary light reflexes	Occipitoparietal regions (PRES, potentially from preeclampsia/eclampsia) [25, 27]
Central, painful visual loss Fundoscopic exam: optic disc pallor	Optic neuritis (MS especially postpartum, NMO, idiopathic)
Positive symptoms	
Fortification spectra, scintillating scotoma, "kaleidoscope" or "broken glass" vision	Migraine
Hallucinations	Occipital lobe focal seizures
Mixed or variable symptoms	
Blurred or decreased vision, spots, color defects Fundoscopic exam: vascular narrowing, segmental vasospasm. Cotton wool spots, hemorrhages, disc edema, emboli, retinal infarction. Elschnig spots – red or yellow spots with dark centers due to choroid infarction (may need indocyanine green angiography to see)	Preeclampsia/eclampsia
Papilledema – may be accompanied with diplopia, pulse-synchronous tinnitus, decreased visual acuity [22, 36]	Increased intracranial pressure

(continued)

Table 20.2 (continued)

Visual change	Possible diagnosis
With thunderclap headache ± diplopia	Pituitary apoplexy, cerebral venous sinus thrombosis
With positional headache (worse laying down)	Idiopathic intracranial hypertension (formerly pseudotumor cerebri)

MS multiple sclerosis, *NMO* neuromyelitis optica
[a]Blurry vision due to a progesterone-induced refractory problem is considered normal in pregnancy

Table 20.3 Common presentations of weakness and possible diagnoses

Weakness presentation	Description
Acute, unilateral (face and arm, or face, arm, and leg), aphasia, gaze deviation, depressed level of consciousness	Acute ischemic or hemorrhagic stroke
Bilateral, proximal extremity or bulbar weakness, diplopia, dysphagia, dysarthria	Myasthenia gravis
Acute, variable, segmental or unilateral, may include sensory loss or pain	Multiple sclerosis
Ascending weakness and numbness, ± bulbar, respiratory, or facial weakness or ophthalmoplegia. Areflexia, dysautonomia	AIDP, CIDP

AIDP acute inflammatory demyelinating polyradiculoneuropathy, *CIDP* chronic inflammatory demyelinating polyradiculoneuropathy

The most serious peripheral nervous system disease causing weakness in the pregnant patient is acute inflammatory demyelinating polyradiculoneuropathy (AIDP), also known as Guillain-Barre syndrome (GBS). It is characterized by ascending weakness and numbness, potentially leading to paralysis and respiratory distress or failure. Another emergency cause of peripheral nervous system weakness is myasthenia gravis (MG), which is characterized by fluctuating weakness, in the extremities or in the facial, extraocular, or bulbar muscles. MG can also precipitate loss of airway control and respiratory failure. Further details on these diagnoses can be found on Chap. 8.

The central nervous system causes of weakness include acute ischemic stroke (AIS), intracerebral hemorrhage (ICH), and multiple sclerosis (MS). AIS and ICH occur acutely and typically causes unilateral weakness that may be accompanied by numbness, aphasia, dysarthria, diplopia or gaze deviation, incoordination, or gait changes. Weakness associated to MS is variable and may affect the entire hemibody or just one myotome. MS flares can be accompanied by numbness or pain, optic neuritis (or other acute visual changes), or brainstem findings.

Features useful to discriminate the cause of weakness are displayed on Table 20.3.

Seizures in pregnancy can occur because of three reasons:

- Breakthrough seizures from chronic epilepsy
- Emergence of seizures from a previous unknown seizure disorder with breakthrough due to a lowered seizure threshold from pregnancy
- Seizures secondary to other neurological disorders associated with pregnancy

Though breakthrough seizures in a patient with known epilepsy may not represent neurological emergencies, new onset seizures should be thoroughly worked up and could represent manifestations of PRES or intracerebral hemorrhage (ICH). In addition, both convulsive and nonconvulsive status epilepticus may emerge and require emergent management. Seizure mimics in the pregnant population are more extensive than in the general population due to the increased risk of developing nonepileptic hyperkinetic movement disorders during pregnancy and puerperium. For example, the rhythmic movements of tremor or the contorted postures of dystonia may resemble focal motor seizures.

Diagnosis and Management of Specific Neurological Emergencies

Preeclampsia and Eclampsia

Preeclampsia/eclampsia is a common condition in pregnancy (7.5% of pregnancies worldwide) [5], with a heterogeneous presentation and variable neurological consequences. It is not a disease exclusive to pregnancy, as it can emerge up to 6 weeks postpartum.

Preeclampsia is defined by the triad of hypertension (>140/90 mmHg), proteinuria (>300 mg per day), and peripheral edema. The pathophysiology is unknown but may be due to placental hypoperfusion and hypoxia, leading to release of antiangiogenic factors, impairing maternal endothelium and causing vascular permeability (accounting for proteinuria and peripheral edema) and vasoconstriction (accounting for hypertension). The neurological consequences of preeclampsia are numerous and include seizure (which elevates the diagnosis from preeclampsia to eclampsia), PRES, reversible cerebral vasoconstriction syndrome/postpartum angiopathy (RCVS/PPA), AIS, and ICH. Other systemic symptoms include hemolytic anemia, elevated liver enzymes, and low platelets (the combination of which constitutes HELLP syndrome), disseminated intravascular coagulopathy, pulmonary edema, myocardial infarction, renal failure, and placental abruption [6] (Table 20.4).

Table 20.4 Clinical features and management of preeclampsia, PRES, and PPA/RCVS

Disease	Clinical features	Diagnostics	Therapeutics	Prognosis
Preeclampsia	Hypertension Proteinuria Peripheral edema	≥140/90 mmHg ≥300 mg/day	First-line antihypertensive – labetalol and hydralazine	Accounts for 10–15% of maternal deaths worldwide, <1% in developed nations
Eclampsia	Preeclampsia + seizures		Magnesium sulfate	
HELLP	Hemolytic anemia Transaminitis Thrombocytopenia (can cause ICH or SAH)	Schistocytes Total bilirubin >1.2 mg/dL, AST >2 times of upper limit of normal platelet count ≤100,000 cells/μL	Delivery Platelet transfusion may temporize condition	Good if delivery <48 hours of onset; 1% mortality rate
PRES	Headache, confusion, cortical blindness, Balint syndrome	White matter predominant MRI T2 and FLAIR hyperintensities, typically with posterior predilection	Blood pressure management	Favorable but variable depending on comorbid conditions (ICH, SAH)
PPA/RCVS	Thunderclap headache, encephalopathy, focal deficits, seizures, vomiting, photophobia	Multifocal "string of beads" stenosis of large and/or medium cerebral blood vessels Cerebral vascular border-zone T2/FLAIR hyperintensities or DWI changes (if ischemia present)	Headache control, seizure control (magnesium sulfate), stroke management, blood pressure management, supportive care	Typically favorable and reversible, but occasionally fulminant

GTC generalized tonic-clonic, *HELLP* hemolysis, elevated liver enzymes, low platelets, *PRES* posterior reversible encephalopathy syndrome, *PPA* postpartum angiopathy, *RCVS* reversible cerebral vasoconstriction syndrome, *MRI* magnetic resonance imaging, *FLAIR* fluid attenuated inversion recovery, *AST* aspartate aminotransferase

Posterior Reversible Encephalopathy Syndrome and Postpartum Angiopathy

PRES and PPA can be serious potential consequences of preeclampsia/eclampsia [7]. Both conditions can occur even if all criteria for preeclampsia/eclampsia are not met [8].

If preeclampsia/eclampsia is a syndrome of "leaky" systemic blood vessels, PRES is a result of abnormal "leaky" blood vessels of the brain. The resulting vasogenic edema occurs predominantly in the posterior circulation (perhaps due to less prominent sympathetic activity in the posterior circulation) but can arise in the frontal white matter or basal ganglia [9]. Symptoms typically appear in the second or third trimester and usually progress over the course of hours to days. They can be vague or localizing to the occipital lobes or brainstem and include headache, encephalopathy, cortical vision changes, and seizures (typically generalized tonic-clonic seizures). In many cases, PRES can be identified on head computed tomography (CT), though magnetic resonance imaging (MRI) is more sensitive and specific. On CT, PRES appears as patchy hypodensities predominantly on the white matter (though gray matter is often involved) that do not respect one vascular distribution [10]. Similarly, MRI T2/FLAIR sequences show hyperintensities in the affected areas. Diffusion-weighted imaging (DWI) sequences are typically negative, and gadolinium enhancement on T1 sequences is variable. Occasionally, areas of hemorrhage can be identified, particularly on susceptibility-weighted imaging (SWI) or gradient echo (GRE) sequences, and vasospasm (particularly of the posterior cerebral and basilar arteries) can be seen on angiography. The mainstay of treatment is supportive care and removing the inciting agent or condition (e.g., gradually controlling hypertension).

PPA is a form of RCVS that can occur up to 4–6 weeks postpartum. It is likely due to the vasoconstrictive consequences of preeclampsia/eclampsia. In addition to preeclampsia/eclampsia, PPA is associated with serotonergic agents (ergot derivatives and selective serotonin reuptake inhibitors). Presentation is usually more abrupt than PRES and includes thunderclap headache or sudden onset of neurological symptoms. Vasoconstriction can be treated with calcium channel blockers such as nimodipine and verapamil, though there are no controlled trials. Magnesium sulfate should be administered when combined with eclampsia. PPA can be associated with intracerebral hemorrhage, ischemic stroke, and subarachnoid hemorrhage, and a fulminant form has been described [11].

For seizures associated with eclampsia, PRES, or PPA, magnesium sulfate is the mainstay of therapy [12–14]. Magnesium is administered as a bolus (4–6 g) followed by continuous infusion. Biomarkers of magnesium toxicity include loss of deep tendon reflexes, depressed respiration, and oliguria. Calcium gluconate should be administered if magnesium toxicity is suspected.

Cerebrovascular Disease

Several physiological changes during pregnancy can predispose women to developing AIS and ICH.

- Hemodynamic changes – vascular dilatation and hypervolemia cause relative venous stasis.

- Vascular changes – blood vessel remodeling, reduction in collagen and elastin with increased contractile force [15].
- Hypercoagulability – increased levels of procoagulant factors I, VII, VIII, IX, X, XII, and XIII, as well as estrogen [16]. Decreased in coagulation inhibitors antithrombin III and protein S.

Thus, pregnancy-related changes affect all elements of the Virchow's triad (hemostasis, vascular injury, and hypercoagulability) and predispose pregnant women to systemic and cerebral thrombosis. The most commonly identified causes of AIS are cardioembolism and venous sinus thrombosis. A substantial proportion of ischemic strokes during pregnancy remain cryptogenic despite exhaustive investigations (20–44%) [15, 17, 18].

Acute Ischemic Stroke

The presentation, workup, and management of AIS in the pregnant patient are similar to that of nonpregnant patients. AIS should be considered whenever a patient develops acute neurological deficits, especially those consistent with known stroke syndromes. Specific radiographic considerations will be discussed later in the chapter, but it is imperative to conduct appropriate neuroimaging. Non-contrast CT of the head is the fastest test for ruling out hemorrhage and may disclose early ischemic changes and signs suggestive of venous sinus occlusion with venous infarction. CT angiogram (CTA) and CT perfusion (CTP) can be used to determine presence of a large vessel occlusion (LVO) and the volumes of ischemia core and surrounding penumbra. MRI does not use radiation and can give a more detailed picture of the stroke core and penumbra, though it takes longer to complete, and it is usually less readily available. Noninvasive angiograms may also demonstrate vasoconstriction in patients with PPA/RCVS.

Typical AIS laboratory investigations should be completed, including hemoglobin A1C and lipid panel. Additional laboratory studies may include erythrocyte sedimentation rate (ESR), C-reactive protein (CRP), liver transaminases, and thyroid-stimulating hormone (TSH). A thorough cardiac workup should include echocardiography with agitated saline bubble study to evaluate for a patent foramen ovale with a right-to-left shunt.

In addition to prothrombin time (PT), partial thromboplastin time (PTT), and international normalized ration (INR), inherited or acquired hypercoagulopathies may need to be excluded in certain cases, especially in the setting of cerebral venous thrombosis. Tests include the following:

- Antiphospholipid (anticardiolipin) antibody panel
- Prothrombin G20210A mutation
- Factor V Leiden mutation

- Beta-2 glycoprotein I antibodies
- Methylenetetrahydrofolate reductase (MTHFR) mutation
- Hemoglobin electrophoresis

Yet, some coagulation test results may be abnormal during pregnancy and in the acute phase of AIS (especially in the setting of thrombolysis or anticoagulation) without necessarily representing a pathogenic process. They include the following:

- Protein C
- Protein S
- Antithrombin III (deficiency)

There are no randomized controlled studies on the use of IV recombinant tissue plasminogen activator (rTPA) in pregnant patients. Several case series have demonstrated comparable success to that observed in the general population [19, 20]. Although tPA does not cross the placental barrier, it does pose a risk of placental hemorrhage and consequent miscarriage. For this reason, it is often reserved as salvage therapy for major and disabling strokes. A multidisciplinary team, including obstetrics and neonatology, should be involved in discussing the risks and benefits of intravenous thrombolysis with the pregnant patient.

Endovascular thrombectomy has emerged as standard of care for stroke patients with large vessel occlusions, with or without IV thrombolysis [21]. It has become an attractive option for treating AIS in the pregnant patient. To date, there are five published reports on thrombectomy for AIS during pregnancy. These reports indicate that mechanical thrombectomy can be used safely in pregnant patients and, when recanalization is achieved, can result in excellent functional recovery [22–26]. Refer to Chap. 9 for a more detailed discussion on the diagnosis and management of AIS.

Cerebral Venous Sinus Thrombosis

Cerebral venous sinus thrombosis (CVST) can present with headache (thunderclap), seizures, focal neurological deficits, nausea and vomiting, and decreased level of consciousness. Evaluation includes cerebral imaging, including non-contrasted or contrasted head CT, CT venography, MRI, or MR venography, to identify a venous thrombus or filling defect and any associated conditions such as hemorrhage (intraparenchymal, subarachnoid, intraventricular, or subdural), edema, ischemia, and hydrocephalus.

Mainstay of therapy is full heparin anticoagulation, even if hemorrhage is already present [27]. Endovascular thrombectomy has not been well studied in CVST but may be useful in selected cases [28]. Further details on this topic can be found on Chap. 10.

Hemorrhagic Strokes

Pregnancy increases the risk of hemorrhagic stroke substantially (relative risk 2.5 during pregnancy, 28.5 in the early postpartum period). The most common causes of hemorrhage are preeclampsia/eclampsia, arteriovenous malformation (AVM), cerebral aneurysm, and CVST.

Historical data for AVM bleeding risk has been inconsistent [29], but recent reports support an increased hemorrhagic risk during pregnancy [30]. AHA guidelines recommend that if a woman has a known AVM and anticipates pregnancy, the AVM should be treated before pregnancy. These guidelines also recommend that if a pregnant woman is found to have an incidental AVM, it should be treated postpartum. An AVM that bleeds during pregnancy should be considered for treatment before delivery, depending on location and severity [31, 32].

Aneurysmal subarachnoid hemorrhage (aSAH) carries a high mortality and morbidity rate in the general population, but in pregnant patients, maternal and fetal mortality can be as high as 35% and 17%, respectively, if the aneurysm is secured, and 63% and 27%, respectively, if the aneurysm is not secured [33]. Therefore, the priority is to secure the ruptured aneurysm either by surgical clipping or endovascular coiling. Due to the increased risk of aneurysm rupture and the high mortality rate, it is recommended to have a low threshold to prophylactically treat concomitant unruptured aneurysms in pregnant patients.

Chapters 11 and 12 provide detailed discussions on ICH and aSAH.

Status Epilepticus

Status epilepticus (SE) is rare in pregnancy [34] but can occur during all pregnancy stages, including labor and puerperium. SE poses life-threatening risk to not only the mother but also to the fetus as sympathetic hyperactivity can provoke placental vasoconstriction. Many anti-seizure medications are teratogenic and contraindicated in pregnancy. The most appropriate treatment algorithm for the treatment of SE in pregnancy has not been established.

The primary causes of SE in pregnant patients are PRES, eclampsia, and CVST. Other causes include history of symptomatic epilepsy (e.g., from mesial temporal sclerosis), withdrawal of anti-seizure medication, intracranial hemorrhage, and autoimmune encephalitis (anti-NMDAR encephalitis) [34–36]. Most patients have convulsive SE, though 18–57% can have either focal SE or nonconvulsive SE (NCSE) [34, 35].

Amniotic embolism is a rare cause of seizures and acute neurological decline. Amniotic embolism can occur in pregnancy, during delivery, or postpartum, and the most common presentation is cardiopulmonary collapse, though neurological manifestations are common. Encephalopathy is the most prevalent feature, but seizures, hypoxia, and stroke can occur. In fact, up to 50% of cases can present with seizure.

Morbidity and mortality are high, and up to 85% of survivors can have neurological morbidity. Systemic treatment is supportive, and seizures should be managed aggressively when present.

When SE occurs during pregnancy, maternal outcome is generally good; yet, 24–43% can have functional sequelae [34, 35]. The baby may be born without complications, but the risks of preterm labor, low-birth weight, respiratory distress, anoxic brain injury, and intraventricular hemorrhage are increased. These rates are higher in women with refractory SE [34].

Though there are no guidelines for treatment of SE in pregnant patients, benzodiazepines are typically used as the first-line treatment. Among second-line anti-seizure drugs, levetiracetam and fosphenytoin are most commonly prescribed. Because of pharmacokinetic changes that may occur in pregnancy, monitoring serum levels of the anti-seizure is recommended. Patients who are refractory to these drugs are placed on IV anesthesia, usually midazolam or propofol. As mentioned in the preeclampsia/eclampsia section, magnesium sulfate is the treatment of choice for eclampsia-related seizures. A list of anti-seizure medications with the most important safety considerations is provided on Table 20.5. For a more detailed discussion on the management of acute seizures and SE, please refer to Chap. 2.

Immunological Diseases

AIDP is an autoimmune disorder characterized by ascending flaccid weakness, areflexia, albuminocytologic dissociation in the cerebrospinal fluid, and diffusely slowing of nerve conduction velocities on electrophysiological studies. AIDP may occur during pregnancy, though epidemiological data indicate similar incidence as in the general age-matched population. It can progress to produce ophthalmoplegia, dysarthria, dysphagia, ataxia, autonomic instability, and neuromuscular respiratory insufficiency (short, shallow breaths, nasal flaring, paradoxical breathing, and variable use of accessory breathing muscles depending on the extent of the disease). Objective respiratory function measurements of forced vital capacity and maximal inspiratory and expiratory pressures should be recorded with bedside spirometry. Endotracheal Tracheal intubation and mechanical ventilation should be pursued without delay in patients with signs of respiratory failure.

Treatment options aim to reduce the immune response. Plasma exchange and IV immunoglobulin have similar efficacy and are considered safe during pregnancy [37]. Labor may be induced early [37], but termination of pregnancy is not advised as maternal and neonatal outcomes are typically good. Both general and local anesthesia has been used successfully, but depolarizing neuromuscular blockage should be avoided.

MG is a chronic autoimmune disease of the neuromuscular junction. The hallmark of presentation is fluctuating weakness of the oculobulbar and appendicular muscles. During pregnancy, MG remains most often stable but can worsen in 20–30% of patients [38, 39]. Like AIDP, the most concerning consequence is

Table 20.5 Characteristics of common anti-seizure drugs and considerations before administering in a pregnant patient [44]

Drug	Dose	FDA pregnancy class	Maternal and fetal risks
Benzodiazepines			
Diazepam	0.15 mg/kg IV, 10 mg max per dose	D	Hypotension, respiratory distress
Midazolam	0.2 mg/kg IM, 10 mg max	D	
Lorazepam	0.1 mg/kg IV, 4 mg max per dose	D	
Anti-seizure drugs			
Levetiracetam	40–60 mg/kg IIV	C	
Fosphenytoin	20 mg PE/kg IV	D	Hypotension, arrhythmias
Lacosamide	200–400 mg IV	N/A	PR interval prolongation, hypotension
Topiramate	200–400 mg NG/PO	D (previously C)	Facial clefts, metabolic acidosis
Valproic acid	40 mg/kg IV	X	Congenital malformations (spina bifida, hypospadias) Hyperammonemia, pancreatitis, thrombocytopenia, hepatotoxicity
Phenobarbital	20 mg/kg IV	D	Cardiac defects, mental retardation Hypotension, respiratory depression, decreased level of consciousness
Anesthetics			
Midazolam (continuous)	0.2 mg/kg followed by 0.2–5 mg/kg/min	D	Respiratory depression, hypotension, tachyphylaxis
Propofol	20–80 mcg/kg/min	B	Hypotension, respiratory distress, cardiac failure, rhabdomyolysis, metabolic acidosis, renal failure
Ketamine	1–5 mg/kg/hr	N/A	Hypertension, tachycardia
Pentobarbital	5–10 mg/kg (<50 mg/min) followed by 1–5 mg/kg/hr	D	Hypotension, respiratory depression, cardiac depression, paralytic ileus, infection/pneumonia
Thiopental	2–7 mg/kg (<50 mg/min)	C	Hypotension, respiratory depression, cardiac depression

N/A not assigned

respiratory failure from weakness of breathing muscles and aspiration from bulbar muscle weakness and weak cough.

Treatment includes pyridostigmine, prednisone, IVIg, and plasma exchange. As in AIDP, IVIg and plasma exchange have been safely used in pregnancy. Chronic immunomodulators such as cyclosporine, mycophenolate mofetil, azathioprine, rituximab, and methotrexate should not be used until after delivery.

Maternal and fetal outcomes in MG are good. Though fatigability could emerge during the second stage of labor, vaginal deliveries are not absolutely contraindicated. If surgical intervention is warranted, regional anesthesia is preferred to general anesthesia, and nondepolarizing neuromuscular blockade is contraindicated.

In patients with MG and eclampsia, magnesium sulfate should be used judiciously as it prevents acetylcholine release. As an alternative, phenytoin can be used for eclamptic seizures. If magnesium sulfate must be given, ventilator support may be needed.

Chapter 8 provides more in-depth discussions on AIDP and MG exacerbation.

Considerations for Diagnostic Workup

Several of the conditions discussed in this chapter require diagnostic tests that raise safety concerns in pregnant patients. Exposure to radiation from CT is a frequent concern. Head CT should be completed if indicated, but MRI is preferred if available. Using lead shields over the mother's abdomen and pelvis is advisable. In the case of digitally subtracted angiography (DSA), minimizing number of views, reducing high-dose acquisition time, optimal collimator placement, and pulse radiation can be helpful in reducing radiation exposure. Using a radial access may also reduce radiation exposure [25]. Expected degrees of radiation exposure by radiation modality are shown on Table 20.6. Possible effects on the fetus are shown on Table 20.7. As seen on these tables, the levels of radiation exposure expected to occur during routine neuroimaging are well below the threshold for serious concern. That said, concern for radiation-related fetal complications is greater during the first trimester.

Iodinated contrast crosses the placental barrier, but no studies have shown fetal harm. There is a hypothetical risk of fetal and neonatal thyroid dysfunction [40]. It is typical to check neonatal thyroid function if iodine contrast had to be administered to the pregnant mother; however, iodinated contrast should only be used if it will affect management.

Table 20.6 Fetal radiation exposure based on radiographic modality [41, 45]

Fetal exposure	Radiation (mGy)
Background radiation during term pregnancy	2.3
Head or neck CT	0.001–0.01
Cervical spine X-ray (AP)	<0.001
Lumbar spine X-ray	1.0–10
DSA (transradial approach)	~1.0
Chest X-ray (2 views)	0.0005–0.01
Chest CT/CTA	0.01–0.66
Abdominal X-ray	0.1–3.0
Abdominal CT	1.3–35
Pelvic CT	10–50

AP anteroposterior, *DSA* digitally subtracted angiography

Table 20.7 Fetal complications by levels of radiation exposure [43, 46]

Amount of radiation exposure to fetus	Potential complication
<50 mGy	No appreciable fetal risk of spontaneous abortion, developmental malformations, or cognitive deficiencies to radiation
10–20 mGy	Childhood leukemia increases from 3.6 per 10,000 children to 5 per 10,000 children
50–100 mGy	May cause anatomical or cognitive changes but has not been proven
>100 mGy	Significant risk of spontaneous abortion, anatomical malformations, and diminished IQ, depending on the timing of gestation

MRI has the advantage of avoiding ionizing radiation. There are theoretical risks of teratogenicity, amniotic fluid heating, and fetal acoustic damage. Yet, there is no evidence to support any of these concerns [41]. Gadolinium contrast should only be used if the results will change management. In small studies, gadolinium showed no risk of perinatal or neonatal adverse outcomes [42]. However, a larger epidemiological study showed a higher risk of stillbirths, neonatal deaths, rheumatologic, inflammatory, and infiltrative skin conditions in the offspring of women who had MRI with gadolinium during pregnancy as compared to those without (though rates were overall low) [41, 42]. Gadolinium can cross the placental barrier, such that it can stay in the fetal circulation longer than in the mother's, amplifying concern for possible adverse effects.

Cardinal Messages
- Neurological emergencies during pregnancy, though rare, have a broad differential diagnosis, and a complete history and exam are needed to narrow down the possibilities.
- Preeclampsia/eclampsia is a heterogeneous disease that can cause several neurological complications. Correction of hypertension can help treat PRES, and calcium channel blockade may be helpful for RCVS/PPA.
- Intravenous thrombolysis and particularly mechanical thrombectomy can be offered to pregnant women with AIS, especially if symptoms are severely disabling.
- Benzodiazepines, levetiracetam, fosphenytoin, and propofol are most commonly used for status epilepticus.
- Rapidly progressive weakness should prompt consideration for GBS or MG. IVIg and plasma exchange can be used safely during pregnancy.
- Optimal management of neurological emergencies in pregnant women demands the combined expertise of a multidisciplinary team including specialists in obstetrics, neonatology, neurology/neurocritical care, and, when necessary, neurosurgery.

References

1. Frontera JA, Ahmed W. Neurocritical care complications of pregnancy and puerperum. J Crit Care. 2014;29(6):1069–81.
2. Cripe SM, Frederick IO, Qiu C, Williams MA. Risk of preterm delivery and hypertensive disorders of pregnancy in relation to maternal co-morbid mood and migraine disorders during pregnancy. Paediatr Perinat Epidemiol. 2011;25(2):116–23.
3. Lynch KM, Brett F. Headaches that kill: a retrospective study of incidence, etiology and clinical features in cases of sudden death. Cephalalgia. 2012;32(13):972–8.
4. Aromaa M, Rautava P, Helenius H, Sillanpaa ML. Prepregnancy headache and the well-being of mother and newborn. Headache. 1996;36(7):409–15.
5. Wallis AB, Saftlas AF, Hsia J, Atrash HK. Secular trends in the rates of preeclampsia, eclampsia, and gestational hypertension, United States, 1987–2004. Am J Hypertens. 2008;21(5):521–6.
6. Bushnell C, McCullough LD, Awad IA, Chireau MV, Fedder WN, Furie KL, et al. Guidelines for the prevention of stroke in women: a statement for healthcare professionals from the American Heart Association/American Stroke Association. Stroke. 2014;45(5):1545–88.
7. Singhal AB. Postpartum angiopathy with reversible posterior leukoencephalopathy. Arch Neurol. 2004;61(3):411–6.
8. Roth C, Ferbert A. The posterior reversible encephalopathy syndrome: what's certain, what's new? Pract Neurol. 2011;11(3):136–44.
9. Fugate JE, Rabinstein AA. Posterior reversible encephalopathy syndrome: clinical and radiological manifestations, pathophysiology, and outstanding questions. Lancet Neurol. 2015;14(9):914–25. Epub 2015 Jul 13
10. Bartynski WS. Posterior reversible encephalopathy syndrome, part 1: fundamental imaging and clinical features. AJNR Am J Neuroradiol. 2008;29(6):1036–42.
11. Fugate JE, Wijdicks EF, Parisi JE, Kallmes DF, Cloft HJ, Flemming KD, Giraldo EA, Rabinstein AA. Fulminant postpartum cerebral vasoconstriction syndrome. Arch Neurol. 2012;69(1):111–7.
12. Raps EC, Galetta SL, Broderick M, Atlas SW. Delayed peripartum vasculopathy: cerebral eclampsia revisited. Ann Neurol. 1993;33(2):222–5.
13. Which anticonvulsant for women with eclampsia? Evidence from the Collaborative Eclampsia Trial. Lancet. 1995;345(8963):1455–63.
14. Lucas MJ, Leveno KJ, Cunningham FG. A comparison of magnesium sulfate with phenytoin for the prevention of eclampsia. N Engl J Med. 1995;333(4):201–5.
15. Hull AD, Long DM, Longo LD, Pearce WJ. Pregnancy-induced changes in ovine cerebral arteries. Am J Phys. 1992;262(1 Pt 2):R137–43.
16. Koellhoffer EC, McCullough LD. The effects of estrogen in ischemic stroke. Transl Stroke Res. 2013;4(4):390–401.
17. Sibai B, Dekker G, Kupferminc M. Pre-eclampsia. Lancet. 2005;365(9461):785–99.
18. Sibai BM. Etiology and management of postpartum hypertension-preeclampsia. Am J Obstet Gynecol. 2012;206(6):470–5.
19. Wiese KM, Talkad A, Mathews M, Wang D. Intravenous recombinant tissue plasminogen activator in a pregnant woman with cardioembolic stroke. Stroke. 2006;37(8):2168–9.
20. Murugappan A, Coplin WM, Al-Sadat AN, McAllen KJ, Schwamm LH, Wechsler LR, et al. Thrombolytic therapy of acute ischemic stroke during pregnancy. Neurology. 2006;66(5):768–70.
21. Nogueira RG, Jadhav AP, Haussen DC, Bonafe A, Budzik RF, Bhuva P, et al. Thrombectomy 6 to 24 hours after stroke with a mismatch between deficit and infarct. N Engl J Med. 2018;378(1):11–21.
22. Aaron S, Shyamkumar NK, Alexander S, Babu PS, Prabhakar AT, Moses V, et al. Mechanical thrombectomy for acute ischemic stroke in pregnancy using the penumbra system. Ann Indian Acad Neurol. 2016;19(2):261–3.

23. Zhu F, Gory B, Mione G, Humbertjean L, Derelle AL, Richard S. Combined reperfusion therapy to treat cryptogenic acute ischemic stroke during the first trimester of pregnancy: case report and literature review. Ther Clin Risk Manag. 2018;14:1677–83.
24. Watanabe TT, Ichijo M, Kamata T. Uneventful pregnancy and delivery after thrombolysis plus thrombectomy for acute ischemic stroke: case study and literature review. J Stroke Cerebrovasc Dis. 2019;28:70–5.
25. Shah SS, Snelling BM, Brunet MC, Sur S, McCarthy D, Stein A, et al. Transradial mechanical thrombectomy for proximal Mca occlusion in a first trimester pregnancy: case report and literature review. World Neurosurg. 2018;120:415.
26. Bhogal P, Aguilar M, AlMatter M, Karck U, Bazner H, Henkes H. Mechanical thrombectomy in pregnancy: report of 2 cases and review of the literature. Interv Neurol. 2017;6(1–2):49–56.
27. Stam J, De Bruijn SF, DeVeber G. Anticoagulation for cerebral sinus thrombosis. Cochrane Database Syst Rev. 2002;(4):CD002005.
28. Kashkoush AI, Ma H, Agarwal N, Panczykowski D, Tonetti D, Weiner GM, et al. Cerebral venous sinus thrombosis in pregnancy and puerperium: a pooled, systematic review. J Clin Neurosci. 2017;39:9–15.
29. Horton JC, Chambers WA, Lyons SL, Adams RD, Kjellberg RN. Pregnancy and the risk of hemorrhage from cerebral arteriovenous malformations. Neurosurgery. 1990;27(6):867–71.. discussion 71–2
30. Porras JL, Yang W, Philadelphia E, Law J, Garzon-Muvdi T, Caplan JM, et al. Hemorrhage risk of brain arteriovenous malformations during pregnancy and puerperium in a North American Cohort. Stroke. 2017;48(6):1507–13.
31. Ogilvy CS, Stieg PE, Awad I, Brown RD Jr, Kondziolka D, Rosenwasser R, et al. Recommendations for the management of intracranial arteriovenous malformations: a statement for healthcare professionals from a special writing group of the Stroke Council, American Stroke Association. Circulation. 2001;103(21):2644–57.
32. Derdeyn CP, Zipfel GJ, Albuquerque FC, Cooke DL, Feldmann E, Sheehan JP, et al. Management of Brain Arteriovenous Malformations: a scientific statement for healthcare professionals from the American Heart Association/American Stroke Association. Stroke. 2017;48(8):e200–e24.
33. Dias MS, Sekhar LN. Intracranial hemorrhage from aneurysms and arteriovenous malformations during pregnancy and the puerperium. Neurosurgery. 1990;27(6):855–65.. discussion 65–6
34. Rajiv KR, Radhakrishnan A. Status epilepticus in pregnancy: etiology, management, and clinical outcomes. Epilepsy Behav. 2017;76:114–9.
35. Lu YT, Hsu CW, Tsai WC, Cheng MY, Shih FY, Fu TY, et al. Status epilepticus associated with pregnancy: a cohort study. Epilepsy Behav. 2016;59:92–7.
36. Wu M, Hao N, Yan B, Chi X, Zhou D. Status epilepticus in pregnant women with epilepsy after valproate adjustment: a case series. Seizure. 2016;43:39–41.
37. Chan LY, Tsui MH, Leung TN. Guillain-Barre syndrome in pregnancy. Acta Obstet Gynecol Scand. 2004;83(4):319–25.
38. Djelmis J, Sostarko M, Mayer D, Ivanisevic M. Myasthenia gravis in pregnancy: report on 69 cases. Eur J Obstet Gynecol Reprod Biol. 2002;104(1):21–5.
39. Batocchi AP, Majolini L, Evoli A, Lino MM, Minisci C, Tonali P. Course and treatment of myasthenia gravis during pregnancy. Neurology. 1999;52(3):447–52.
40. Atwell TD, Lteif AN, Brown DL, McCann M, Townsend JE, Leroy AJ. Neonatal thyroid function after administration of IV iodinated contrast agent to 21 pregnant patients. AJR Am J Roentgenol. 2008;191(1):268–71.
41. Committee on Obstetric P. Committee opinion no. 723: guidelines for diagnostic imaging during pregnancy and lactation. Obstet Gynecol. 2017;130(4):e210–e6.
42. Ray JG, Vermeulen MJ, Bharatha A, Montanera WJ, Park AL. Association between MRI exposure during pregnancy and fetal and childhood outcomes. JAMA. 2016;316(9):952–61.
43. Radiology ACo. ACR manual on contrast media. Version 10.3. 2017.

44. Brophy GM, Bell R, Claassen J, Alldredge B, Bleck TP, Glauser T, et al. Guidelines for the evaluation and management of status epilepticus. Neurocrit Care. 2012;17(1):3–23.
45. Osei EK, Faulkner K. Fetal doses from radiological examinations. Br J Radiol. 1999;72(860):773–80.
46. Wakeford R, Little MP. Risk coefficients for childhood cancer after intrauterine irradiation: a review. Int J Radiat Biol. 2003;79(5):293–309.

Index

A
Acute cerebral venous stroke, *see* Cerebral venous thrombosis
Acute chorea, 340–341
Acute demyelinating diseases
   acute disseminated encephalomyelitis, 321–322
   axial FLAIR imaging, 329–331
   Balo concentric sclerosis, 323–324
   diagnosis of, 329–331
   leukoencephalopathy, differential diagnosis of, 329–330
   management and treatment of, 330
      disease-modifying therapy, 331
      immunosuppressive therapy, 331
      intravenous corticosteroids, 331
      plasma exchange, 331
      supportive therapy, 331
   Marburg disease, 323
   multiple sclerosis, 322–323
   neuromyelitis optica, 324–327
   optic neuritis, 327–328
   prognosis of, 332
   transverse myelitis, 328–329
   tumefactive multiple sclerosis, 324
Acute disseminated encephalomyelitis (ADEM), 321–322
Acute dystonia, 341–342
Acute inflammatory demyelinating polyneuropathy (AIDP), 160, 362, 369
Acute ischemic stroke (AIS)
   brain code, 173
   care after reperfusion therapy, 182–183
   classification and secondary prevention
      cardiac embolism, 185
      cervical dissections, 185
      large vessel disease, 184
      patent foramen ovale, 185
      small vessel disease, 184
      undetermined strokes, 185–186
   collateral circulation, 173
   initial evaluation
      airway, breathing, and circulation, 174
      algorithm, 176–177
      brain CT, 175–176
      capillary glycemia, 176
      coagulation and platelets, 176
      contraindications for intravenous thrombolysis, 174, 175
      medications, 174
      past medical history, 174
      physical examination, 175
      time of symptoms onset, 174
      vascular risk factors, 174
   intravenous thrombolysis, 177–179
   ischemic core and penumbra, 172
   mechanical thrombectomy
      with aphasia and right hemiparesis, 181
      clinical criteria, 180
      DAWN trial, 181
      DEFUSE 3 trial, 181
      ECASS4 and EPITHET trials, 182
      EXTEND trial, 182
      WAKE UP trial, 181–182
   in pregnant patients
      causes of, 366
      coagulation test, 367
      endovascular thrombectomy, 367
      laboratory investigations, 366–367
      non-contrast computed tomography, 366

Acute ischemic stroke (AIS) (cont.)
    salvage therapy, 367
    unilateral weakness, 362
  reperfusion treatments, 174
  secondary brain damage, 173
  stroke with no reperfusion treatment, 183
  stroke with transient symptoms, 183
  transient ischemic attack, 183
Acute Parkinsonism, 337
ADEM, see Acute disseminated encephalomyelitis
AIS, see Acute ischemic stroke
Alberta Stroke Program Early CT Score (ASPECTS), 176
Alcohol, 285
Alteplase-associated intracranial hemorrhage, 179
Altered mental status, 290–291, 351
Alternate cover test, 71–72
American Spinal Injury Association (ASIA) tool, 273, 274
Amniotic embolism, in pregnancy, 368
Analgesic medications, 303
Anesthetic agents, 302, 303
Aneurysmal subarachnoid hemorrhage (aSAH), 368
  assessment of severity, 236
  causes, 232
  clinical grading scale, 236
  clinical presentation, 232–233
  continuous EEG monitoring, 242
  diagnosis
    catheter angiogram, 234
    CT angiogram, 234
    magnetic resonance imaging, 234
    non-contrast brain CT scan, 233–234
  early complications, 232
  fever, 240–241
  hydrocephalus, 234, 235, 241
  hyponatremia, 232, 238, 240
  incidence, 232
  initial stabilization
    antiseizure medication, treatment with, 235
    fluid status, 235
    mechanical ventilation, 234–235
    pressure support ventilation, 235
    synchronized intermittent mandatory ventilation, 235
  management of, 232
    cardiovascular support and fluid, 238
    delayed cerebral ischemia, 238–239
    vasospasm, 238–240
  modified Fisher radiological grading scale, 236, 237
  prognosis, 242
  re-rupture with clinical deterioration, 235–236
  risk factors, 232
  treatment mode
    access to locations with open surgery, 236–237
    catheter cerebral angiogram, 236, 237
    morphology, 237–238
    neurosurgical clipping, 237–238
  vasospasm, prediction of, 236, 237
Aneurysmal third nerve palsy, 99–101
Anisocoria
  dangerous causes of, 95
  Horner syndrome, 95–97
  pharmacologic exposure, 97
  physiologic anisocoria, 97
  third nerve compression, 97
  tonic pupil, 98
Anoxic-ischemic brain injury, 6, 7, 10
Anterior inferior cerebellar artery (AICA) strokes, 72
Antiarrhythmics, 303
Antibiotics, 61, 123, 140, 142, 144, 303, 308–310
Anticholinergic medications, 157, 304, 305, 309, 340, 342
Anticonvulsants, 343
Antidepressant medications, 304–305, 309
Antiepileptic drug therapy, 204
Antiepileptic medications, 223, 304, 310–311, 348
Antiplatelet drugs, 220
Antirejection medications, 305, 311–312
Antiseizure drug (ASD) therapy, 21, 295
Arboviruses, 128, 134–136
Arteriovenous malformation (AVM), 368
Arteritic anterior ischemic optic neuropathy (AAION), 87–88
Arthropod-borne CNS infections, 135
aSAH, see Aneurysmal subarachnoid hemorrhage
Asterixis, 6, 311, 342, 350
Autologous stem cell transplant, 143
Autonomic dysreflexia, 278
Ayahuasca, 288, 290

B

Bacterial and parasitic encephalitis, 137–139
Bacterial meningitis, 61
  ampicillin, 123

Index   379

cerebral spinal fluid studies, 123
independent factors, 124
initial management, 123, 134
intravenous dexamethasone, 123
lumbar puncture, 123
neurologic complications, 124
steroids, 124–125
symptoms, 123
third-generation cephalosporin, 123, 125
Balo concentric sclerosis (BCS), 323–324
Barbiturates, 28, 258, 352
BCS, *see* Balo concentric sclerosis
Benign paroxysmal positional vertigo (BPPV), 69, 70, 78–79
Benzodiazepines, 28
acute alcohol withdrawal, 285
dystonica, 342
myoclonus, 343
neuroleptic malignant syndrome, 338
seizures, 295
status epilepticus, 26
Bevacizumab, 113, 116, 117, 313
BiPAP bilevel positive airway pressure, 159
Bismuth toxicity, 316
Bitemporal hemianopia, 55, 56, 86, 361
Botulism, 103
Brainstem hemorrhage, 225
Brainstem reflexes, 2, 4, 6
Brain tissue hypoxia, 258–260
Brain tumor headache, 58–59
Branch retinal artery occlusion (BRAO), 88–89
Brivaracetam, 31, 39
Bromocriptine, 338

C

Calcineurin inhibitors, 311, 347–348, 352, 353
Calcium channel blockers, 52–53
Cannabinoids
marijuana, 285–286
synthetic, 286
Capillary glycemia, 176
Carbamazepine, 31, 39, 311, 341
Cardiac arrhythmias, 77
Cardiac embolism, 185
Carotid cavernous fistula (CCF), 101–102
Carotid dissection, 95–96
Carotid endarterectomy/stenting, 75
Cathinone, 284
Cavernous sinus thrombosis, 101
CD-19, 118
Central Horner syndrome, 96–97

Central nervous system (CNS) abscesses, 290, 296–297
Central nervous system (CNS) infections
encephalitis
arboviruses, 134–136
bacterial and parasitic encephalitis, 137–139
cytomegalovirus, 133
enterovirus, 134
Epstein-Barr virus, 133
herpes simplex virus, 131–133
Human herpes virus-6, 134
rabies, 136
VZV, 133
human immunodeficiency virus, 146–147
infectious myelitis, 137, 140
meningitis
bacteria, 123–127
fungal, 128–130
tuberculosis, 127–128
viral, 128, 131
neurological complication in transplant patients
categories, 350
causes, 350
clinical manifestations, 349
CSF analysis, 349
imaging studies, 349
lumbar puncture, 349
organisms responsible, 349
by time course posttransplant, 349–350
space-occupying lesions
bacterial abscesses, 140, 142–145
fungal abscesses, 144
parasites, 146
unbiased testing, 140, 141
Central paroxysmal positional vertigo (CPPV), 78
Central retinal artery occlusion (CRAO), 88–89
Cerebellar hemorrhage, *see* Intraparenchymal hemorrhage
Cerebral abscesses, 296–297
Cerebral infarction, 113
Cerebral venous sinus thrombosis (CVST), 367
Cerebral venous thrombosis (CVT), 58, 190
acute management
algorithm, 203
anticoagulation, 202, 204
endovascular therapy, 202, 204
of medical complications, 204
monitoring for neurological deterioration, 201–202

Cerebral venous thrombosis (CVT) (*cont.*)
  thrombolysis, 202, 204
  causes of, 206
  chronic management, 204–205
  clinical outcomes, 205
  clinical presentation, 191–193
  diagnostic evaluation, 200–201
  imaging studies
    computed tomography (*see* Computed tomography)
    conventional angiogram, 196
    CT venogram, 194, 195
    magnetic resonance imaging (*see* Magnetic resonance imaging)
    magnetic resonance venography, 194, 196–198
  pathophysiology, 190–191
  prognosis, 205
  recurrence, 206
  risk factors of, 191–192
  sex-related factors, 191, 193
  signs and symptoms, 193
Cerebrospinal fluid (CSF) analysis, 8–9, 25, 50, 163
Cerebrovascular disease, 19, 71, 190, 365–366
Cervical arterial dissections, 54–55
Cervical dissections, 185
Chemotherapeutic agents, 115, 116, 305–306, 312–313
Chemotherapy-associated encephalopathy, 115
Chimeric antigen receptor T-cell (CAR-T) therapy, 117–118, 315
Cholinesterase-inhibiting medications, 314
Chorea, acute, 340–341
Chronic papilledema, 93
Critical illness myopathy (CIM), 168
Critical illness polyneuropathy (CIP), 168
Clobazam, 28, 35
Clonazepam, 28
CNS infections, *see* Central nervous system (CNS) infections
Coagulopathy, 218
Cocaine, 283, 292
Collateral circulation, 173
Colloid cyst, 56
Coma
  diagnosis, 2
    brain imaging, 7, 8
    checklist, 3
    electroencephalography, 7
    history, 3–4
    lumbar puncture, 8–9
    physical examination, 4–6
  pathophysiology, 2
  prognosis, 10–11
  treatment
    therapeutic principles, 9
    treatable causes, 9, 10
Computed tomography (CT)
  angiogram
    acute ischemic stroke, 366
    aneurysmal subarachnoid hemorrhage, 234
  brain, 108–109, 175
  cerebral venous thrombosis, 194, 195, 367
    intraparenchymal hemorrhage, 199
    isolated subarachnoid hemorrhage, 199, 202
    temporal-occipital intraparenchymal hemorrhage, 199, 201
    venous and sinus abnormalities, 194
  cervical segment stenosis, 54
  hyperdense pituitary mass, 55
  ICH etiology
    arteriography, 224
    venography, 224
  intracranial hypertension, 91
  intraparenchymal hemorrhage, 216
  neurological complications after
    heart transplantation, 353
    liver transplantation, 352
  perfusion, acute ischemic stroke, 366
  posterior reversible encephalopathy syndrome, 365
  severity of edema, 352
Conjugate gaze abnormality, 102
Convulsive status epilepticus, 17
CRAO, *see* Central retinal artery occlusion
Critical illness neuromyopathy (CINM), 168
CVT, *see* Cerebral venous thrombosis
Cyclophosphamide, 115
Cytokine response syndrome (CRS), 117
Cytomegalovirus (CMV), 133
Cytotoxic T-lymphocyte-associated protein 4 (CTLA-4) therapies, 315

D

Dabigatran, 220
Demyelinating diseases
  acute
    acute disseminated encephalomyelitis, 321–322
    Balo concentric sclerosis, 323–324
    diagnosis of, 329–331
    leukoencephalopathy, differential diagnosis of, 329–330
    management and treatment of, 330–331

Index 381

Marburg disease, 323
multiple sclerosis, 322–323
neuromyelitis optica, 324–327
optic neuritis, 327–328
prognosis of, 332
transverse myelitis, 328–329
tumefactive multiple sclerosis, 324
chronic, 320
complications, 320
Depressants, 284
Devic disease, *see* Neuromyelitis optica
Dexamethasone, 109, 110
Diazepam, 31
Diffuse axonal injury (DAI), 247
Dihydroergotamine (DHE), 57
Diplopia/ocular motility disorders, 98–99
aneurysmal third nerve palsy, 99–101
botulism, 103
cavernous sinus thrombosis, 101
CCF, 101–102
dorsal midbrain syndrome, 102–103
monocular diplopia, 104
myasthenia gravis, 104
skew deviation, 103
top of the basilar syndrome, 102
wernicke encephalopathy, 103
Directed rescue therapy, 315
Direct oral anticoagulants (DOACs), 176, 205
Disc edema, 92, 93
Dizziness, 68
acute vestibular syndrome
causes, 70
medical treatments, 75
nystagmus and skew deviation, 71–73
patient management with acute posterior circulation stroke, 75
physical examination, 71
posterior circulation stroke, exam for, 74
rehabilitation, 75
surgical treatments, 75
diagnostic pitfalls, 69–70
differential diagnosis, 68–69
s-EVS, 76–77
t-EVS, 77–79
Dopamine agonist withdrawal syndrome (DAWS), 340
Dopamine-blocking antiemetics, 342
Dopaminergic medications, 314
Dorsal midbrain syndrome, 102–103
Drug-induced movement disorders
neuroleptic malignant syndrome, 337–338
serotonin syndrome, 338–339

Drug reaction with eosinophilia and systemic symptoms (DRESS) syndrome, 310–311
Dysautonomia, 338
Dyschromatopsia, 327
Dysphagia, 226, 338
Dystonia, acute, 341–342

E
Electroconvulsive therapy, 338
Electroencephalography (EEG)
coma, 7
in encephalopathic patient, 351
nonconvulsive seizures in liver transplant patients, 352
seizures, 348, 350–351
Encephalitis
arboviruses, 134–136
bacterial and parasitic encephalitis, 137–139
cytomegalovirus, 133
enterovirus, 134
epstein-barr virus, 133
herpes simplex virus, 131–133
Human herpes virus (HHV)-6, 134
rabies, 136
VZV, 133
Encephalitis, Nonconvulsive Status Epilepticus, Diazepam Resistance, Image Abnormality, Tracheal Intubation (END-IT) score, 44
Encephalopathy, 115, 351, 353
Enterovirus, 134
Epidemiology-Based Mortality Score in Status Epilepticus (EMSE), 43
Epidural spinal cord compression (ESCC), 109–110
Episodic dizziness, 77
Epstein-barr virus (EBV), 133
External ventricular device (EVD), 108–109

F
Factor Xa inhibitors, 219–220
Febrile infection-related epilepsy syndrome (FIRES), 23
Fever
acute disseminated encephalomyelitis, 321
aneurysmal subarachnoid hemorrhage, 240–241
intraparenchymal hemorrhage, 226
Flumazenil, 351
Focal motor, 18

Fosphenytoin, 32, 39
    status epilepticus, 369
Full Outline of UnResponsiveness (FOUR) score, 4, 5, 216
Fungal meningitis, 128–130

G

GABAergic targets, status epilepticus, 28
Gabapentin, 35
Gamma-aminobutyric acid A (GABA$_A$) receptors, 23
Gamma-hydroxybutyric acid (GHB), 287–288
GBS, *see* Guillain-Barré syndrome
Giant cell arteritis (GCA), *see* Temporal arteritis
Glasgow Coma Scale (GCS) score, 216, 236
Glucocorticoids, 80
Graft-*versus*-host disease, 143
Guillain-Barré syndrome (GBS), 362
    acute inflammatory demyelinating polyneuropathy, 160
    acute motor and sensory axonal polyneuropathy, 161
    ascending pattern of weakness, 161
    axolemmal surface antigens in acute motor, 161
    clinical presentation, 163
    common precipitants, 161, 163
    diagnosis, 163
    immunomodulatory therapy, 163
    long-term disability, 166
    Miller-Fisher variants, 160
    molecular mimicry, 161
    oropharyngeal weakness, 161
    systemic complications, 163, 164
    treatment regimens and side effects, 163, 166

H

Hallucinogens
    ayahuasca, 290
    lysergic acid diethylamide, 288–289
    mescaline, 289
    phencyclidine, 289
    psilocybin, 289–290
Headache, 49–50
    acute disseminated encephalomyelitis, 321
    acute/subacute with focal neurologic features, 57–58
        CVT, 58
        hemiplegic migraine, 60
        ischemic strokes, 58
        SMART syndrome, 59, 60
        subdural hematoma headache, 59
    aneurysmal subarachnoid hemorrhage, 233
    cerebral venous thrombosis, 193
    with fever, CNS infections, 349
    persistent headache
        idiopathic intracranial hypertension, 62, 63
        intracranial hypotension, 63–64
        temporal arteritis, 62
    in pregnant patients
        benign cephalalgias/life threating conditions, 358
        characteristics, 358–359
        differential diagnosis, 359
    secondary etiology, 51
    status migrainosus, 64
    subacute-chronic progressive headache, 61
        bacterial meningitis, 61
        intracranial abscess/empyema, 61
    thunderclap headache, 50
        cervical arterial dissections, 54, 55
        colloid cyst and hydrocephalus, 56
        differential diagnosis, 52
        pituitary apoplexy, 55, 56
        PRES, 54
        RCVS, 52–53
        retroclival hematoma, 56
        subarachnoid hemorrhage, 51–52
        trigeminal autonomic cephalalgias, 56–57
Head impulse test (HIT), 71, 72
Head position in Stroke Trial (HeadPoST), 173
Hemiplegic migraine, 60
Hemodynamic management, 254
Hemorrhagic strokes, 368
Heparin and Low Molecular Weight Heparin (LMWH), 220
Herpes simplex virus (HSV), 131–133
Homonymous visual field deficits, 89
Horner syndrome, 74, 95
    carotid dissection, 95–96
    lateral medullary infarction, 96–97
Human herpes virus (HHV)-6, 134
Human immunodeficiency virus (HIV), 146–147
Hydrocephalus, 56, 204, 234, 235, 241
Hyperammonemia, 351
Hyperglycemia, 255
Hyperperfusion syndrome, 353
Hypertensive optic neuropathy, 92–93
Hyperthermia, 254, 298–299
Hyperventilation, 109

Hyponatremia, 232, 238, 240, 255
Hypotension, 254
Hypoxemic hypercarbic respiratory failure, 153–15

I
Idiopathic intracranial hypertension (IIH), 62, 63
Immune reconstitution inflammatory syndrome (IRIS), 147
Immunotherapy, 306–307, 314–315
Infectious myelitis, 137, 140
Inhalants, 288
Interferon-gamma release assay (IGRA), 127
2015 International League Against Epilepsy (ILAE), 17–20
Intracerebral hemorrhage (ICH), *see* Intraparenchymal hemorrhage
Intracranial abscess/empyema, 61
Intracranial hemorrhage, 293–294
Intracranial hypertension management, 91–92, 204, 255–258
 algorithm, 256
 barbiturates, 258
 bispectral index, 257
 first-level measures, 257
 hypertonic lactate, 257
 hyperventilation, 257–258
 indomethacin, 258
 induced hypothermia, 258
 mannitol, 257
 monitoring and treatment, 241
 osmotherapy, 257
 refractory ICH, 258
 side effects, 257
 space-occupying lesions, 256
 ventricular drainage, 256–257
Intracranial hypotension, 63–64
Intranasal midazolam, 28
Intraparenchymal hemorrhage
 algorithm for acute management of, 211
 brain injuries by
  bleeding in, 213
  direct mechanical disruption and distortion, 213
 brainstem hemorrhage, 225
 cerebellar hemorrhage, 225
 clinical presentation of, 216
 initial evaluation and management
  clinical presentation, 216
  determining etiology, 223–224
  diagnostics, 217
  imaging, 216

 life-threatening complications, 214–216
 prehospital evaluation of stroke patients, 213
 secondary brain injury, causes of, 218–223
intraventricular hemorrhage, 224
medical complications, management of
 dysphagia, 226
 fever, 226
 hyperglycemia, 226
 hypoglycemia, 226
 prognosis, 226
neurologic signs and symptoms, 217
primary, 210
secondary brain injury, treatment causes of
 antiplatelet drugs, 220
 coagulopathy, 218, 219
 heparin and low molecular weight heparin, 220
 hydrocephalus, 221
 hypertension, 218
 intracranial hypertension and herniation, 221–223
 seizure treatment, 223
secondary, causes of, 210, 212
supratentorial hemorrhages, 224
treating life-threatening complications, 214
 elevated ICP and/or brain herniation, 215–216
 initial hemodynamic management, 214
 poor airway and breathing, 214
Intraventricular hemorrhage (IVH), 224
Ischemic brain damage, 247
Ischemic stroke, 58, 292–293

J
John Cunningham (JC) virus, 146

K
Ketamine, 29
 infusions, 40
Ketogenic diet, 41
Khat, 284

L
Lacosamide, 32, 39
Lance-Adams syndrome, 343
Large vessel disease, 184
Lateral medullary infarction, 96–97
Levetiracetam, 33, 39, 369

Lorazepam, 33
Lumbar puncture (LP)
  bacterial meningitis, 123
  cerebral abscesses, 296
  CNS infections, 349
  coma, 8–9
  headache, 50
  intracranial hypertension, 91
  intracranial hypotension, 63
  seizures, 350
  status epilepticus, 25
Lysergic acid diethylamide (LSD), 288–289

M

Magnesium sulfate
  eclampsia-related seizures, 369
  myasthenia gravis, 371
  postpartum angiopathy, 365
Magnetic resonance angiography (MRA)
  left internal carotid artery, 96
  left posterior communicating artery aneurysm, 100
  multifocal intracerebral arterial stenoses mimicking vasculitis, 52, 53
  stroke, 75
Magnetic resonance imaging (MRI)
  acute disseminated encephalomyelitis, 328, 329
  aneurysmal subarachnoid hemorrhage, 234
  Balo concentric sclerosis, 324
  brain, 56, 109
    acute chorea, 341
    acute parkinsonism, 337
    idiopathic intracranial hypertension, 62
    necrotic brain tumor, 109
    pituitary apoplexy, 89
    vasogenic edema, 108
    Wernicke encephalopathy, 103
  cerebral venous thrombosis
    focal parenchymal abnormalities, 198–200
    gradient-echo and susceptibility-weighted imaging sequences, 196, 197
    hyperintense region of edema, 199, 201
    intraparenchymal hemorrhage, 199, 200
    signal changes, 194, 195
    temporal-occipital intraparenchymal hemorrhage, 201
    venous and sinus abnormalities, 194–196
  CNS infections, 349

  coma, 7, 8
  complications after liver transplant, 352
  ESCC, 110
  head, 55, 59
  intracranial hypertension, 91, 92
  intraparenchymal hemorrhage, 216
  neck, 54
  neuromyelitis optica, 326, 327
  optic neuritis, 328
  posterior reversible encephalopathy syndrome, 348
  during pregnancy
    advantage, 372
    cerebral venous sinus thrombosis, 367
    with gadolinium, 372
    posterior reversible encephalopathy syndrome, 365
  seizures, 350
  transverse myelitis, 329
  tumefactive multiple sclerosis, 324, 325
  tumor-related epilepsy, 111
Magnetic resonance venography (MRV)
  cerebral venous thrombosis, 367
  gadolinium-enhanced MRV, 196–198
  time of flight technique, 196
  venous and sinus abnormalities, 194, 196–198
ICH etiology, 224
Marburg disease, 323
Marijuana, 285–286
Mass effect, 108–109
MDE, see Movement disorders emergency
Mechanical embolectomy, 114
Mechanical thrombectomy, 75
  with aphasia and right hemiparesis, 181
  clinical criteria, 180
  DAWN trial, 181
  DEFUSE 3 trial, 181
  ECASS4 and EPITHET trials, 182
  EXTEND trial, 182
  WAKE UP trial, 181–182
Mechanical ventilation, 254
Medical therapy
  brain tissue hypoxia, 258–260
  clinical practice guidelines, 255
  general measures, 260
  hemodynamic management, 254
  hyperglycemia, 255
  hyperthermia, 254
  hyponatremia, 255
  hypotension, 254
  intracranial hypertension management, 255–258
  mechanical ventilation, 254

Index 385

normothermia, 254
rapid sequence intubation, 254
regular insulin, 255
restrictive transfusion strategy, 255
shivering, 254
surgical treatment
  asymmetry and abnormality, 261
  bilateral bifrontal decompression, 264, 267
  blood volume, 261, 264
  cisterns, 261
  decompressive hemicraniectomy, 264–266
  deviation of midline, 261
  external elements, 261
  guidelines, 263–264
  methodical interpretation, 261–263
  open/closed fractures, 264
  penetrating cranial injuries, 264, 268
target physiological parameters, 253
Ménière's disease, 76
Meninges, inflammation of, *see* Meningitis
Meningitis
  bacteria, 123–127
  fungal, 128–130
  tuberculosis, 127–128
  viral, 128, 131
Mescaline, 289
Methamphetamine, 283
Methanol, 90
3,4-methylenedioxy methamphetamine (MDMA), 283
MG, *see* Myasthenia gravis
Midazolam, 29, 40
Middle cerebral artery (MCA) aneurysms, 237
Migraine
  acute ischemic strokes, 58
  hemiplegic, 60
  status, 64
  vestibular, 76
  visual change, 360
Monoamine oxidase inhibitors (MAOIs)
  psychosis, 339
  serotonin syndrome, 339
Monocular diplopia, 104
Motor responses, 6
Movement disorders emergency (MDE)
  definition, 336
  hyperkinetic, 336
    acute chorea, 340–341
    acute dystonia, 341–342
    myoclonus, 342–343
    tics status, 343
  hypokinetic, 336

acute parkinsonism, 337
neuroleptic malignant syndrome, 337–338
Parkinson disease, 339–340
serotonin syndrome, 338–339
MS, *see* Multiple sclerosis
Mucormycosis, 90
Multiple sclerosis (MS), 322–323
Muscle relaxants, 307, 315–316
Myasthenia gravis (MG), 104, 166–167
  consequences, 369–370
  magnesium sulfate, 371
  maternal and fetal outcomes, 370
  peripheral nervous system weakness, 362
  surgical intervention, 371
  treatment, 370
Myasthenic crisis, 167
Myelitis, 137, 140
Myoclonic status epilepticus, 18, 342–343
Myoclonus, 6, 342–343

N

Naloxone, 9, 287, 288, 351
National Institutes of Health Stroke Scale (NIHSS) score, 175, 216
Neuroleptic malignant syndrome (NMS)
  causes of, 338
  characteristics, 338
  diagnosis, 338
  incidence, 337
  treatment, 338
Neuromuscular respiratory failure
  critical illness neuromyopathy, 168
  differential diagnosis, 160–161
  Guillain-Barré syndrome
    acute inflammatory demyelinating polyneuropathy, 160
    acute motor and sensory axonal polyneuropathy, 161
    ascending pattern of weakness, 161
    axolemmal surface antigens in acute motor, 161
    clinical presentation, 163
    common precipitants, 161, 163
    diagnosis, 163
    immunomodulatory therapy, 163
    long-term disability, 166
    Miller-Fisher variants, 160
    molecular mimicry, 161
    oropharyngeal weakness, 161
    systemic complications, 163, 164
    treatment regimens and side effects, 163, 166

Neuromuscular respiratory failure (*cont.*)
  historical and exam features, 160, 162
  initial evaluation
    clinical features, 154–155
    diagnostic evaluation, 156–157
    initial management and disposition, 157–160
  Myasthenia gravis, 166–167
  pathophysiology
    hypoxemic hypercarbic respiratory failure, 153–154
    normal respiratory mechanics, 153
    oropharyngeal weakness, 154
Neuromyelitis optica (NMO)
  age and gender factors, 325
  characteristics, 324
  clinical manifestations, 325–326
  diagnostic criteria for, 326, 327
  incidence and prevalence rate, 324
  posterior reversible leukoencephalopathy syndrome, 326
Neuro-oncologic emergencies
  epidural spinal cord compression, 109–110
  mass effect, 108–109
  pituitary apoplexy, 111
  treatment-related neurologic emergencies
    CAR-T, 117–118
    post-radiation vasculopathy, 113–114
    radiation therapy, 111–113
    SMART syndrome, 114–115
    systemic therapies, 115–116
    targeted therapies, 117
  tumor-related epilepsy, 111
Neuro-ophthalmologic urgencies and emergencies
  anisocoria
    dangerous causes of, 95
    Horner syndrome, 95–97
    pharmacologic exposure, 97
    physiologic anisocoria, 97
    third nerve compression, 97
    tonic pupil, 98
  diplopia/ocular motility disorders, 98–99
    aneurysmal third nerve palsy, 99–101
    botulism, 103
    cavernous sinus thrombosis, 101
    CCF, 101–102
    dorsal midbrain syndrome, 102–103
    monocular diplopia, 104
    myasthenia gravis, 104
    skew deviation, 103
    top of the basilar syndrome, 102
    wernicke encephalopathy, 103
  papilledema, 91
    chronic papilledema, 93
    hypertensive optic neuropathy and retinopathy, 92–93
    intracranial hypertension, 91–92
    pseudopapilledema, 94
  vision loss
    GCA, arteritic anterior ischemic optic neuropathy from, 87–88
    mucormycosis, 90
    non-emergent differentials, 90
    pituitary apoplexy, 89
    retinal artery occlusion and stroke, 88–89
    toxic optic neuropathy, 90
Neuro-otologic emergencies, 68
  dizziness, 68
    AVS, 70–75
    diagnostic pitfalls, 69–70
    differential diagnosis, 68–69
    s-EVS, 76–77
    t-EVS, 77–79
  SSNHL, 68
Neurosyphilis, 127
New-onset refractory status epilepticus (NORSE), 22–23
NMO, *see* Neuromyelitis optica
NMS, *see* Neuroleptic malignant syndrome
Non-contrast computed tomography
  brain CT, 233–234
  head
    cerebellar hemorrhage with mass effect, 221, 222
    hydrocephalus, 221, 222
    intraventricular hemorrhage, 221, 222
    seizures, 350
    volume of hematoma, 221
  ICH etiology, 224
  posterior reversible encephalopathy syndrome, 348
  status epilepticus, 26
Nonconvulsive status epilepticus (NCSE), 18, 21–22
Normothermia, 254
Nystagmus testing, 71–73

O

Ocular motility disorders, 98–99
  aneurysmal third nerve palsy, 99–101
  botulism, 103
  carotid cavernous fistula, 101–102
  cavernous sinus thrombosis, 101
  dorsal midbrain syndrome, 102–103
  monocular diplopia, 104

Index 387

myasthenia gravis, 104
skew deviation, 103
top of the basilar syndrome, 102
wernicke encephalopathy, 103
ON, *see* Optic neuritis (ON)
Opiates
   heroin, 287
   Kratom, 287
   prescription, 286–287
Optic neuritis (ON)
   clinical manifestation, 327
   diagnosis of, 328
   dyschromatopsia, 327
   incidence, 327
   with unilateral ocular pain, 325
Orolingual angioedema, 179
Orthostatic hypotension, 78, 79
Osmotic demyelination, 352
Osmotic diuretics, 109
Oxcarbazepine, 36, 304
Oxygen reactivity index (ORx), 251

P

Pallid disc edema, 87
Papilledema, 91
   hypertensive optic neuropathy and retinopathy, 92–93
   intracranial hypertension, 91–92
   non-emergency differential diagnoses
      chronic papilledema, 93
      pseudopapilledema, 94
Paracetamol (Acetaminophen) Stroke (PAIS) trial, 173
Paralytics, 307
Parinaud syndrome, 102–103
Parkinson disease (PD) complications
   acute psychosis, impulse control disorders, 339–340
   dopamine agonist withdrawal syndrome, 340
Parkinsonism, acute, 337
Patent foramen ovale (PFO), 185
Pentobarbital, 30
Perampanel, 36
Persistent headache
   idiopathic intracranial hypertension, 62, 63
   intracranial hypotension, 63–64
   temporal arteritis, 62
Phencyclidine (PCP), 289
Phenobarbital, 28, 34
Phenytoin, 34, 39, 235, 242, 304, 311, 351, 371
Photophobia, 123
Pituitary apoplexy, 55, 56, 89
   neuro-oncologic emergencies, 111
Pneumococcal meningitis, 124, 126
Posterior reversible encephalopathy syndrome (PRES), 54, 116, 311, 347–348, 350, 351, 360
   abnormal leaky blood vessels of brain, 365
   clinical features, 364
   imaging studies, 365
Postpartum angiopathy (PPA)
   associated with serotonergic agents, 365
   clinical features, 364
   clinical presentation, 365
   treatment, 365
   vasoconstrictive consequences, 365
Powassan virus encephalitis, 135, 136
PPA, *see* Postpartum angiopathy
Preeclampsia and eclampsia
   clinical features, 364
   definition, 363
   management, 364
   neurological consequences, 363
   pathophysiology, 363
Pregabalin, 36, 277
Pregnancy
   clinical presentation
      headache, 358–359
      seizures, 363
      visual change, 359–360
      weakness, 360, 362
   diagnostic tests
      computed tomography imaging, 371
      digitally subtracted angiography, 371
      fetal radiation exposure complication, 371, 372
      magnetic resonance imaging studies, 371, 372
   neurological emergency
      acute ischemic stroke, 366–367
      cerebral venous sinus thrombosis, 367
      cerebrovascular disease, 365–366
      hemorrhagic strokes, 368
      immunological diseases, 369–371
      posterior reversible encephalopathy syndrome, 364–365
      postpartum angiopathy, 364–365
      preeclampsia/eclampsia, 363–364
      status epilepticus, 368–369
PRES, *see* Posterior reversible encephalopathy syndrome
Pressure reactivity index (PRx), 251
Presyncopal episodes, 77
Programmed cell death receptor 1 (PD-1) inhibitors, 315

Progressive multifocal leukoencephalopathy (PML), 146
Prolonged refractory status epilepticus (PRSE), 22
Prolonged super refractory status epilepticus (PSRSE), 22
Propofol, 30, 40, 241, 302, 303, 370
Propofol infusion syndrome (PRIS), 40
Pseudopapilledema, 94
Psilocybin, 289–290

R
Rabies, 136
Radiation-induced necrosis, 112
Radiation-induced vasculopathy, 113–114
Radiation necrosis, 113
Radiation therapy, 111–113
Ramsay Hunt syndrome, 71
Recreational substances
  alcohol, 285
  cannabinoids
    marijuana, 285–286
    synthetic, 286
  cathinone, 284
  cocaine, 283
  depressants, 284
  gamma-hydroxybutyric acid, 287–288
  hallucinogens
    ayahuasca, 290
    lysergic acid diethylamide, 288–289
    mescaline, 289
    phencyclidine, 289
    psilocybin, 289–290
  methamphetamine, 283
  3,4-methylenedioxy methamphetamine, 283
  opiates
    heroin, 287
    Kratom, 287
    prescription, 286–287
  stimulants, 282–283
  symptom-based approach
    altered mental status, 290–291
    CNS abscesses, 296–297
    hyperthermia, 298–299
    intracranial hemorrhage, 293–294
    ischemic stroke, 292–293
    seizures, 295–296
Reflex syncope, 77
Refractory status epilepticus (RSE), 22, 24
Rehabilitation, 75
Relative afferent pupillary defect (RAPD), 86
Retinal artery occlusion, 88–89
Retinopathy, 92–93
Retroclival hematoma, 56
Reversible cerebral vasoconstriction syndrome (RCVS), 52–53
Reversible posterior leukoencephalopathy syndrome (RPLS), *see* Posterior reversible encephalopathy syndrome
Rhabdomyolysis, 338
Rocky Mountain spotted fever, 137

S
Salzburg Consensus Criteria, 21
SE, *see* Status epilepticus
Seizures, 295–296, 363
Sentinel hemorrhage, 233
Serotonin syndrome, 317
  causes of, 338, 339
  clinical symtoms, 338–339
  drug interactions, 339
  incidence, 338
Sheehan's syndrome, 89
Skew deviation, 71–73
  diplopia/ocular motility disorders, 103
Small vessel disease, 184
Spinal epidural abscesses, 296
Spontaneous episodic vestibular syndrome (s-EVS), 76–77
Status epilepticus (SE), 16
  anti-seizure medications, 369, 370
  causes of, 368
  definitions and classifications
    FIRES, 23
    ILAE, 17–20
    NCSE, 21–22
    NORSE, 22–23
    PRSE, 22
    PSRSE, 22
    RSE, 22
    SRSE, 22
  epidemiology, 23–24
  etiologies, 19–20
  evaluation and diagnosis, 24–26
  life-threatening risk, 368
  maternal outcome, 369
  morbidity and mortality rate, 369
  pathophysiology, 23
  prognosis, 42–44
  risk factors, 369
  systemic effects, 41–42
  treatment, 26–28, 369

Index   389

ASD targets and classification, 28, 38
dosing, pharmacokinetic data and
    considerations of therapeutic
    agents, 29–37
GABAergic targets, 28
glutamatergic targets, 40–41
synaptic vesicle targets, 39
tiered approach, 26–27
voltage-dependent sodium channel
    targets, 39
Status Epilepticus Severity Score (STESS), 43
Status migrainosus, 64
Steroid therapy, 315
Stimulants, 282–283
Stroke, 88–89, 292–293
    complication after heart transplantation, 353
    intraparenchymal hemorrhage (*see* Intraparenchymal hemorrhage)
Stroke Hyperglycemia Insulin Network Effort
    (SHINE) trial, 173
Stroke like migraine attacks after radiation
    herapy (SMART) syndrome, 59, 60, 114–115
Subacute-chronic progressive headache, 61
    bacterial meningitis, 61
    intracranial abscess/empyema, 61
Subacute edema, 75
Subarachnoid hemorrhage, 51–52
Subdural hematoma headache, 59
Sudden sensorineural hearing loss (SSNHL), 68, 79–80
Super refractory status epilepticus (SRSE), 22, 24
Synthetic cannabinoids, 286
Synthetic cathinones (bath salts), 284
Syphilitic meningitis, 125–126

T
TBI, *see* Traumatic brain injury
Temporal arteritis, 62
Testrictive transfusion strategy, 255
Third nerve compression, 97
Third ventricular colloid cyst, 57
Thunderclap headache, 50
    cervical arterial dissections, 54, 55
    colloid cyst and hydrocephalus, 56
    differential diagnosis, 52
    pituitary apoplexy, 55, 56
    PRES, 54
    RCVS, 52–53
    retroclival hematoma, 56

subarachnoid hemorrhage, 51–52
trigeminal autonomic cephalalgias, 56–57
TM, *see* Transverse myelitis
TMS, *see* Tumefactive multiple sclerosis
Tonic pupil, 98
Topiramate, 37, 370
Top of the basilar syndrome, 102
Toxic optic neuropathy, 90
Transient ischaemic attack (TIA), 76, 77
Transplant patients, 346–347
    CNS infections
        categories, 350
        caused by, 350
        clinical manifestations, 349
        CSF analysis, 349
        imaging studis, 349
        lumbar puncture, 349
        organisms responsible, 349
        by time course posttransplant, 349–350
    encephalopathy, 351
    with immunosuppressive medications
        antiepileptic drugs, 348
        calcineurin inhibitors, 347–348
        corticosteroids, 347
        diagnostic evaluation, 348
        encephalopathy, 348
        risk factors, 348
        seizures, 348
    organ-specific emergency
        heart transplantion, 353
        kidney transplantion, 353–354
        liver transplantion, 352
        lung transplantion, 353
    seizures
        AED therapy, 351
        EEG monitoring, 348, 350–351
        focal, 350
        generalized, 350
        imaging studies, 350
        lumbar puncture and CSF analysis, 350
Transverse myelitis (TM)
    causes of, 328
    classification, 328
    diagnosis, 329
    incidence, 328
    symptoms and signs of, 328
Traumatic brain injury (TBI)
    definition, 246
    initial assessment, 249, 250
    medical therapy
        brain tissue hypoxia, 258–260
        clinical practice guidelines, 255
        general measures, 260

Traumatic brain injury (TBI) (cont.)
  hemodynamic management, 254
  hyperglycemia, 255
  hyperthermia, 254
  hyponatremia, 255
  hypotension, 254
  intracranial hypertension management, 255–258
  mechanical ventilation, 254
  normothermia, 254
  rapid sequence intubation, 254
  regular insulin, 255
  restrictive transfusion strategy, 255
  shivering, 254
  surgical treatment, 260–268
  target physiological parameters, 253
 multimodal neuromonitoring, 251–252
 pathophysiology, 247
  brain oxygenation, 250–251
  cerebral blood flow, 249
  cerebral metabolism, 250–251
  intracranial pressure, 250
  systemic derangements, 251
 prevalence, 246
 primary injury, 247
 prognosis, 265–266
 secondary insults, 247–248
 tertiary insults, 248–249
Traumatic spinal cord injury
 autonomic dysreflexia, 278
 emergency management, 275, 276
 inducing blood pressure augmentation, 275, 276
 intestinal dilatation, 277
 monitoring spinal cord perfusion pressure, 275
 neuropathic pain, 277
 pathophysiology, 272
 physical examination, 273–274
 prognosis, 278
 radiological evaluation, 274–275
 spasticity, 278
 systemic complications, 277
Trigeminal autonomic cephalalgias, 56–57
Triggered episodic vestibular syndrome (t-EVS), 77–79
Tuberculous meningitis, 127–128
Tumefactive multiple sclerosis (TMS), 324, 325

V
Valproate, 35
Varicella zoster virus (VZV), 133
Vertigo, 69
Vestibular migraine, 76
Vestibular neuritis, 70–73, 75
Vestibulo-ocular reflex (VOR), 72
Vigabatrin, 37
Viral meningitis, 128, 131
Vision loss, 204
 GCA, arteritic anterior ischemic optic neuropathy from, 87–88
 mucormycosis, 90
 non-emergent differentials, 90
 pituitary apoplexy, 89
 retinal artery occlusion and stroke, 88–89
 toxic optic neuropathy, 90
Visual change, in pregnant patients
 clinical presentation, 360
 differential diagnosis, 360, 361
 features, 360
 ophthalmologic examination, 359
 red flags, 360
 Wernicke encephalopathy, 360
Visual loss, 86
Vitamin deficiencies, 316
Vitamin K antagonist (VKA), 204, 219

W
Warfarin, 176, 218
Weakness, in pregnant patients
 causes of, 363
 central nervous system, 362
 characteristics, 360
 peripheral nervous system disease, 362
 presentations of, 362
Weber and Rinne tests, 80
Wernicke encephalopathy, 103, 116, 360
West Nile virus, 134, 135, 162
World Federation of Neurological Surgeons scoring system (WFNS), 236

X
Xanthochromia, 52, 234